Arthritis Sourcebook

Basic Consumer Health Information about Specific Forms of Arthritis and Related Disorders, Including Rheumatoid Arthritis, Osteoarthritis, Gout, Polymyalgia Rheumatica, Psoriatic Arthritis, Spondyloarthropathies, Juvenile Rheumatoid Arthritis, and Juvenile Ankylosing Spondylitis; Along with Information about Medical, Surgical, and Alternative Treatment Options, and Including Strategies for Coping with Pain, Fatigue, and Stress

Edited by Allan R. Cook. 575 pages. 1998. 0-7808-0201-2. $78.

Back & Neck Disorders Sourcebook

Basic Information about Disorders and Injuries of the Spinal Cord and Vertebrae, Including Facts on Chiropractic Treatment, Surgical Interventions, Paralysis, and Rehabilitation, Along with Advice for Preventing Back Trouble

Edited by Karen Bellenir. 548 pages. 1997. 0-7808-0202-0. $78.

"The strength of this work is its basic, easy-to-read format. Recommended."
— *Reference and User Services Quarterly, Winter '97*

Blood & Circulatory Disorders Sourcebook

Basic Information about Blood and Its Components, Anemias, Leukemias, Bleeding Disorders, and Circulatory Disorders, Including Aplastic Anemia, Thalassemia, Sickle-Cell Disease, Hemochromatosis, Hemophilia, Von Willebrand Disease, and Vascular Diseases; Along with a Special Section on Blood Transfusions and Blood Supply Safety, a Glossary, and Source Listings for Further Help and Information

Edited by Karen Bellenir and Linda M. Shin. 575 pages. 1998. 0-7808-0203-9. $78.

Brain Disorders Sourcebook

Basic Consumer Health Information about Strokes, Epilepsy, Amyotrophic Lateral Sclerosis (ALS/Lou Gehrig's Disease), Parkinson's Disease, Brain Tumors, Cerebral Palsy, Headache, Tourette Syndrome, and More; Along with Statistical Data, Treatment and Rehabilitation Options, Coping Strategies, Reports on Current Research Initiatives, a Glossary, and Resource Listings for Additional Help and Information

Edited by Karen Bellenir. 600 pages. 1999. 0-7808-0229-2. $78.

Burn

*Basic In...
Scalds, ...
and Su...
ments, ... Surgery,
Prevention Suggestions, and First Aid*

Edited by Allan R. Cook. 600 pages. 1999. 0-7808-0204-7. $78.

Cancer Sourcebook, 1st Edition

Basic Information on Cancer Types, Symptoms, Diagnostic Methods, and Treatments, Including Statistics on Cancer Occurrences Worldwide and the Risks Associated with Known Carcinogens and Activities

Edited by Frank E. Bair. 932 pages. 1990. 1-55888-888-8. $78.

"Written in nontechnical language. Useful for patients, their families, medical professionals, and librarians."
— *Guide to Reference Books, '96*

"Designed with the non-medical professional in mind. Libraries and medical facilities interested in patient education should certainly consider adding the *Cancer Sourcebook* to their holdings. This compact collection of reliable information . . . is an invaluable tool for helping patients and patients' families and friends to take the first steps in coping with the many difficulties of cancer."
— *Medical Reference Services Quarterly, Winter '91*

"Specifically created for the nontechnical reader . . . an important resource for the general reader trying to understand the complexities of cancer."
— *American Reference Books Annual, '91*

"This publication's nontechnical nature and very comprehensive format make it useful for both the general public and undergraduate students." — *Choice, Oct '90*

New Cancer Sourcebook, 2nd Edition

Basic Information about Major Forms and Stages of Cancer, Featuring Facts about Primary and Secondary Tumors of the Respiratory, Nervous, Lymphatic, Circulatory, Skeletal, and Gastrointestinal Systems, and Specific Organs; Statistical and Demographic Data; Treatment Options; and Strategies for Coping

Edited by Allan R. Cook. 1,313 pages. 1996. 0-7808-0041-9. $78.

"This book is an excellent resource for patients with newly diagnosed cancer and their families. The dialogue is simple, direct, and comprehensive. Highly recommended for patients and families to aid in their understanding of cancer and its treatment."
— *Booklist Health Sciences Supplement, Oct '97*

"The amount of factual and useful information is extensive. The writing is very clear, geared to general readers. Recommended for all levels." — *Choice, Jan '97*

Continues next page

Cancer Sourcebook, 3rd Edition

Basic Information about Major Forms and Stages of Cancer, Featuring Facts about Primary and Secondary Tumors of the Respiratory, Nervous, Lymphatic, Circulatory, Skeletal, and Gastrointestinal Systems, and Specific Organs, Statistical and Demographic Data, Treatment Options, and Strategies for Coping

Edited by Edward J. Prucha. 800 pages. 1999. 0-7808-0227-6. $78.

Cancer Sourcebook for Women

Basic Information about Specific Forms of Cancer That Affect Women, Featuring Facts about Breast Cancer, Cervical Cancer, Ovarian Cancer, Cancer of the Uterus and Uterine Sarcoma, Cancer of the Vagina, and Cancer of the Vulva; Statistical and Demographic Data; Treatments, Self-Help Management Suggestions, and Current Research Initiatives

Edited by Allan R. Cook and Peter D. Dresser. 524 pages. 1996. 0-7808-0076-1. $78.

". . . written in easily understandable, non-technical language. Recommended for public libraries or hospital and academic libraries that collect patient education or consumer health materials."
— *Medical Reference Services Quarterly, Spring '97*

"Would be of value in a consumer health library. . . . written with the health care consumer in mind. Medical jargon is at a minimum, and medical terms are explained in clear, understandable sentences."
— *Bulletin of the MLA, Oct '96*

"The availability under one cover of all these pertinent publications, grouped under cohesive headings, makes this certainly a most useful sourcebook."
— *Choice, Jun '96*

"Presents a comprehensive knowledge base for general readers. Men and women both benefit from the gold mine of information nestled between the two covers of this book. Recommended."
— *Academic Library Book Review, Summer '96*

"This timely book is highly recommended for consumer health and patient education collections in all libraries." — *Library Journal, Apr '96*

Cancer Sourcebook for Women, 2nd Edition

Basic Information about Specific Forms of Cancer That Affect Women, Featuring Facts about Breast Cancer, Cervical Cancer, Ovarian Cancer, Cancer of the Uterus and Uterine Sarcoma, Cancer of the Vagina, and Cancer of the Vulva, Statistical and Demographic Data, Treatments, Self-Help Management Suggestions, and Current Research Initiatives

Edited by Edward J. Prucha. 600 pages. 1999. 0-7808-0226-8. $78.

Cardiovascular Diseases & Disorders Sourcebook

Basic Information about Cardiovascular Diseases and Disorders, Featuring Facts about the Cardiovascular System, Demographic and Statistical Data, Descriptions of Pharmacological and Surgical Interventions, Lifestyle Modifications, and a Special Section Focusing on Heart Disorders in Children

Edited by Karen Bellenir and Peter D. Dresser. 683 pages. 1995. 0-7808-0032-X. $78.

". . . comprehensive format provides an extensive overview on this subject." — *Choice, Jun '96*

". . . an easily understood, complete, up-to-date resource. This well executed public health tool will make valuable information available to those that need it most, patients and their families. The typeface, sturdy non-reflective paper, and library binding add a feel of quality found wanting in other publications. Highly recommended for academic and general libraries. "
— *Academic Library Book Review, Summer '96*

Communication Disorders Sourcebook

Basic Information about Deafness and Hearing Loss, Speech and Language Disorders, Voice Disorders, Balance and Vestibular Disorders, and Disorders of Smell, Taste, and Touch

Edited by Linda M. Ross. 533 pages. 1996. 0-7808-0077-X. $78.

"This is skillfully edited and is a welcome resource for the layperson. It should be found in every public and medical library."
— *Booklist Health Sciences Supplement, Oct '97*

Congenital Disorders Sourcebook

Basic Information about Disorders Acquired during Gestation, Including Spina Bifida, Hydrocephalus, Cerebral Palsy, Heart Defects, Craniofacial Abnormalities, Fetal Alcohol Syndrome, and More, Along with Current Treatment Options and Statistical Data

Edited by Karen Bellenir. 607 pages. 1997. 0-7808-0205-5. $78.

"Recommended reference source." — *Booklist, Oct '97*

Consumer Issues in Health Care Sourcebook

Basic Information about Health Care Fundamentals and Related Consumer Issues, Including Exams and Screening Tests, Physician Specialties, Choosing a Doctor, Using Prescription and Over-the-Counter Medications Safely, Avoiding Health Scams, Managing Common Health Risks in the Home, Care Options for Chronically or Terminally Ill Patients, and a List of Resources for Obtaining Help and Further Information

Edited by Karen Bellenir. 592 pages. 1998. 0-7808-0221-7. $78.

Continues in back end sheets

Diet and Nutrition
SOURCEBOOK

Second Edition

Health Reference Series

AIDS Sourcebook, 1st Edition

AIDS Sourcebook, 2nd Edition

Allergies Sourcebook

Alternative Medicine Sourcebook

Alzheimer's, Stroke & 29 Other Neurological Disorders Sourcebook

Alzheimer's Disease Sourcebook, 2nd Edition

Arthritis Sourcebook

Back & Neck Disorders Sourcebook

Blood & Circulatory Disorders Sourcebook

Brain Disorders Sourcebook

Burns Sourcebook

Cancer Sourcebook, 1st Edition

New Cancer Sourcebook, 2nd Edition

Cancer Sourcebook, 3rd Edition

Cancer Sourcebook for Women

Cancer Sourcebook for Women, 2nd Edition

Cardiovascular Diseases & Disorders Sourcebook

Communication Disorders Sourcebook

Congenital Disorders Sourcebook

Consumer Issues in Health Care Sourcebook

Contagious & Non-Contagious Infectious Diseases Sourcebook

Death & Dying Sourcebook

Diabetes Sourcebook, 1st Edition

Diabetes Sourcebook, 2nd Edition

Diet & Nutrition Sourcebook, 1st Edition

Diet & Nutrition Sourcebook, 2nd Edition

Domestic Violence Sourcebook

Ear, Nose & Throat Disorders Sourcebook

Endocrine & Metabolic Disorders Sourcebook

Environmentally Induced Disorders Sourcebook

Ethical Issues in Medicine Sourcebook

Fitness & Exercise Sourcebook

Food & Animal Borne Diseases Sourcebook

Gastrointestinal Diseases & Disorders Sourcebook

Genetic Disorders Sourcebook

Head Trauma Sourcebook

Health Insurance Sourcebook

Healthy Aging Sourcebook

Immune System Disorders Sourcebook

Kidney & Urinary Tract Diseases & Disorders Sourcebook

Learning Disabilities Sourcebook

Medical Tests Sourcebook

Men's Health Concerns Sourcebook

Mental Health Disorders Sourcebook

Ophthalmic Disorders Sourcebook

Oral Health Sourcebook

Pain Sourcebook

Physical & Mental Issues in Aging Sourcebook

Pregnancy & Birth Sourcebook

Public Health Sourcebook

Rehabilitation Sourcebook

Respiratory Diseases & Disorders Sourcebook

Sexually Transmitted Diseases Sourcebook

Skin Disorders Sourcebook

Sleep Disorders Sourcebook

Sports Injuries Sourcebook

Substance Abuse Sourcebook

Women's Health Concerns Sourcebook

Workplace Health & Safety Sourcebook

Health Reference Series

Second Edition

Diet and Nutrition SOURCEBOOK

Basic Consumer Health Information about Dietary Guidelines, Recommended Daily Intake Values, Vitamins, Minerals, Fiber, Fat, Weight Control, Dietary Supplements, and Food Additives; Along with Special Sections on Nutrition Needs throughout Life and Nutrition for People with Such Specific Medical Concerns as Allergies, High Blood Cholesterol, Hypertension, Diabetes, Celiac Disease, Seizure Disorders, Phenylketonuria (PKU), Cancer, and Eating Disorders, and Including Reports on Current Nutrition Research and Source Listings for Additional Help and Information

Edited by
Karen Bellenir

Omnigraphics, Inc.

Penobscot Building / Detroit, MI 48226

Bibliographic Note

Because this page cannot legibly accommodate all the copyright notices, the Bibliographic Note portion of the Preface constitutes an extension of the copyright notice.

Beginning with books published in 1999, each volume of the *Health Reference Series* on a new topic will be individually titled and called a "First Edition." Subsequent updates will carry sequential edition numbers. To help avoid confusion and to provide maximum flexibility in our ability to respond to informational needs, the practice of consecutively numbering each volume will be discontinued.

Edited by Karen Bellenir

Health Reference Series

Karen Bellenir, *Series Editor*
Peter D. Dresser, *Managing Editor*
Joan Margeson, *Research Associate*
Dawn Matthews, *Verification Assistant*
Margaret Mary Missar, *Research Coordinator*
Jenifer Swanson, *Research Associate*

Omnigraphics, Inc.

Matthew P. Barbour, *Manager, Production and Fulfillment*
Laurie Lanzen Harris, *Vice President, Editorial Director*
Peter E. Ruffner, *Vice President, Administration*
James A. Sellgren, *Executive Vice President, Operations and Finance*
Jane J. Steele, *Marketing Consultant*

Frederick G. Ruffner, Jr., Publisher

Library of Congress Cataloging-in-Publication Data

Diet and nutrition sourcebook : basic consumer health
    information about dietary guidelines — / edited by
    Karen Bellenir. — 2nd ed.
        p. cm. — (Health reference series)
    First ed. published in 1996 edited by Dan R. Harris.
    Includes bibliographical references and index.
    ISBN 0-7808-0228-4 (lib. bdg. : alk. paper)
    1. Nutrition. I. Bellenir, Karen II. Series
RA784.D534 1999   99-17687
613.2 — dc21   CIP

∞

This book is printed on acid-free paper meeting the ANSI Z39.48 Standard. The infinity symbol that appears above indicates that the paper in this book meets that standard.

Printed in the United States

Table of Contents

Part II: Nutrition Needs throughout Life

Part III: Nutrition for People with Specific Medical Concerns

Part IV: Weight Control

Part V: Dietary Supplements and Food Additives

Part VI: Nutrition Research

Part VII: Additional Help and Information

Preface

Many Americans struggle to achieve dietary balance. According to a report from the National Academy of Science's Institute of Medicine, dieting Americans spend more than $33 billion annually on weight-reduction products, including diet foods and drinks. Yet, studies over the last two decades by the National Center for Health Statistics show that obesity, a disorder associated with overeating, is actually on the rise. Today, approximately 35 percent of women and 31 percent of men age 20 and older are considered obese, up from approximately 30 percent and 25 percent, respectively, in 1980.

Disorders associated with undereating also plague some segments of the population. Anorexia nervosa, a disorder of self-starvation, afflicts an estimated one in every hundred young women and girls. In addition, some statistics indicate that up to 40 percent of older adults receive inadequate amounts of three or more nutrients, and as many as 50 percent of nursing home residents in the United States may be malnourished.

This *Sourcebook* contains information about basic dietary principles and guidelines for people of all ages and for people with specific medical concerns, including food allergies, high blood cholesterol, hypertension, diabetes, celiac disease, seizure disorders, phenylketonuria (PKU), cancer, and eating disorders. In addition, it provides information about developments that have occurred in the field of nutrition science since the publication of the first edition of *Diet and Nutrition Sourcebook* in 1996.

About This Book

How to Use This Book

This book is divided into parts and chapters. Parts focus on broad areas of interest. Chapters are devoted to single topics within a part.

Part I: Nutrition Fundamentals presents basic information about essential vitamins, minerals, and other nutrients. It describes healthy dietary patterns and includes information about reports issued by the National Academy of Science, Institute of Medicine, Food and Nutrition Board updating previously established recommended dietary allowances.

Part II: Nutrition Needs throughout Life describes the human body's changing dietary needs from infancy through childhood, adolescence, and adulthood. Individual chapters address the special concerns of parents, adults living alone, and older adults.

Part III: Nutrition for People with Specific Medical Concerns addresses the unique problems faced by people undergoing treatment for diseases and disorders with dietary implications. These include food allergies, high blood cholesterol, hypertension, diabetes, celiac disease, seizure disorders, phenylketonuria (PKU), cancer, and eating disorders.

Part IV: Weight Control provides fundamental information for people with concerns about controlling body weight through dietary modification. For more in-depth information about obesity, including its medical consequences, treatment strategies, and reports on current research initiatives, see *Obesity Sourcebook,* a forthcoming volume in the *Health Reference Series.*

Part V: Dietary Supplements and Food Additives offers answers to commonly asked questions about the safety and efficacy of such supplements as vitamins, minerals, and fluoride, and additives including fat substitutes, low-calorie sweeteners, monosodium glutamate, artificial coloring, and preservatives. A separate chapter cautions consumers about products that make unsubstantiated health claims.

Part VI: Nutrition Research presents information about nutrient and micronutrient excesses, deficiencies, and imbalances. Individual chapters highlight some recent studies concerning the interrelationship between nutrients and immune function, the possible connection between dietary choices and asthma, and the role selenium may play in cancer prevention.

Part VII: Additional Help and Information includes a glossary of dietary and nutrition terms, a description of federal nutritional support programs, a guide to finding accurate nutrition advice on the internet, a list of available nutrition resources, and a directory of organizations able to provide additional information.

Bibliographic Note

This volume contains documents and excerpts from publications issued by the following U.S. government agencies: National Cancer Institute (NCI); National Heart, Lung, and Blood Institute (NHLBI); National Institute of Child Health and Human Development (NICHD); National Institute of Dental Research (NIDR); National Institute of Diabetes and Digestive and Kidney Diseases (NIDDK); National Institute on Alcohol Abuse and Alcoholism (NIAAA); Office of Alternative Medicine (OAM); U.S. Administration on Aging (AoA); U.S. Department of Agriculture (USDA); and U.S. Food and Drug Administration (FDA).

In addition, this volume contains copyrighted documents from the following organizations: American Dietetic Association; International Food Information Council; National Academy of Sciences, Institute of Medicine, Food and Nutrition Board; Stanford University School of Medicine; and the University of Iowa Hospitals and Clinics. Articles from the following journals are also included: *Archives of Internal Medicine; Food Insight; RN; The Johns Hopkins Medical Letter Health After 50*; and *Tufts University Health and Nutrition Letter*. Full citation information is provided on the first page of each chapter. Every effort has been made to secure all necessary rights to reprint the copyrighted material. If any omissions have been made, please contact Omnigraphics to make corrections for future editions.

Acknowledgements

In addition to the many organizations listed above that provided the material presented in this volume, special thanks are due to researchers Joan Margeson, Margaret Mary Missar, and Jenifer Swanson, permissions specialist Maria Franklin, verification assistant Dawn

Matthews, indexer Edward J. Prucha, and document engineer Bruce Bellenir.

Note from the Editor

This book is part of Omnigraphics' *Health Reference Series*. The series provides basic consumer health information about a broad range of medical concerns. It is not intended to serve as a tool for diagnosing illness, in prescribing treatments, or as a substitute for the physician/patient relationship. All persons concerned about medical symptoms or the possibility of disease are encouraged to seek professional care from an appropriate health care provider.

Our Advisory Board

The *Health Reference Series* is reviewed by an Advisory Board comprised of librarians from public, academic, and medical libraries. We would like to thank the following board members for providing guidance to the development of this series:

Nancy Bulgarelli,
William Beaumont Hospital Library, Royal Oak, MI

Karen Morgan,
Mardigian Library, University of Michigan, Dearborn, MI

Rosemary Orlando,
St. Clair Shores Public Library, St. Clair Shores, MI

Health Reference Series *Update Policy*

The inaugural book in the *Health Reference Series* was the first edition of *Cancer Sourcebook* published in 1992. Since then, the *Series* has been enthusiastically received by librarians and in the medical community. In order to maintain the standard of providing high-quality health information for the lay person, the editorial staff at Omnigraphics felt it was necessary to implement a policy of updating volumes when warranted.

Medical researchers have been making tremendous strides, and the challenge to stay current with the most recent advances is one our editors take seriously. Each decision to update a volume will be made on an individual basis. Some of the considerations will include how much new information is available and the feedback we receive from people who use the books. If there's a topic you would like to see added to the update list, or an area of medical concern you feel has not been adequately addressed, please write to:

Editor
Health Reference Series
Omnigraphics, Inc.
2500 Penobscot Bldg.
Detroit, MI 48226

The commitment to providing on-going coverage of important medical developments has also led to some technical changes in the *Health Reference Series*. Beginning with books published in 1999, each volume on a new topic will be individually titled and called a "First Edition." Subsequent updates will carry sequential edition numbers. To help avoid confusion and to provide maximum flexibility in our ability to respond to informational needs, the practice of consecutively numbering each volume will be discontinued.

Part One

Nutrition Fundamentals

Chapter 1

Dietary Guidelines for Americans

Diet Is Important to Health at All Stages of Life

Healthful diets help children grow, develop, and do well in school. They enable people of all ages to work productively and feel their best. Food choices also can help to reduce the risk for chronic diseases, such as heart disease, certain cancers, diabetes, stroke, and osteoporosis, that are leading causes of death and disability among Americans. Good diets can reduce major risk factors for chronic diseases—factors such as obesity, high blood pressure, and high blood cholesterol.

Foods Contain Energy

People require energy and certain other essential nutrients. These nutrients are essential because the body cannot make them and must obtain them from food. Essential nutrients include vitamins, minerals, certain amino acids, and certain fatty acids. Foods also contain other components such as fiber that are important for health. Although each of these food components has a specific function in the body, all of them together are required for overall health. People need calcium to build and maintain strong bones, for example, but many other nutrients also are involved.

Excerpted from *Nutrition and Your Health: Dietary Guidelines for Americans, Fourth Edition*, U.S. Department of Agriculture (USDA) and U.S. Department of Health and Human Services (DHHS), 1995.

3

The carbohydrates, fats, and proteins in food supply energy, which is measured in calories. Carbohydrates and proteins provide about 4 calories per gram. Fat contributes more than twice as much—about 9 calories per gram. Alcohol, although not a nutrient, also supplies energy—about 7 calories per gram. Foods that are high in fat are also high in calories. However, many lowfat or nonfat foods can also be high in calories.

Calorie needs vary by age and level of activity. Many older adults need less food, in part due to decreased activity, relative to younger, more active individuals. People who are trying to lose weight and eating little food may need to select more nutrient-dense foods in order to meet their nutrient needs in a satisfying diet. Nearly all Americans need to be more active, because a sedentary lifestyle is unhealthful. Increasing the calories spent in daily activities helps to maintain health and allows people to eat a nutritious and enjoyable diet.

What Is a Healthful Diet?

Healthful diets contain the amounts of essential nutrients and calories needed to prevent nutritional deficiencies and excesses. Healthful diets also provide the right balance of carbohydrate, fat, and protein to reduce risks for chronic diseases, and are a part of a full and productive lifestyle. Such diets are obtained from a variety of foods that are available, affordable, and enjoyable.

Research has shown that certain diets raise risks for chronic diseases. Such diets are high in fat, saturated fat, cholesterol, and salt and they contain more calories than the body uses. They are also low in grain products, vegetables, fruit, and fiber.

The Food Guide Pyramid and the Nutrition Facts Label serve as educational tools to put the Dietary Guidelines into practice. The Pyramid translates the Recommended Dietary Allowances (RDAs) and the Dietary Guidelines into the kinds and amounts of food to eat each day. The Nutrition Facts Label is designed to help you select foods for a diet that will meet the Dietary Guidelines. Most processed foods now include nutrition information. However, nutrition labels are not required for foods like coffee and tea (which contain no significant amounts of nutrients), certain ready-to-eat foods like unpackaged deli and bakery items, and restaurant food. Labels are also voluntary for many raw foods—your grocer may supply this information for the fish, meat, poultry, and raw fruits and vegetables that are consumed most frequently.

Eat a Variety of Foods

To obtain the nutrients and other substances needed for good health, vary the foods you eat. Foods contain combinations of nutrients and other healthful substances. No single food can supply all nutrients in the amounts you need. For example, oranges provide vitamin C but no vitamin B_{12}; cheese provides vitamin B_{12} but no vitamin C. To make sure you get all of the nutrients and other substances needed for health, choose the recommended number of daily servings from each of the five major food groups displayed in the Food Guide Pyramid. Use foods from the base of the Food Guide Pyramid as the foundation of your meals.

Choose Foods from Each of Five Food Groups

The Food Guide Pyramid illustrates the importance of balance among food groups in a daily eating pattern. Most of the daily serv-

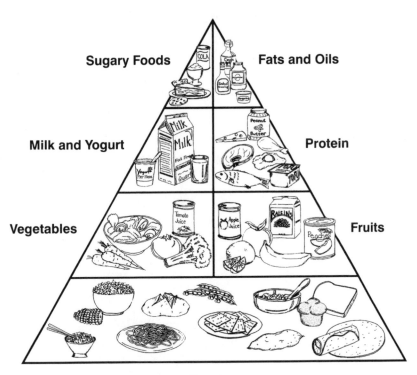

Figure 1.1. *Food Guide Pyramid*

5

ings of food should be selected from the food groups that are the largest in the picture and closest to the base of the Pyramid.

- Choose most of your foods from the grain products group (6-11 servings), the vegetable group (3-5 servings), and the fruit group (2-4 servings).

- Eat moderate amounts of foods from the milk group (2-3 servings) and the meat and beans group (2-3 servings).

COOKIES

Nutrition Facts

Serving Size 3 cookies (34g/1.2 oz)
Servings Per Container About 5

Serving Size reflects the amount typically eaten by many people.

Amount Per Serving		
Calories 180	Calories from Fat 90	

	% Daily Value*
Total Fat 10g	**15%**
Saturated Fat 3.5g	**18%**
Polyunsaturated Fat 1g	
Monounsaturated Fat 5g	
Cholesterol 10mg	**3%**
Sodium 80mg	**3%**
Total Carbohydrate 21g	**7%**
Dietary Fiber 1g	**4%**
Sugars 11g	
Protein 2g	

Vitamin A 0%	•	Vitamin C 0%	
Calcium 0%	•	Iron 4%	
Thiamin 6%	•	Riboflavin 4%	
Niacin 4%			

The list of nutrients covers those most important to the health of today's consumers.

*Percent Daily Values are based on a 2,000 calorie diet. Your daily values may be higher or lower depending on your calorie needs:

		Calories	2,000	2,500
Total Fat	Less than		65g	80g
Sat Fat	Less than		20g	25g
Cholesterol	Less than		300mg	300mg
Sodium	Less than		2,400mg	2,400mg
Total Carbohydrate			300g	375g
Dietary Fiber			25g	30g

Ingredients: Unbleached enriched wheat flour [flour, niacin, reduced iron, thiamin mononitrate (vitamin B₁)], sweet chocolate (sugar, chocolate liquor, cocoa butter, soy lecithin added as an emulsifier, vanilla extract), sugar, partially hydrogenated vegetable shortening (soybean, cottonseed and/or canola oils), nonfat milk, whole eggs, cornstarch, egg whites, salt, vanilla extract, baking soda, and soy lecithin.

Calories from Fat are now shown on the label to help consumers meet dietary guidelines that recommend people get no more than 30 percent of the calories in their overall diet from fat.

% Daily Value (DV) shows how a food in the specified serving size fits into the overall daily diet. By using the %DV you can easily determine whether a food contributes a lot or a little of a particular nutrient. And you can compare different foods with no need to do any calculations.

Figure 1.2. Example of Nutrition Facts Label

- Choose sparingly foods that provide few nutrients and are high in fat and sugars.

Note: A range of servings is given for each food group. The smaller number is for people who consume about 1,600 calories a day, such as many sedentary women. The larger number is for those who consume about 2,800 calories a day, such as active men.

What Counts as a "Serving"?

Grain Products Group (bread, cereal, rice, and pasta)

- 1 slice of bread
- 1 ounce of ready-to-eat cereal
- ½ cup of cooked cereal, rice, or pasta

Vegetable Group

- 1 cup of raw leafy vegetables
- ½ cup of other vegetables—cooked or chopped raw
- ¾ cup of vegetable juice

Fruit Group

- 1 medium apple, banana, orange
- ½ cup of chopped, cooked, or canned fruit
- ¾ cup of fruit juice

Milk Group (milk, yogurt, and cheese)

- 1 cup of milk or yogurt
- 1½ ounces of natural cheese
- 2 ounces of processed cheese

Meat and Beans Group (meat, poultry, fish, dry beans, eggs, and nuts)

- 2-3 ounces of cooked lean meat, poultry, or fish
- ½ cup of cooked dry beans or 1 egg counts as 1 ounce of lean meat. Two tablespoons of peanut butter or 1/3 cup of nuts count as 1 ounce of meat.

Some foods fit into more than one group. Dry beans, peas, and lentils can be counted as servings in either the meat and beans group or vegetable group. These "cross over" foods can be counted as servings from

7

either one or the other group, but not both. Serving sizes indicated here are those used in the Food Guide Pyramid and based on both suggested and usually consumed portions necessary to achieve adequate nutrient intake. They differ from serving sizes on the Nutrition Facts Label, which reflect portions usually consumed.

What about Vegetarian Diets?

Some Americans eat vegetarian diets for reasons of culture, belief, or health. Most vegetarians eat milk products and eggs, and as a group, these lacto-ovo-vegetarians enjoy excellent health. Vegetarian diets are consistent with the *Dietary Guidelines for Americans* and can meet Recommended Dietary Allowances for nutrients. You can get enough protein from a vegetarian diet as long as the variety and amounts of foods consumed are adequate. Meat, fish, and poultry are major contributors of iron, zinc, and B vitamins in most American diets, and vegetarians should pay special attention to these nutrients.

Vegans eat only food of plant origin. Because animal products are the only food sources of vitamin B_{12}, vegans must supplement their diets with a source of this vitamin. In addition, vegan diets, particularly those of children, require care to ensure adequacy of vitamin D and calcium, which most Americans obtain from milk products.

Foods Vary in Their Amounts of Calories and Nutrients

Some foods such as grain products, vegetables, and fruits have many nutrients and other healthful substances but are relatively low in calories. Fat and alcohol are high in calories. Foods high in both sugars and fat contain many calories but often are low in vitamins, minerals, or fiber.

People who do not need many calories or who must restrict their food intake need to choose nutrient-rich foods from the five major food groups with special care. They should obtain most of their calories from foods that contain a high proportion of essential nutrients and fiber.

Growing Children, Teenage Girls, and Women Have Higher Needs for Some Nutrients

Many women and adolescent girls need to eat more calcium-rich foods to get the calcium needed for healthy bones throughout life. By selecting lowfat or fat-free milk products and other lowfat calcium sources, they can obtain adequate calcium and keep fat intake from being too high. Young children, teenage girls, and women of childbearing age should also eat enough iron-rich foods, such as lean meats and whole-grain or enriched white bread, to keep the body's iron stores at adequate levels.

Some Good Sources of Calcium

- Most foods in the milk group: milk and dishes made with milk, such as puddings and soups made with milk; cheeses such as Mozzarella, Cheddar, Swiss, and Parmesan; and yogurt (Some foods in this group are high in fat, cholesterol, or both. Choose lower fat, lower cholesterol foods most often. Read the labels.)

- Canned fish with soft bones such as sardines, anchovies, and salmon

- Dark-green leafy vegetables, such as kale, mustard greens, and turnip greens, and pak-choi

- Tofu, if processed with calcium sulfate. Read the labels.

- Tortillas made from lime-processed com. Read the labels.

Note: Does not include complete list of examples.

Some Good Sources of Iron

- Meats-beef, pork, lamb, and liver and other organ meats*

- Poultry-chicken, duck, and turkey, especially dark meat; liver*

- Fish—shellfish, like clams, mussels, and oysters; sardines; anchovies; and other fish*

- Leafy greens of the cabbage family, such as broccoli, kale, turnip greens, collards

- Legumes, such as lima beans and green peas; dry beans and peas, such as pinto beans, black-eyed peas, and canned baked beans

- Yeast-leavened whole-wheat bread and rolls

- Iron-enriched white bread, pasta, rice, and cereals. Read the labels.

*Some foods in this group are high in fat, cholesterol, or both. Choose lean, lower fat, lower cholesterol foods most often. Read the labels.

Note: Does not include complete list of examples.

Choose a Diet with Plenty of Grain Products, Vegetables, and Fruits

Grain products, vegetables, and fruits are key parts of a varied diet. They are emphasized in this guideline because they provide vitamins, minerals, complex carbohydrates (starch and dietary fiber), and other substances that are important for good health. They are also generally low in fat, depending on how they are prepared and what is added to them at the table. Most Americans of all ages eat fewer than the recommended number of servings of grain products, vegetables, and fruits, even though consumption of these foods is associated with a substantially lower risk for many chronic diseases, including certain types of cancer.

Most fruits and vegetables are excellent sources of vitamin C, vitamin B_6, carotenoids, including those which form vitamin A, and folate. The antioxidant nutrients found in plant foods (e.g., vitamin C, carotenoids, vitamin E, and certain minerals) are presently of great interest to scientists and the public because of their potentially beneficial role in reducing the risk for cancer and certain other chronic diseases. Scientists are also trying to determine if other substances in plant foods protect against cancer.

Folate, also called folic acid, is a B vitamin that, among its many functions, reduces the risk of a serious type of birth defect. Minerals such as potassium, found in a wide variety of vegetables and fruits, and calcium, found in certain vegetables, may help reduce the risk for high blood pressure.

Fiber is found only in plant foods like whole-grain breads and cereals, beans and peas, and other vegetables and fruits. Because there are different types of fiber in foods, choose a variety of foods daily. Eating a variety of fiber-containing plant foods is important for proper bowel function, can reduce symptoms of chronic constipation, diverticular disease, and hemorrhoids, and may lower the risk for heart disease and some cancers. However, some of the health benefits associated with a high-fiber diet may come from other components present in these foods, not just from fiber itself. For this reason, fiber is best obtained from foods rather than supplements.

Some Good Sources of Carotenoids

- Dark-green leafy vegetables (such as spinach, collards, kale, mustard greens, turnip greens), broccoli, carrots, pumpkin and calabasa, red pepper, sweet potatoes, and tomatoes

- Fruits like mango, papaya, cantaloupe

Note: Does not include complete list of examples.

Some Good Sources of Folate

- Dry beans (like red beans, navy beans, and soybeans), lentils, chickpeas, cow peas, and peanuts

- Many vegetables, especially leafy greens (spinach, cabbage, brussels sprouts, romaine, looseleaf lettuce), peas, okra, sweet corn, beets, and broccoli

- Fruits such as blackberries, boysenberries, kiwifruit, oranges, plantains, strawberries, orange juice, and pineapple juice

Note: Does not include complete list of examples.

Choose a Diet Low in Fat, Saturated Fat, and Cholesterol

Some dietary fat is needed for good health. Fats supply energy and essential fatty acids and promote absorption of the fat-soluble vitamins A, D, E, and K. Most people are aware that high levels of saturated fat and cholesterol in the diet are linked to increased blood cholesterol levels and a greater risk for heart disease. More Americans are now eating less fat, saturated fat, and cholesterol-rich foods than in the recent past, and fewer people are dying from the most common form of heart disease. Still, many people continue to eat high-fat diets, the number of overweight people has increased, and the risk of heart disease and certain cancers (also linked to fat intake) remains high. This guideline emphasizes the continued importance of choosing a diet with less total fat, saturated fat, and cholesterol.

Some foods and food groups in the Food Guide Pyramid are higher in fat than others. Fats and oils, and some types of desserts and snack foods that contain fat provide calories but few nutrients. Many foods in the milk group and in the meat and beans group (which includes eggs and nuts, as well as meat, poultry, and fish) are also high in fat, as are some processed foods in the grain group. Choosing lower fat options among these foods allows you to eat the recommended servings from these groups and increase the amount and variety of grain products, fruits, and vegetables in your diet without going over your calorie needs.

Fat, whether from plant or animal sources, contains more than twice the number of calories of an equal amount of carbohydrate or protein. Choose a diet that provides no more than 30 percent of total calories from fat. The upper limit on the grams of fat in your diet will depend on the calories you need. Cutting back on fat can help you consume fewer calories. For example, at 2,000 calories per day, the suggested upper limit of calories from fat is about 600 calories. Sixty-five grams of fat contribute about 600 calories (65 grams of fat x 9 calories per gram = about 600 calories). On the Nutrition Facts Label, 65 grams of fat is the Daily Value for a 2,000-calorie intake.

Maximum Total Fat Intake at Different Calorie Levels

- At 1,600 calories: 53 grams total fat
- At 2,200 calories: 73 grams total fat
- At 2,800 calories: 93 grams total fat

For a Diet Low in Fat, Saturated Fat, and Cholesterol

Fats and Oils

- Use fats and oils sparingly in cooking and at the table.

- Use small amounts of salad dressings and spreads such as butter, margarine, and mayonnaise. Consider using lowfat or fat-free dressings for salads.

- Choose vegetable oils and soft margarines most often because they are lower in saturated fat than solid shortenings and animal fats, even though their caloric content is the same.

- Check the Nutrition Facts Label to see how much fat and saturated fat are in a serving; choose foods lower in fat and saturated fat.

Grain Products, Vegetables, and Fruits

- Choose lowfat sauces with pasta, rice, and potatoes.

- Use as little fat as possible to cook vegetables and grain products.

- Season with herbs, spices, lemon juice, and fat-free or lowfat salad dressings.

Meat, Poultry, Fish, Eggs, Beans, and Nuts

- Choose two to three servings of lean fish, poultry, meats, or other protein-rich foods, such as beans, daily. Use meats labeled "lean" or "extra lean." Trim fat from meat; take skin off poultry. (Three ounces of cooked lean beef or chicken without skin—a piece the size of a deck of cards—provides about 6 grams of fat; a piece of chicken with skin or untrimmed meat of that size may have as much as twice this amount of fat.) Most beans and bean products are almost fat-free and are a good source of protein and fiber.

- Limit intake of high-fat processed meats such as sausages, salami, and other cold cuts; choose lower fat varieties by reading the Nutrition Facts Label.

- Limit the intake of organ meats (three ounces of cooked chicken liver have about 540 mg of cholesterol); use egg yolks in moderation (one egg yolk has about 215 mg of cholesterol). Egg whites contain no cholesterol and can be used freely.

Milk and Milk Products

- Choose skim or lowfat milk, fat-free or lowfat yogurt, and lowfat cheese.

- Have two to three lowfat servings daily. Add extra calcium to your diet without added fat by choosing fat-free yogurt and lowfat milk more often. (One cup of skim milk has almost no fat; 1 cup of 1 percent milk has 2.5 grams of fat; 1 cup of 2 percent milk has 5 grams, one teaspoon, of fat; and 1 cup of whole milk has 8 grams of fat.) If you do not consume foods from this group, eat other calcium-rich foods.

Advice on Dietary Fat for Children

Advice in the previous sections does not apply to infants and toddlers below the age of 2 years. After that age, children should gradually adopt a diet that, by about 5 years of age, contains no more than 30 percent of calories from fat. As they begin to consume fewer calories from fat, children should replace these calories by eating more grain products, fruits, vegetables, and lowfat milk products or other calcium-rich foods and beans, lean meat, poultry, fish, or other protein-rich foods.

Choose a Diet Moderate in Sugars

Sugars are carbohydrates. Dietary carbohydrates also include the complex carbohydrates starch and fiber. During digestion all carbohydrates except fiber break down into sugars. Sugars and starches occur naturally in many foods that also supply other nutrients. Examples of these foods include milk, fruits, some vegetables, breads, cereals, and grains. Americans eat sugars in many forms, and most people like their taste. Some sugars are used as natural preservatives, thickeners, and baking aids in foods; they are often added to foods during processing and preparation or when they are eaten. The body cannot tell the difference between naturally occurring and added sugars because they are identical chemically.

Scientific evidence indicates that diets high in sugars do not cause hyperactivity or diabetes. The most common type of diabetes occurs in overweight adults. Avoiding sugars alone will not correct overweight. To lose weight reduce the total amount of calories from the food you eat and increase your level of physical activity.

On a food label, sugars include: brown sugar, corn sweetener, fructose, fruit juice concentrate, glucose (dextrose), high-fructose corn syrup, honey, invert sugar, lactose, molasses, raw sugar, [table] sugar (sucrose), and syrup. A food is likely to be high in sugars if one of these terms appears first or second in the ingredients list, or if several of them are listed.

Sugar substitutes such as sorbitol, saccharin, and aspartame are ingredients in many foods. Most sugar substitutes do not provide significant calories and therefore may be useful in the diets of people concerned about calorie intake. Foods containing sugar substitutes, however, may not always be lower in calories than similar products that contain sugars. Unless you reduce the total calories you eat, the use of sugar substitutes will not cause you to lose weight.

Both sugars and starches can promote tooth decay. The more often you eat foods that contain sugars and starches, and the longer these foods are in your mouth before you brush your teeth, the greater the risk for tooth decay. Thus, frequent eating of foods high in sugars and starches as between-meal snacks may be more harmful to your teeth than eating them at meals and then brushing. Regular daily dental hygiene, including brushing with a fluoride toothpaste and flossing, and an adequate intake of fluoride, preferably from fluoridated water, will help you prevent tooth decay.

Choose a Diet Moderate in Salt and Sodium

Sodium and sodium chloride—known commonly as salt—occur naturally in foods, usually in small amounts. Salt and other sodium-containing ingredients are often used in food processing. Some people add salt and salty sauces, such as soy sauce, to their food at the table, but most dietary sodium or salt comes from foods to which salt has already been added during processing or preparation. Although many people add salt to enhance the taste of foods, their preference may weaken with eating less salt.

In the body, sodium plays an essential role in regulation of fluids and blood pressure. Many studies in diverse populations have shown that a high sodium intake is associated with higher blood pressure. Most evidence suggests that many people at risk for high blood pressure reduce their chances of developing this condition by consuming less salt or sodium. Some questions remain, partly because other factors may interact with sodium to affect blood pressure.

Following other guidelines in the *Dietary Guidelines for Americans* may also help prevent high blood pressure. An important example is the guideline on weight and physical activity. The role of body weight in blood pressure control is well documented. Blood pressure increases with weight and decreases when weight is reduced. The guideline to consume a diet with plenty of fruits and vegetables is relevant because fruits and vegetables are naturally lower in sodium and fat and may help with weight reduction and control. Consuming more fruits and vegetables also increases potassium intakes which may help to reduce blood pressure. Increased physical activity helps lower blood pressure and control weight. Alcohol consumption has also been associated with high blood pressure. Another reason to reduce salt intake is the fact that high salt intakes may increase the amount of calcium excreted in the urine and, therefore, increase the body's need for calcium.

Some Good Sources of Potassium

- Vegetables and fruits in general, especially: potatoes and sweet potatoes; spinach, swiss chard, broccoli, winter squashes, and parsnips; dates, bananas, cantaloupes, mangoes, plantains, dried apricots, raisins, prunes, orange juice, and grapefruit juice; dry beans, peas, and lentils

- Milk and yogurt are good sources of potassium and have less sodium than cheese; cheese has much less potassium and usually has added salt.

Note: Does not include complete list of examples.

If You Drink Alcoholic Beverages, Do So in Moderation

Alcoholic beverages supply calories but few or no nutrients. The alcohol in these beverages has effects that are harmful when consumed in excess. These effects of alcohol may alter judgment and can lead to dependency and a great many other serious health problems. Alcoholic beverages have been used to enhance the enjoyment of meals by many societies throughout human history. If adults choose to drink alcoholic beverages, they should consume them only in moderation

What Is Moderation?

Moderation is defined as no more than one drink per day for women and no more than two drinks per day for men. Count as a drink:

- 12 ounces of regular beer (150 calories)
- 5 ounces of wine (100 calories)
- 1.5 ounces of 80-proof distilled spirits (100 calories)

Where Do Vitamin, Mineral, and Fiber Supplements Fit in?

Supplements of vitamins, minerals, or fiber also may help to meet special nutritional needs. However, supplements do not supply all of the nutrients and other substances present in foods that are important to health. Supplements of some nutrients taken regularly in large amounts are harmful. Daily vitamin and mineral supplements at or below the Recommended Dietary Allowances are considered safe, but are usually not needed by people who eat the variety of foods depicted in the Food Guide Pyramid.

Sometimes supplements are needed to meet specific nutrient requirements. For example, older people and others with little exposure to sunlight may need a vitamin D supplement. Women of childbearing age may reduce the risk of certain birth defects by consuming folate-rich foods or folic acid supplements. Iron supplements are recommended for pregnant women. However, because foods contain many nutrients and other substances that promote health, the use of supplements cannot substitute for proper food choices.

Enriched and Fortified Foods Have Essential Nutrients Added to Them

National policy requires that specified amounts of nutrients be added to enrich some foods. For example, enriched flour and bread contain added thiamin, riboflavin, niacin, and iron; skim milk, lowfat milk, and margarine are usually enriched with vitamin A; and milk is usually enriched with vitamin D. Fortified foods may have one or several nutrients added in extra amounts. The number and quantity of nutrients added vary among products. Fortified foods may be useful for meeting special dietary needs. Read the ingredient list to know which nutrients are added to foods. How these foods fit into your total diet will depend on the amounts you eat and the other foods you consume.

Chapter 2

Why Do We Need Vitamins and Minerals?

Vitamins

Why Do We Need Vitamin A?

Vitamin A, a fat-soluble vitamin, is involved in the formation and maintenance of healthy skin, hair, and mucous membranes. Vitamin A helps us to see in dim light and is necessary for proper bone growth, tooth development, and reproduction. The U.S. RDA[1] for vitamin A is 1,000 retinol equivalents per day.[2] (Retinol is the form of Vitamin A found in mammals.)

Why Do We Need Vitamin B₁ (Thiamin)?

Thiamin, a water-soluble vitamin, helps the body release energy from carbohydrates during metabolism. Thus, persons who expend more energy and have a higher intake of calories need more thiamin than those who eat fewer calories. Thiamin also plays a vital role in the normal functioning of the nervous system. The U.S. RDA[1] for thiamin is 1.5 milligrams per day.[2] Newly released DRI levels are 1.2 milligrams per day for males over the age of 13, 1.0 milligrams for females aged 14 to 18, and 1.1 milligrams for females over the age of 18.[3]

Excerpted from *Good Sources of Nutrients*, a set of 17 fact sheets produced by the U.S. Department of Agriculture, Human Nutrition Information Service, January 1990; additions and updated information on Dietary Reference Intakes (DRIs) added by the editor in 1998.

Why Do We Need Vitamin B₂ (Riboflavin)?

Riboflavin, a water-soluble vitamin, helps the body release energy from protein, fat, and carbohydrates during metabolism. The U.S. RDA[1] for riboflavin is 1.7 milligrams per day.[2] Newly released DRI levels are 1.3 milligrams per day for males over the age of 13, 1.0 milligrams for females aged 14 to 18, and 1.1 milligrams for females over the age of 18.[3]

Why Do We Need Vitamin B₆?

Vitamin B₆ a water-soluble vitamin, helps use protein to build body tissue and aids in the metabolism of fat. The need for Vitamin B₆ is directly related to protein intake. As the intake of protein increases, the need for Vitamin B₆ increases. The U.S. RDA[1] for vitamin B₆ is 2 milligrams per day.[2] Newly released DRI levels are 1.3 milligrams per day for males between the ages of 14 and 50; 1.7 milligrams for males aged 51 and older; 1.2 milligrams for females aged 14 to 18; 1.3 for females aged 19 to 50; and 1.5 for females aged 51 and older.[3]

Why Do We Need Vitamin B₁₂?

Vitamin B₁₂, a water-soluble vitamin, aids in forming red blood cells and in building genetic material. Vitamin B₁₂ also helps in the functioning of the nervous system and in metabolizing protein and fat in the body. The U.S. RDA[1] for vitamin B₁₂ is 6 micrograms per day.[2] The newly released DRI level is 2.4 micrograms per day for males and females over the age of 18.[3]

Why Do We Need Folate?

Folate (also called folacin or folic acid), a water-soluble vitamin of the B complex, helps the body form red blood cells and aids in the formation of genetic material within every body cell. Folate deficiency has been linked to neural tube birth defects. The U.S. RDA[1] for folate is 400 micrograms per day.[2] The DRI level for pregnant women is 600 micrograms per day.[3]

Why Do We Need Niacin?

Niacin (also called nicotinic acid), a water-soluble vitamin of the B complex, helps the body release energy from protein, fat, and carbohydrate during metabolism. The U.S. RDA[1] for niacin is 20 milligrams per day.[2] Newly released DRI levels are 16 milligrams per day for males over the age of 13, and 14 milligrams for females over the age of 13.[3]

Why Do We Need Vitamin C?

Vitamin C (also called ascorbic acid), a water-soluble vitamin, is important in forming collagen, a protein that gives structure to bones, cartilage, muscle, and blood vessels. It also helps to maintain capillaries, bones, and teeth and aids in the absorption of iron. The U.S. RDA[1] for vitamin C is 60 milligrams per day.[2]

Why Do We Need Vitamin D?

Vitamin D, a fat-soluble vitamin, is necessary for bone and tooth formation. Newly released DRIs recommend 5 micrograms per day for males and females under the age of 51. For males and females between the ages of 51 and 70, 10 micrograms are recommended; for males and females over the age of 70, 15 micrograms are recommended.[3]

Why Do We Need Vitamin E?

Vitamin E, a fat-soluble vitamin, protects vitamin A and essential fatty acids from oxidation in the body cells and prevents breakdown of body tissues. The U.S. RDA[1] for vitamin E is 10 milligrams per day.[2]

Minerals

Why Do We Need Calcium?

Calcium, a mineral, is used for building bones and teeth and in maintaining bone strength. Calcium is also used in muscle contraction, blood clotting, and maintenance of cell membranes. The U.S. RDA[1] for calcium is 1,000 milligrams per day.[2] Newly released DRI levels are 1300 milligrams per day for males and females between the ages of 9 and 18, 1,000 milligrams for people between the ages of 19 and 50, and 1,200 milligrams for people over the age of 50.[4]

Why Do We Need Copper?

Copper, a mineral, is necessary (along with iron) for the formation of hemoglobin. It also helps keep bones, blood vessels, and nerves healthy. The U.S. RDA[1] for copper is 2 milligrams per day.[2]

Why Do We Need Iron?

Iron, a mineral, functions primarily as a carrier of oxygen in the body, both as a part of hemoglobin in the blood and of myoglobin in the muscles. The U.S. RDA[1] for iron is 19 milligrams per day.[2]

Why Do We Need Magnesium?

Magnesium, a mineral, is used in building bones, manufacturing proteins, releasing energy from muscle storage, and regulating body temperature. The U.S. RDA[1] for magnesium is 400 milligrams per day.[2] Newly released DRI levels are 410 milligrams per day for males between the ages of 14 and 18, 400 milligrams per day for males between the ages of 19 and 30, 420 milligrams for males over the age of 30; 360 milligrams for females between the ages of 14 and 18, 310 milligrams for females between the ages of 19 and 30, and 320 milligrams for females over the age of 30.[4]

Why Do We Need Phosphorus?

Phosphorus, a mineral, helps build strong bones and teeth. Phosphorus is also involved in the release of energy from fat, protein, and carbohydrates during metabolism, and in the formation of genetic material, cell membranes, and many enzymes. The U.S. RDA[1] for phosphorus is 1,000 milligrams per day.[2] Newly released DRI levels are 1250 milligrams per day for both males and females between the ages of 9 and 18 and 700 milligrams per day for people over 18 years of age. [4]

Why Do We Need Potassium?

Potassium, a mineral, assists in muscle contraction and in maintaining fluid and electrolyte balance in body cells. Potassium is also important in sending nerve impulses as well as releasing energy from protein, fat, and carbohydrates during metabolism. The Food and Nutrition Board of the National Academy of Sciences has estimated the minimum requirement for potassium for men and women over 18 years of age to be 2,000 milligrams per day.

Why Do We Need Zinc?

Zinc, a mineral, plays an important role in the formation of protein in the body and thus assists in wound healing, blood formation, and general growth and maintenance of all tissues. Zinc is a component of many enzymes and thus is involved in most metabolic processes. The U.S. RDA[1] for zinc is 15 milligrams per day.[2]

Dietary Fiber

Why Do We Need Dietary Fiber?

Dietary fiber is a complex mixture of plant materials that are resistant to breakdown (digestion) by the human digestive system. There are two major kinds of dietary fiber—insoluble (cellulose, hemicellulose, lignin) and soluble (gums, mucilages, pectins). Insoluble fiber is most frequently found in whole-grain products such as whole-wheat bread. Foods containing soluble fibers are fruits, vegetables, dry beans and peas, and some cereals such as oats.

Insoluble fiber promotes normal elimination by providing bulk for stool formation and thus hastening the passage of the stool through the colon. Insoluble fiber also helps to satisfy appetite by creating a full feeling. Some studies indicate that soluble fibers may play a role in reducing the level of cholesterol in the blood.

The Food and Nutrition Board of the National Academy of Sciences has not set a Recommended Dietary Allowance (RDA) for dietary fiber. However, the importance of dietary fiber has been stressed by several health organizations and the Federal government. The Dietary Guidelines for Americans published jointly by the U.S. Departments of Agriculture and Health and Human Services recommend eating foods that have adequate amounts of fiber, and one organization, the National Cancer Institute, recommends 20 to 30 grams of fiber per day with an upper limit of 35 grams.

Notes

1. U.S. Recommended Daily Allowances (RDAs) are based on the 1968 Recommended Dietary Allowances for 24 sex-age categories set by the Food and Nutrition Board of the National Academy of Sciences. The Food and Nutrition Board is reviewing its recommendations and publishing a series of new guidelines for Dietary Reference Intakes (DRIs).

2. The U.S. RDA is given for adults (except pregnant or lactating women) and children over 4 years of age.

3. DRIs for the B vitamins, folate, and other related nutrients were announced in 1998 by the Food and Nutrition Board of

the National Academy of Sciences. The levels listed are for the ages given. Unless otherwise specified, recommendations for women are for non-pregnant, non-lactating women.

4. DRIs for calcium, phosphorus, magnesium and other related nutrients were announced in 1997 by the Food and Nutrition Board of the National Academy of Sciences. The levels listed are for the ages given. Unless otherwise specified, recommendations for women are for non-pregnant, non-lactating women.

Chapter 3

New Report Recasts Dietary Requirements for Calcium and Related Nutrients

Americans and Canadians at risk of osteoporosis should consume between 1,000 and 1,300 milligrams of calcium per day, according to a new report[1] from the Institute of Medicine (IOM) aimed at decreasing the risk of chronic disease through nutrition. The first in a series of reports on Dietary Reference Intakes (DRIs)—which will update and expand the Recommended Dietary Allowances (RDAs) set by the National Academy of Sciences since 1941—reviews calcium, phosphorus, magnesium, vitamin D, and fluoride, which are related to the health of bones and to other body functions. The report recommends intake levels for U.S. and Canadian individuals and population groups, and for the first time, sets maximum-level guidelines to reduce the risk of adverse health effects from over consumption of a nutrient.

"Our understanding of the relationship between nutrition and chronic disease has progressed to the point where we can now begin to recommend intakes that are thought to help people achieve measurable physical indicators of good health," said Vernon Young, chair of the IOM's Standing Committee on Dietary Reference Intakes and professor of nutritional biochemistry, Massachusetts Institute of Technology, Cambridge. "The new DRIs represent a major leap forward in nutrition science—from a primary concern for the prevention of deficiency to an emphasis on beneficial effects of healthy eating."

National Academy of Sciences, Institute of Medicine, Food and Nutrition Board, Press Release dated August 13, 1997; reprinted with permission.

Unlike the RDAs, which established the minimal amounts of nutrients needed to be protective against possible nutrient deficiency, the new values are designed to reflect the latest understanding about nutrient requirements based on optimizing health in individuals and groups. The new recommendations—which include four categories of reference intakes—were made by a group of more than 30 U.S. and Canadian scientists who examined the results of hundreds of nutritional studies on both the beneficial aspects of nutrients and the hazards of taking too much of a nutrient. Where the scientific evidence allowed, the committee made recommendations aimed at helping individuals at different stages of life obtain enough of a nutrient to promote bone strength and to maintain normal nutritional status. Six additional reports—on folate and B vitamins, antioxidants, macronutrients, trace elements, electrolytes and water, and other food components—will follow.

Indicators of Good Health

Below are highlights describing each nutrient examined by the committee.

- **Calcium** recommendations were set at levels associated with maximum retention of body calcium, since bones that are calcium rich are known to be less susceptible to fractures. In addition to calcium consumption, other factors that are thought to affect bone retention of calcium and risk of osteoporosis include high rates of growth in children during specific periods, hormonal status, exercise, genetics, and other diet components.

- **Phosphorus**, an important nutrient for bone and soft tissue growth, is so prevalent in various foods that near starvation or a metabolic disorder is required to produce deficiency. Different from former RDAs, phosphorus values in the report are not derived in relation to calcium. The values recommended are considered sufficient to support normal bone growth and metabolism at various ages.

- **Magnesium** works with many enzymes to regulate body temperature, allow nerves and muscles to contract, and synthesize proteins. Although some researchers have argued that magnesium recommendations should be based on relationships with the risk of cardiovascular disease, the report does not find enough data available at this time to do so. The levels recommended, although somewhat higher, do not differ substantially from the most recent RDAs but are higher than current Canadian recommendations.

- **Vitamin D** used by the body comes mostly through exposure to the sun. Vitamin D deficiency can exacerbate osteoporosis and other bone problems in adults. The levels recommended in the report—which are greater than those recommended in previous RDAs for people over the age of 50—are estimated to provide enough vitamin D even for individuals with limited sun exposure. Dietary intake of vitamin D is unnecessary for individuals who spend adequate amounts of time in the sun.

- **Fluoride** is found naturally in some community water systems, and is added to water in other areas to reduce dental decay. The levels recommended in the DRIs have been shown to reduce tooth decay without causing marked fluorosis, a discoloration of the teeth that could occur in children who use dental products with fluoride in addition to fluoridated water.

The greatest disparity between recommended values and current dietary patterns is in calcium, which in American and Canadian diets comes primarily from dairy products. Data from surveys indicate that many do not consume the amount of calcium recommended in the report. While many may be consuming sufficient intakes to meet their requirements, the recommendations are intended to provide general guidance to vulnerable individuals and population groups in order to reduce the likelihood that they will develop osteoporosis.

Although the report does not prescribe a means for increasing individual consumption of calcium, it suggests that possible methods for doing so include educating consumers to eat more calcium-rich foods, fortifying foods, and recommending dietary supplements. Individuals who wish to increase their calcium can consume more low- or non-fat dairy products, or fortified food products. According to the report, taking supplements such as calcium tablets may be appropriate for those at high risk of health problems due to low calcium intake.

Dietary Reference Intakes

Dietary Reference Intakes (DRIs) include:

- **Recommended Dietary Allowance:** The intake that meets the nutrient need of almost all of the healthy individuals in a specific age and gender group. The RDA should be used in guiding individuals to achieve adequate nutrient intake aimed at decreasing the risk of chronic disease. It is based on estimating an average requirement plus an increase to account for the variation within a particular group. The amount of scientific evidence available allowed the committee to calculate RDAs for phosphorus and magnesium.

- **Adequate Intake:** When sufficient scientific evidence is not available to estimate an average requirement, Adequate Intakes (AIs) have been set. Individuals should use the AI as a goal for intake where no RDAs exist. The AI is derived though experimental or observational data that show a mean intake which appears to sustain a desired indicator of health, such as calcium retention in bone for most members of a population group. For example, AIs have been set for infants through one year of age using the average observed nutrient intake of populations of breast-fed infants as the standard. The committee set AIs for calcium, vitamin D, and fluoride.

- **Estimated Average Requirement:** The intake that meets the estimated nutrient need of half the individuals in a specific group. This figure is to be used as the basis for developing the RDA and is to be used by nutrition policy-makers in the evaluation of the adequacy of nutrient intakes of the group and for planning how much the group should consume.

- **Tolerable Upper Intake Level:** The maximum intake by an individual that is unlikely to pose risks of adverse health effects in almost all healthy individuals in a specified group. This figure is not intended to be a recommended level of intake, and there is no established benefit for individuals to consume nutrients at levels above the RDA or AI. For most nutrients, this figure refers to total intakes from food, fortified food, and nutrient supplements.

About the Institute of Medicine

The Institute of Medicine is a private, non-profit organization that provides health policy advice under a congressional charter granted to the National Academy of Sciences. This study was funded by the Food and Drug Administration, the U.S. Department of Agriculture, Health Canada, and the U.S. National Institutes of Health. A list of committee members can be found at http://www2.nas.edu/new/276a.htm.

Table 3.1. Criteria and Dietary Reference Intake Values for Calcium by Life Stage

Life-Stage Group[1]	Criterion	AI (mg/day)
0 to 6 months	Human milk content	210
6 to 12 months	Human milk + solid food	270
1 through 3 years	Extrapolation of maximal calcium retention from 4 through 8 years	500
4 through 8 years	Maximal calcium retention	800
9 through 13 years	Maximal calcium retention	1,300
14 through 18 years	Maximal calcium retention	1,300
19 through 30 years	Maximal calcium retention	1,000
31 through 50 years	Calcium balance	1,000
51 through 70 years	Maximal calcium retention	1,200
> 70 years	Extrapolation of maximal calcium retention from 51 through 70 years	1,200
Pregnancy		
<19 years	Bone mineral mass	1,300
19 through 50 years	Bone mineral mass	1,000
Lactation		
<19 years	Bone mineral mass	1,300
19 through 50 years	Bone mineral mass	1,000

[1]*All groups except Pregnancy and Lactation are males and females.*

29

Table 3.2. Criteria and Dietary Reference Intake Values for Phosphorus by Life-Stage Group

Life-State Group[1]	Criterion	EAR (mg/day)	RDA (mg/day)	AI (mg/day)
0 to 6 months	Human milk content	—	—	100
6 to 12 months	Human milk + solid food	—	—	275
1 through 3 years	Factorial approach	380	460	—
4 through 8 years	Factorial approach	405	500	—
9 through 13 years	Factorial approach	1,055	1,250	—
14 through 18 years	Factorial approach	1,055	1,250	—
19 through 30 years	Serum P(i)[2]	580	700	—
31 through 50 years	Serum P(i)	580	700	—
51 through 70 years	Extrapolation of serum P(i) from 19 through 50 years	580	700	—
> 70 years	Extrapolation of serum P(i) from 19 through 50 years	580	700	—
Pregnancy				
<19 years	Factorial approach	1,055	1,250	—
19 through 50 years	Serum P(i)	580	700	—
Lactation				
<19 years	Factorial approach	1,055	1,250	—
19 through 50 years	Serum P(i)	580	700	—

[1]*All groups except Pregnancy and Lactation are males and females.*
[2]*Serum inorganic phosphate concentration.*

Table 3.3. Criteria and Dietary Reference Intake Values for Magnesium by Life-Stage Group

Life Stage Group	Criterion	EAR (mg/day) Male/Female	RDA (mg/day) Male/Female	AI (mg/day) Male/Female
0 to 6 months	Human milk content	—/—	—/—	30/30
6 to 12 months	Human milk + solid food	—/—	—/—	75/75
1 through 3 years	Extrapolation of balance from older children	65/65	80/80	
4 through 8 years	Extrapolation of balance from older children	110/110	130/130	
9 through 13 years	Balance studies	200/200	240/240	
14 through 18 years	Balance studies	340/300	410/360	
19 through 30 years	Balance studies	330/255	400/310	
31 through 50 years	Balance studies	350/265	420/320	
51 through 70 years	Balance studies	350/265	420/320	
> 70 years	Intracellular studies; decreases in adsorption	350/265	420/320	
Pregnancy				
<19 years	Gain in lean mass	—/335	—/400	
19 through 30 years	Gain in lean mass	—/290	—/350	
31 through 50 years	Gain in lean mass	—/300	—/360	
Lactation				
<19 years	Balance studies	—/300	—/360	
19 through 30 years	Balance studies	—/255	—/310	
31 through 50 years	Balance studies	—/265	—/320	

Table 3.4. Criteria and Dietary Reference Intake Values for Vitamin D by Life-Stage Group

Life-Stage Group[1]	Criterion	AI (micrograms/day)[2,3]
0 to 6 months	Serum25(OH)D	5
6 to 12 months	Serum25(OH)D	5
1 through 3 years	Serum25(OH)D	5
4 through 8 years	Serum25(OH)D	5
9 through 13 years	Serum25(OH)D	5
14 through 18 years	Serum25(OH)D	5
19 through 30 years	Serum25(OH)D	5
31 through 50 years	Serum25(OH)D	5
51 through 70 years	Serum25(OH)D	10
> 70 years	Serum25(OH)D	15
Pregnancy		
<19 years	Serum25(OH)D	5
19 through 50 years	Serum25(OH)D	
Lactation		
<19 years	Serum25(OH)D	5
19 through 50 years	Serum25(OH)D	

[1]*All groups except Pregnancy and Lactation are males and females*
[2]*As cholecalciferol. 1 micrograms cholecalciferol = 40 IU vitamin D.*
[3]*In the absence of adequate exposure to sunlight.*

Table 3.5. Criteria and Dietary Reference Intake Values for Fluoride by Life-Stage Group

Life-Stage Group	Criterion	AI (mg/day) Male/Female
0 to 6 months	Human milk content	0.01/0.01
6 to 12 months	Caries prevention	0.5/0.5
1 through 3 years	Caries prevention	0.7/0.7
4 through 8 years	Caries prevention	1.1/1.1
9 through 13 years	Caries prevention	2.0/2.0
14 through 18 years	Caries prevention	3.2/2.9
19 through 30 years	Caries prevention	3.8/3.1
31 through 50 years	Caries prevention	3.8/3.1
51 through 70 years	Caries prevention	3.8/3.1
> 70 years	Caries prevention	3.8/3.1
Pregnancy		
<19 years	Caries prevention	—/2.9
19 through 50 years	Caries prevention	—/3.1
Lactation		
<19 years	Caries prevention	—2.9
19 through 50 years	Caries prevention	—/3.1

Table 3.6. Tolerable Upper Intake Levels (UL), by Life-Stage Group

Life-State Group	Calcium (g/day)	Phosphorus (g/day)	Magnesium[1] (mg/day)	Vitamin D (Micrograms/day)[2]	Fluoride (mg/day)
0 to 6 months	ND[3]	ND	ND	25	.07
6 to 12 months	ND	ND	ND	25	.09
1 through 3 years	2.5	3	65	50	1.3
4 through 8 years	2.5	3	110	50	2.2
9 through 18 years	2.5	4	350	50	10
19 through 70 years	2.5	4	350	50	10
> 70 years	2.5	3	350	50	10
Pregnancy					
<19 years	2.5	3.5	350	50	10
19 through 50 years	2.5	3.5	350	50	10
Lactation					
<19 years	2.5	4	350	50	10
19 through 50 years	2.5	4	350	50	10

[1]The UL for magnesium represents intake from a pharmacological agent only and does not include intake from food and water.

[2]As cholecalciferol. a g cholecalciferol = 40 IU vitamin D.

[3]ND. Not determinable due to lack of data of adverse effects in this age group and concern with regard to lack of ability to handle excess amounts. Source of intake should be from food only in order to prevent high levels of intake.

Note

1. For pricing and availability information about the report *Dietary Reference Intakes for Calcium, Phosphorus, Magnesium, Vitamin D, and Fluoride*, contact the National Academy Press (202) 334-3313 or 1-800-624-6242.

Chapter 4

New Dietary Requirements for B Vitamins and Choline

Women who might become pregnant need 400 micrograms of folic acid per day to reduce their risk of having a child with neural tube defects, according to the latest report[1] on Dietary Reference Intakes (DRIs) from the Institute of Medicine. The report—the second in a new series by American and Canadian scientists—provides Recommended Dietary Allowances (RDAs) and other dietary reference values for B vitamins, of which folate is one, and choline. It says that all adult men and women need 400 micrograms of folate in their diet—a level that many in the United States have not met, according to surveys completed before January of this year, when many foods began to be fortified with folic acid, a synthetic form of folate. But it emphasized the special needs of childbearing women.

"Research over the past decade strongly indicates that women capable of becoming pregnant should eat a varied diet and also take extra folic acid, especially in the month just prior to conception and the first month of pregnancy," said committee chair Roy M. Pitkin, professor emeritus of obstetrics and gynecology at University of California, Los Angeles. "They can best get folic acid from fortified cereal grains or from a supplement."

Since fortification of enriched cereal grains began, folic acid can be found in enriched bread, pasta, flour, crackers, breakfast cereal, rice, and many other foods in the United States. To reduce the risk of

"Adults Need to Increase Intake of Folate; Some Women Should Take More," National Academy of Sciences, Institute of Medicine, Food and Nutrition Board, Press Release dated April 7, 1998; reprinted with permission.

neural tube defects, women capable of becoming pregnant should consume 400 micrograms of folic acid daily from fortified foods, vitamin supplements, or a combination of the two, the report says. This is in addition to the naturally occurring folate they obtain from a varied diet. Whether these women can rely totally on the folate in food is uncertain, since research has involved giving only additional amounts of folic acid.

Neural tube defects such as spina bifida result from a disruption during the development of the fetus's central nervous system in the first month of pregnancy, when most women do not realize they are pregnant. A common type of congenital malformation of the central nervous system, neural tube defects may appear as incomplete closure of the spinal column or even the absence of part of the brain. In the United States and Canada they occur in about one birth per 1,000.

The report also says that although most Americans and Canadians get sufficient vitamin B_{12} in their food, between 10 percent and 30 percent of older adults have lost the ability to adequately absorb the naturally occurring form of B_{12} found in food. People over age 50 should meet most of their recommended intake with synthetic B_{12} from fortified foods or vitamin supplements.

New Dietary Standards

The committee's report on Dietary Reference Intakes expands on the Recommended Dietary Allowances set periodically by the National Academy of Sciences since 1941. Five additional reports on antioxidants, trace elements, electrolytes and water, macronutrients, and other food components will follow. Dietary Reference Intakes contain four categories of recommendations, including some values intended to help individuals optimize their health and some to help them avoid consuming too much of a nutrient.

In addition to folate, the report recommends individual intakes for thiamin, riboflavin, niacin, vitamins B_6 and B_{12}, pantothenic acid, biotin, and choline. Where possible, it also specifies intake levels above which health problems might occur. Except for folate, recommended intakes for these vitamins have not changed substantially since the last group of recommendations was published in the United States in 1989 and in Canada in 1990. Most Americans and Canadians already meet their requirements for these vitamins through their diet.

A great deal of research in the past two decades has centered on the roles that B vitamins may play in reducing the risk of cardiovascular disease, cancers, or various psychiatric or mental disorders. Although such research is provocative and promising, it is not yet solid enough to serve as the basis for setting recommendations for nutrient intake, the report says. Therefore, rather than set recommended intake levels to reduce the risk of these diseases, the committee based its recommended intake levels on values shown to guard against anemia or other conditions that can develop when these vitamins are lacking.

Research has shown that consumption of folate and vitamin B_6 can reduce elevated levels of homocysteine in the blood, and some studies have linked lower homocysteine concentrations with a decreased risk of cardiovascular disease. But there is conflicting evidence about whether increasing folate or B_6 intake leads directly to a lower incidence of vascular and heart disease. Likewise, data showing that increased folate may protect against colorectal cancer do not provide conclusive evidence of a benefit, the report says.

Upper Levels Set

The committee set the tolerable upper intake level for vitamin B_6 at 100 milligrams per day for adults. Intakes above this amount could cause sensory neuropathy, a nerve disorder that can lead to pain, numbness, and weakness in the limbs. Likewise, adults with vitamin B_{12} deficiency who take excess folic acid place themselves at greater risk of progressive, crippling neurologic damage. For folic acid, the committee set the tolerable upper intake level for adults at 1,000 micrograms, or 1 milligram, per day.

Individuals who consume too much niacin have been shown to feel a flush, warm sensation, itching, and other symptoms. The committee set the tolerable upper intake level for niacin at 35 milligrams per day. Some individuals who take high-dose, over-the-counter niacin supplements may exceed this amount regularly. The tolerable upper level for choline was set at 3.5 grams per day for adults. Intakes above that level could cause hypotension, or low blood pressure, and a fishy body odor in some people.

Because the committee was unable to identify studies conducted on the adverse effects of taking large doses of many of the B vitamins, it did not set upper limits for thiamin, riboflavin, vitamin B_{12}, pantothenic acid, and biotin. Due to the lack of data, the committee urged extra caution with regard to excessive consumption of these vitamins.

Table 4.1. Recommended Levels for Individual Intake, 1998, B Vitamins and Choline

Life-Stage Group	thia-min mg/d	ribo-flavin mg/d	niacin mg/d[a]	B$_6$ mg/d	folate µg/d[b]	B$_{12}$ µg/d	panto-thenic acid mg/d	biotin µg/d	choline[c] mg/d
Infants									
0-5 mo	0.2*	0.3*	2*	0.1*	65*	0.4*	1.7*	5*	125*
6-11 mo	0.3*	0.4*	3*	0.3*	80*	0.5*	1.8*	6*	150*
Children									
1-3 yr	0.5	0.5	6	0.5	150	0.9	2*	8*	200*
4-8 yr	0.6	0.6	8	0.6	200	1.2	3*	12*	250*
Males									
9-13 yr	0.9	0.9	12	1.0	300	1.8	4*	20*	375*
14-18 yr	1.2	1.2	16	1.3	400	2.4	5*	25*	550*
19-30 yr	1.2	1.3	16	1.3	400	2.4	5*	30*	550*
31-50 yr	1.2	1.3	16	1.3	400	2.4	5*	30*	550*
51-70 yr	1.2	1.3	16	1.7	400	2.4[d]	5*	30*	550*
> 70 yr	1.2	1.3	16	1.7	400	2.4[d]	5*	30*	550*
Females									
9-13 yr	0.9	0.9	12	1.0	300	1.8	4*	20*	375*
14-18 yr	1.0	1.0	14	1.2	400[e]	2.4	5*	25*	400*
19-30 yr	1.1	1.1	14	1.3	400[e]	2.4	5*	30*	425*
31-50 yr	1.1	1.1	14	1.3	400[e]	2.4	5*	30*	425*
51-70 yr	1.1	1.1	14	1.5	400[e]	2.4[d]	5*	30*	425*
> 70 yr	1.1	1.1	14	1.5	400	2.4[d]	5*	30*	425*
Pregnancy									
all ages	1.4	1.4	18	1.9	600[f]	2.6	6*	30*	450*
Lactation									
all ages	1.5	1.6	17	20	500	2.8	7*	35*	550*

Table 4.1. Recommended Levels for Individual Intake, 1998, B Vitamins and Choline, Notes.

Note: This table presents Recommended Dietary Allowances (RDAs) in bold type and Adequate Intakes (AIs) in ordinary type followed by an asterisk (*). RDAs and AIs may both be used as goals for individual intake. RDAs are set to meet the needs of almost all (97 to 98 percent) individuals in a group. For healthy breastfed infants, the AI is the mean intake. The AI for other life stage groups is believed to cover their needs, but lack of data or uncertainty in the data prevent clear specification of this coverage.

[a]As niacin equivalents. 1 mg of niacin = 60 mg of tryptophan.
[b]As dietary folate equivalents (DFE). 1 DFE = 1 µg food folate = 0.6 µg of folic acid (from fortified food or supplement) consumed with food = .05 µg of synthetic (supplemental) folic acid taken on an empty stomach.
[c]Although AIs have been set for choline, there are few data to assess whether a dietary supply of choline is needed at all stages of the life cycle, and it may be that the choline requirement can be met by endogenous synthesis at some of these stages.
[d]Since 10 to 30 percent of older people may malabsorb food-bound B_{12}, it is advisable for those older than 50 years to meet their RDA mainly by taking foods fortified with B_{12} or a B_{12}-containing supplement.
[e]In view of evidence linking folate intake with neural tube defects in the fetus, it is recommended that all women capable of becoming pregnant consumer 400 µg of synthetic folic acid from fortified foods and/or supplements in addition to intake of food folate from a varied diet.
[f]It is assumed that women will continue taking 400 µg of folic acid until their pregnancy is confirmed and they enter prenatal care, which ordinarily occurs after the end of the periconceptional period—the critical time for formation of the neural tube.

About the Institute of Medicine

The Institute of Medicine is a private, non-profit organization that provides health policy advice under a congressional charter granted to the National Academy of Sciences. This study was funded by the U.S. Department of Health and Human Services, the National Institutes of Health, the Centers for Disease Control and Prevention, Health Canada, the Institute of Medicine, and the Dietary Reference Intakes Corporate Donors Fund. Contributors to the fund include Roche Vitamins Inc., Mead Johnson Nutrition Group, Daiichi Fine Chemicals Inc., Kemin Foods Inc., M&M Mars, Weider Nutrition Group, and Natural Source Vitamin E Association. This news release, along with a list of committee members, and the full chart of dietary recommendations are available on the World Wide Web at www.nas.edu.

Note

1. For pricing and availability information about the report *Dietary Reference Intakes for Thiamin, Riboflavin, Niacin, Vitamin B6, Folate, Vitamin B12, Pantothenic Acid, Biotin, and Choline*, contact the National Academy Press (202) 334-3313 or 1-800-624-6242.

Chapter 5

The Salt Controversy

For such a simple substance, common table salt has had a very complex past. Once scarce, salt was as precious as gold, valued as a chemical agent used to clean, dye, soften leather, and bleach. But more importantly, early humans recognized salt—sodium chloride, or NaCl—as a necessary part of their diets and an element worth fighting for.

Now modern technology has made salt readily available and at a price almost anyone can afford. As a result, many of us take salt and its merits for granted. But scientists keep salt in the news by debating its role in a healthful diet. At times, discussion and controversy threaten to obscure salt's importance and to confuse thoughtful consumers.

To begin with, the terms "salt" and "sodium" are often used interchangeably. Since sodium has been linked to health problems and sodium is most commonly eaten as salt, measuring salt intake has been an easy way to determine how much sodium people actually consume, explains Food and Drug Administration's Ellen Anderson, Ph.D., physical chemist in the Office of Food Labeling. But recent data suggest that sodium in other forms—such as in sodium bicarbonate (baking soda)—causes no health problem, so that salt itself—as sodium and chloride—could after all be what is so undesirable in large amounts.

At odds, too, are the scientists who do not agree on salt's impact on blood pressure: Does it contribute to high blood pressure? Should salt intake be restricted?

FDA Consumer, November-December 1997.

In the spring of 1995, a report on the results of a four-year observational study in a population with high blood pressure suggested that a link exists between a low-salt diet and a higher risk of heart attack. The study, conducted by Michael Alderman, M.D., professor and chairman of the Department of Epidemiology and Social Medicine at the Albert Einstein College of Medicine of Yeshiva University in New York, was published in *Hypertension*, a journal of the American Heart Association.

While some noted his findings with interest, other experts challenged the study: Only a single urine sample was used to determine usual dietary salt consumption, similar results were not seen in women, and, most importantly, many important risk factors for heart attacks were not well measured and could have accounted for the higher risk factors.

But an even greater furor occurred a year later, when two well-respected medical journals tackled the subject of salt and blood pressure. The *British Medical Journal* dedicated part of its May 18, 1996, issue to the topic, publishing both sides of the debate, as editorials, papers, articles, and commentaries. One article, authored by Richard Hanneman, president of the Salt Institute in Alexandria, Va., challenged evidence of a correlation between salt intake and elevated blood pressure found in two studies by the Intersalt Cooperative Research Group, an international team of investigators who collected and analyzed data on salt and high blood pressure and released their findings in 1988.

Almost immediately afterwards, the *Journal of the American Medical Association (JAMA)* published a meta-analysis (a study in which the results of available clinical studies are pooled, then analyzed) in its May 22-29 issue that suggested restricting dietary sodium intake had only a minimal effect on blood pressure. However, the authors concluded that for younger people with normal blood pressure, a diet high in salt is harmless. *JAMA*'s press release failed to note that an accompanying editorial by Claude Lenfant, M.D., director of the National Institutes of Health's National Heart, Lung, and Blood Institute, took issue with the study's methods and conclusions.

The New York Times immediately picked up the story and, in the early-June food section article "Salt is Regaining Favor and Savor," added that many chefs are using a variety of designer salts—fancy sea salt among them—in their upscale cooking.

Almost unanimously, scientists and authorities called the *JAMA* study flawed, saying among other things, that the study was too limited; it included a subgroup of people who had normal blood pressure and were not fed consistent hospital-controlled diets, and it included trials that lasted too short a time.

Need for Salt

The one fact no one challenges is that the human body needs salt to function. Sodium is the main component of the body's extracellular fluids and it helps carry nutrients into the cells. Sodium also helps regulate other body functions, such as blood pressure and fluid volume, and sodium works on the lining of blood vessels to keep the pressure balance normal.

"You cannot exist without sodium," says Alicia Moag-Stahlberg, a research nutritionist at Northwestern University Medical School in Chicago and a spokeswoman for the American Dietetic Association. "But the amount we need is minor."

The National Research Council of the National Academy of Sciences in Washington, D.C., has determined that the recommended safe minimum daily amount is about 500 milligrams of sodium with an upper limit of 2,400 milligrams. However, the council has said that lowering sodium intake to 1,800 milligrams would probably be healthier.

Many Americans are consuming even higher amounts of salt, up to 6,000 milligrams a day, points out Moag-Stahlberg, with possible harmful effects. "Many people argue that a healthy kidney can get rid of it [the excess], but in many cases, that happens at the expense of losing calcium," she says. It's possible that the habitual high intake of salt produces physiological changes in the kidney, which increases the risk of high blood pressure. For women, as some studies now suggest, this habitual lack of calcium may eventually be linked to the bone disease of old age, osteoporosis, in which long-term calcium loss causes bones to weaken and break easily.

Our ancestors, often living in salt-poor environments, were not faced with these modern-day health problems. Jeremiah Stamler, M.D., professor emeritus of Preventive Medicine, Northwestern University Medical School, Chicago, says that humans are adapted to low-salt intake "with the kidneys and the gastrointestinal tract functioning efficiently for preserving sodium. So how come we started adding salt to our food?"

About 6,000 to 8,000 years ago, our ancestors went from gathering food and hunting to cultivating crops and raising animals. To survive, they needed to preserve and to stockpile foods for the long winter months. "You can dry vegetables and dry meats," Stamler says. "But the other way to preserve food is to salt it." However, adding salt to food did more than cut bacterial growth. It added a whole new dimension to the pleasures of eating: Salt adds flavor and heightens existing flavors, even in sweets, and salt helps process basic raw ingredients into other food products. Of these, cheese is perhaps one of the most familiar examples, since salt is necessary in its formation.

For Americans today, eating preserved and processed foods has become a way of life. According to Regina Hildwine, technical regulatory affairs, the National Food Processors Association, Washington, D.C., it is almost impossible to prepare a meal without using some processed food. Besides, not only is salt one of the four taste categories—salty, sweet, sour, and bitter—salt offers certain technical advantages in the kitchen. Two examples: It reduces the boiling point of water, which helps heat penetrate into cooking foods, and it helps condition dough in baked products. And, adds Richard Hanneman, the biggest advantage of using salt is that it enhances other flavors.

But some scientists are concerned about the amount of salt in processed foods. "Seventy-five percent of the sodium consumed is in processed foods," says Anderson. "What the food industry includes during processing, we can't take out."

Stamler agrees. "If we reduce our salt intake [at the table]," he says, "that won't solve the problem. There's salt in bread, processed meat, cheese, canned vegetables—these are all hidden sources of salt." Fortunately, FDA's food labeling helps consumers monitor their sodium intake in processed foods. But, says Anderson, in restaurant foods, and that includes fast-food chains and Chinese restaurants, the "sodium levels can be very high."

New regulations that went into effect in May 1997 offer consumers some help with restaurant fare. The regulations apply the Nutrition Labeling and Education Act (NLEA) of 1990 to restaurant menu items that carry a claim about the food's nutritional content or health benefits.

Scientists Look at Salt

Scientists' suspicions about salt are not new. As Jeffrey Cutler, M.D., director of the Clinical Applications and Prevention Program, National Heart, Lung, and Blood Institute, points out, physicians in China back in 2,500 B.C. warned patients that if they used too much salt in their food, their "pulse" would harden.

"And since then," says Cutler, "scientists have refined that conclusion and there is scientific support for it. We have learned to measure blood pressure better than measuring the pulse and to quantify salt intake, and we have learned all the scientific experimental designs to study salt intake. The conclusion is still there. The higher the salt intake, the higher the prevalence of hypertension." Higher-than-normal blood pressure may lead to heart attacks, kidney disease, and strokes.

Cutler estimates that persistent high blood pressure—conventionally defined as readings of 140/90 or above—is one of the most common health conditions, affecting nearly 50 million Americans. People at greatest risk for high blood pressure are those with a family history, the elderly, middle-aged men, and middle-aged Black women.

Yet everyone is vulnerable, says Stamler, because blood pressure normally rises with age, a fact corroborated by numerous studies, and high-salt intake contributes to that rise. "The fundamental conclusion is that salt relates to high blood pressure independent of other factors affecting blood pressure, like alcohol and obesity," he says. "There is such a massive body of evidence," he adds, including the 1988 Surgeon General's report on nutrition, the National Academy of Sciences' report on diet and health, and the Intersalt research group.

We don't know exactly how salt works to elevate blood pressure, says Anderson. But the best guess is that too much salt causes the sodium channels (structures that move sodium into and out of cells) to work too hard and gradually the channels begin to fail. This process is irreversible, so that by old age, even if people cut back on salt, their kidneys can no longer flush extra amounts of salt from the body without an increase in blood pressure.

Salt may also be linked to other health problems. "One of the aspects of salt that has been neglected," says Stamler, "is the growing evidence that high-salt intake is bad news for other problems ... such as aggravating asthma, gastric cancer, kidney stones, osteoporosis ... a wide range of problems."

Regulating Salt Intake

FDA is not advising people on how high or low their salt intake should be, says Ida Yoder, a chemist with FDA's over-the-counter drug products division. "By appropriate labeling, we are attempting to inform the public and those who want to keep their sodium intake down as to the amount of sodium they are consuming. The sodium labeling regulations for both foods and over-the-counter drugs require sodium content labeling for those products that contain a certain amount of sodium."

Following a salt-restricted diet will, for many people, be what the doctor orders. And while many people say they crave salt and use it liberally in their food, restricting salt intake is only really a matter of making some adjustments, says Anderson. "If people make a concerted effort to reduce salt intake," she says, "initially they notice that things don't taste salty enough. But if they go through a transition period and then go back to foods they used to like, they find them too salty."

In the end, wise consumers will choose diets of moderation in all things. The Dietary Guidelines, developed jointly by the U.S. Department of Health and Human Services and Department of Agriculture, stresses just that when discussing daily needs for salt, pointing out that eating less salt is not harmful and can be recommended for the healthy normal adult.

Tips on Reducing Salt Intake

Alicia Moag-Stahlberg, a research nutritionist at Northwestern University Medical School in Chicago and spokeswoman for the American Dietetic Association, offers the following tips for those who want to reduce salt intake:

- Take stock of the sources of salt in your diet, such as restaurant meals, salt-based condiments, and convenience foods. Some of these are really loaded with salt.

- Read the labels when shopping. Look for lower sodium in cereals, crackers, pasta sauces, canned vegetables, or any foods with low-salt options.

- If you think your meals are high in sodium, balance them by adding high-potassium foods, such as fresh fruits and vegetables.

- Ask about salt added to food, especially at restaurants. Most restaurant chefs will omit salt when requested.

- If you need to salt while cooking, add the salt at the end; you will need to add much less. The longer the food cooks, the more the salty flavor is muted and at the end, the final taste is on the top layer.

— by Alexandra Greeley

Alexandra Greeley is a writer in Reston, Va.

Chapter 6

Bone Builders

Unearthed skeletons from ancient times testify to the durability of bone long after other bodily tissue turns to dust. Living bone in the body, however, can lose mineral and fracture easily if neglected—a disorder called osteoporosis, or porous bones. One in two women and one in eight men over 50 suffer such fractures, including sometimes life-threatening hip fractures.

But during your preteen and teenage years, you can reduce your risk of fractured bones later in life with calcium-rich foods and physical activity.

Bone Behavior

Your body's 206 living bones continually undergo a buildup, breakdown process called remodeling.

The body starts to form most of its bone mass before puberty, the beginning of sexual development, building 75 to 85 percent of the skeleton during adolescence. Women reach their peak bone mass by around age 25 to 30, while men build bone until about age 30 to 35. The amount of peak bone mass you reach depends largely on your genes. Then gradually, with age, the breakdown outpaces the buildup, and in late middle age bone density lessens when needed calcium is withdrawn from bone for such tasks as blood clotting and muscle contractions, including beating by the heart.

FDA Consumer, September-October 1997.

"You can't do anything about the genes you're dealt," says Mona Calvo, Ph.D., a calcium expert for the Food and Drug Administration. "As a teenager, though, you can make the most of things you do control that can build your bones and help reduce the risk of fractures when you are older."

Supporting the skeleton with healthful habits now so it can support you later in life is especially important if you have an increased risk of osteoporosis—for example, if you're female or have a thin, small-boned frame. These habits are proper diet, exercise, and avoiding bone risks—lifestyle choices that are bad for bones—like smoking.

Eat Your Way to Strong Bones

The main mineral in bones is calcium, one of whose functions is to add strength and stiffness to bones, which they need to support the body. To lengthen long bones during growth, the body builds a scaffold of protein and fills this in with calcium-rich mineral. From the time you're 11 until you're 24, you need about 1,200 milligrams (mg) of calcium each day.

Adolescent bodies are tailor-made to "bone up" on calcium. Calvo says that with the start of puberty, "your body is at a higher capacity to absorb and retain calcium."

Bone also needs vitamin D, to move calcium from the intestine to the bloodstream and into bone. You can get vitamin D from short, normal day-to-day exposure of your arms and legs to sun and from foods fortified with the vitamin. Also needed are vitamin A, vitamin C, magnesium and zinc, as well as protein for the growing bone scaffold.

Mother Nature provides many foods with these nutrients. One stands out, however, as "almost a perfect package," according to Calvo. "Milk is rich in calcium and high-quality protein. Nearly all U.S. milk has vitamins D and A added. And it has magnesium and zinc."

Still, as excellent as milk is for bones, it and other dairy products are not the only foods that contain calcium. All groups in the Food Guide Pyramid, in fact, offer calcium sources—from the pyramid's grain-based foods that you need the most of, to the produce and high-protein groups in the middle, and even to the fats and sweets "use sparingly" group at the top. The importance of choosing calcium sources from the different food groups is that each group offers its unique package of other nutrients as well.

To learn how much calcium is in a food, you can read the food label's Nutrition Facts panel. Look for the "percent Daily Value" (% DV) set by FDA for calcium. The calcium DV is 1,000 mg. But if you are 11 to 24 years old, your growing bones need more—the recommended 1,200 mg. So, each day's calcium % DVs in the foods you eat should add up to 120 percent.

Because many foods are now fortified with calcium, your investigation of labels may turn up surprising sources. To identify foods with at least 10% DV of calcium per serving, FDA allows these terms on their labels:

- 20% DV or more: "High in Calcium," "Rich in Calcium," "Excellent Source of Calcium"

- 10% to 19% DV: "Contains Calcium," "Provides Calcium," "Good Source of Calcium"

- 10% DV calcium or more added: "Calcium-Enriched," "Calcium-Fortified," "More Calcium."

An easy daily plan is to drink a calcium source at every meal and eat one calcium food as a snack, says Ruth Welch, a registered dietitian with FDA.

If the lactose sugar in dairy products causes problems like gas, bloating or diarrhea, try lactose-reduced or lactose-free milk. When fortified, these products can have up to 50% DV for calcium in one serving. Also available are lactase drops and tablets, which can help you digest dairy products like ice milk, yogurt, and cheese.

Get Enough Weight-Bearing Exercise

Growing bone is especially sensitive to the impact of weight and pull of muscle during exercise, and responds by building stronger, denser bones. That's why it's especially important when you're growing a lot to be physically active on a regular basis.

And as far as bone is concerned, Calvo says impact activity like jumping up and down appears to be the best. "But the important thing is to get off the couch and get moving at some activity. It really is a matter of 'Use it now, or lose it later'."

Such activities include sports and exercise, including football, basketball, baseball, jogging, dancing, jumping rope, inline skating, skateboarding, bicycling, ballet, hiking, skiing, karate, swimming, rowing a canoe, bowling, and weight-training. And when your parents make you mow the lawn, rake leaves, or wash and wax the car, they're doing your muscles and bones a favor.

FDA's Welch adds, "Day-to-day activities that start in the teen years, like walking the dog or using stairs instead of elevators, can become life-long habits for healthy bones."

Avoid Bone Risks

Some habits in the teenage years can steal calcium from your bones or increase the need for it, weakening the skeleton for life.

Skipping meals is risky for bone, Welch says. In our three-meal-a-day society, skipping a meal may reduce by a third your chance of getting your 120% DV for calcium—simply by eliminating one occasion to eat.

Replacing milk with nondairy drinks like soda pop or fruit-flavored teas or drinks is another eating habit that prevents bones from getting the calcium and other nutrients they need.

In a survey comparing 1994 daily beverage intakes with those in the late 1970s, the U.S. Department of Agriculture found a switch from milk to other drinks among young people:

• Milk drinkers among teenagers dropped from three-fourths to little more than half.

• Two to three times more children and teenagers drank non-citrus fruit juices.

• Teenage boys nearly tripled their intake of soft drinks, three-fourths of them drinking about 34 ounces; two-thirds of teenage girls drank 23 ounces.

Alcohol abuse and cigarette smoking can hurt bone. Calvo says, "Alcohol abuse can cause loss of calcium, magnesium and zinc in the urine. Many who abuse alcohol also have poor diets and malnourished, weaker bones." Cigarette smoke is also toxic to bone and can influence how much exercise you get because it affects your stamina, she says.

Eating disorders can weaken bone. The repeated vomiting in bulimia and extreme dieting in the appetite disorder anorexia can upset the body's balance of calcium and important hormones like bone-protective estrogen, decreasing bone density. And extreme exercising by young women with or without eating disorders can postpone or stop menstruation, when blood levels of estrogen are reduced.

Small Changes for Big Benefits

As a disorder of aging, osteoporosis may seem far away for worry when you're 15. But, small changes today for better bones tomorrow may be more important than you might guess.

Laura Bacharach, M.D., of Stanford University, wrote in Nutrition & the M.D. last year that adolescents who make "even a 5 percent gain in bone mass can reduce the risk of osteoporosis by 40 percent." And this is in addition to "immediate benefits of feeling stronger and more fit now with these changes!"

"Calcium! Do You Get It?"

Unlike boys, growing girls typically have low calcium intakes. Concerned about the low intakes, the Food and Drug Administration recently developed a pilot education program, funded by the agency's Office of Women's Health, just for girls ages 11 to 14. "Calcium! Do You Get It?" encourages girls to get enough calcium and exercise for healthy bones and to carry these healthy behaviors throughout life.

Girls Don't Get Enough Calcium

Between the ages 11 and 24, people need at least 1,200 milligrams (mg) of calcium every day. A 1995 survey by the U.S. Department of Agriculture, however, found that girls and young women 12 to 19 got only 777 mg of the mineral daily, overall. Intake by boys and young men in the same age group was 1,176 mg daily.

Daily calcium intake by preteen girls was far short of the recommended level also in 1990-1992 and fell with age, wrote Ann Albertson, M.S., R.D., and others recently in the *Journal of Adolescent Health*. Calcium consumption was only 781 mg at ages 11 to 12, 751 at ages 13 to 14, and a mere 602 mg—barely half what it should be—at ages 15 to 18.

Why Is Calcium Intake in Girls and Young Women So Low?

USDA's Agricultural Economic Report No. 746 gives some clues. Compared with other children, female adolescents:

- drink the least amount of fluid milk
- have the highest tendency to skip morning meals, which offer the most calcium because of milk and cereals

• have the highest share of calories from fast-food places, which have a calcium density much lower than foods prepared at home, schools or restaurants.

Eat Enough Calcium and a Balanced Diet, Too

To get enough calcium for growing bones, each day you need to eat foods whose % Daily Value for calcium adds up to 120 percent. Because the amount of calcium in foods can vary, read the food label check the % DV for calcium in what you eat.

So your body will have all the other nutrients it needs, too, be sure to eat the recommended number of servings from the food groups that make up the Food Guide Pyramid:

• Grain Products Group: 6-11 servings
• Vegetables Group: 3-5 servings
• Fruits Group: 2-4 servings
• Milk Products Group: 2-3 servings
• Meat and Bean Group: 2-3 servings
• Fats, Oils, and Sweets: Use sparingly

As shown in the lists below, each group includes foods that provide calcium. The food examples are listed by their serving size and %DV for calcium. (Source: "Calcium! Do You Get It?" pilot education program funded by FDA's Office of Women's Health.)

Grain Products

• Waffles (4-inch square): 2 waffles = 20% DV
• Pancakes (5-inch): pancakes = 20% DV
• Calcium-fortified cereal: 1 cup = 15% DV
• Calcium-fortified bread: 1 slice = 8% DV
• Corn tortilla: 3 tortillas = 8% DV
• Bread: 1 slice = 4% DV

Vegetables

• Collards: 1/2 cup = 20% DV
• Turnip greens: 2/3 cup = 15% DV
• Kale: 2/3 cup = 10% DV
• Bok choy: 1/2 cup = 10% DV
• Broccoli: 1 stalk = 6% DV
• Carrot: 1 medium carrot = 2% DV

Fruits

- Calcium-fortified orange juice: 1 cup = 30% DV
- Dried figs: 2 figs = 6% DV
- Orange: 1 orange = 4% DV
- Kiwi: 2 kiwis = 4% DV
- Strawberries: 8 berries = 2% DV

Milk Products

- Nonfat milk, calcium-fortified: 1 cup = 40% DV
- Yogurt: 1 cup = 35% DV
- Milk, whole, 2%, 1%, skim: 1 cup = 30% DV
- Cheese: 1 ounce = 20% DV
- Cheese spread: 2 Tbsp. = 15% DV
- Pudding: 1/2 cup = 10% DV
- Frozen yogurt: 1/2 cup = 10% DV
- Cottage cheese: 1/2 cup = 6% DV

Meat and Beans

- Calcium-processed tofu: 3 oz. = 60% DV
- Dry-roasted almonds: 1/4 cup = 10% DV
- Scrambled eggs: 2 eggs = 8% DV
- Baked beans with sauce: 1/2 cup = 8% DV
- Black-eyed peas: 1/2 cup = 2% DV

Fats, Oils and Sweets

- Milk chocolate: 1.5-ounce bar = 8% DV

Mixed Dishes

- Cheese pizza (12-inch): 1/4 pizza = 25% DV
- Macaroni and cheese: 1 cup = 25% DV
- Grilled cheese sandwich: 1 sandwich = 25% DV
- Lasagna: 1 cup = 25% DV
- Soups prepared with milk: 1 cup = 15% DV
- Chili con carne with beans: 1 cup = 10% DV
- Taco with cheese: 1 taco = 10% DV
- Tuna salad sandwich: 1 sandwich = 8% DV
- Chicken noodle soup: 1 cup = 2% DV

Want More Information?

Dairy Council of California
1101 National Drive, Suite B
Sacramento, CA 95834
http://www.dairycouncilofca.org/

National Osteoporosis Foundation
P.O. Box 96616
Washington, DC 20077-7456
http://www.nof.org/

Osteoporosis and Related Bone Diseases—National Resource Center
1150 17th St., NW, Suite 500
Washington, DC 20036
(1-800) 624-BONE
(202) 223-0344 TDD
http://www.osteo.org

—by Dixie Farley

Dixie Farley is a staff writer for FDA Consumer.

Chapter 7

Dietary Fiber

More Benefits of 'Roughage' Are Discovered

Because it causes gas, bloating, and other uncomfortable side effects, fiber may be the Rodney Dangerfield of food constituents. But with more and more research showing that a high-fiber diet may help prevent cancer, heart disease, and other serious ailments, roughage has started to get some respect.

The problem is that most Americans don't get enough fiber to realize its potential benefits. The typical American eats only about 11 grams of fiber a day, according to the American Dietetic Association. Health experts recommend a minimum of 20 to 30 grams of fiber a day for most people.

The Food and Drug Administration has recognized fiber's importance by requiring it to be listed on the Nutrition Facts panel of food labels along with other key nutrients and calories. And, based on scientific evidence, the agency has approved four claims related to fiber intake and lowered risk of heart disease and cancer.

The most recent claim, approved in January 1997, allows food companies to state on product labels that foods with soluble fiber from whole oats may reduce heart disease risk when eaten as part of a diet low in saturated fat and cholesterol. Foods covered include rolled oats, oat bran, and whole-oat flour.

Reprinted from "Bulking Up Fiber's Healthful Reputation," *FDA Consumer*, July-August 1997; Pub. No. (FDA) 97-2313.

FDA concluded that the beta-glucan soluble fiber of whole oats is the primary component responsible for lowering total and LDL (low-density lipoprotein), or "bad," blood cholesterol in diets including these foods at appropriate levels. This conclusion is based on a scientific review showing a link between the soluble fiber in whole-oat foods and a reduction in coronary heart disease risk.

The other three claims, allowed since 1993, are:

- Diets low in fat and rich in fiber-containing grain products, fruits, and vegetables may reduce the risk of some types of cancer.

- Diets low in saturated fat and cholesterol and rich in fruits, vegetables, and grain products that contain fiber, particularly soluble fiber, may reduce the risk of coronary heart disease.

- Diets low in fat and rich in fruits and vegetables, which are low-fat foods and may contain fiber or vitamin A (as beta-carotene) and vitamin C, may reduce the risk of some cancers.

Found only in plant foods, such as whole grains, fruits, vegetables, beans, nuts, and seeds, fiber is composed of complex carbohydrates. Some fibers are soluble in water and others are insoluble. Most plant foods contain some of each kind.

Some foods containing high levels of soluble fiber are dried beans, oats, barley, and some fruits, notably apples and citrus, and vegetables, such as potatoes. Foods high in insoluble fiber are wheat bran, whole grains, cereals, seeds, and the skins of many fruits and vegetables.

Fiber's Health Benefits

What can fiber do for you? Numerous epidemiologic (population-based) studies have found that diets low in saturated fat and cholesterol and high in fiber are associated with a reduced risk of certain cancers, diabetes, digestive disorders, and heart disease. However, since high-fiber foods may also contain antioxidant vitamins, phytochemicals, and other substances that may offer protection against these diseases, researchers can't say for certain that fiber alone is responsible for the reduced health risks they observe, notes Joyce Saltsman, a nutritionist with FDA's Office of Food Labeling. "Moreover, no one knows whether one specific type of fiber is more beneficial than another since fiber-rich foods tend to contain various types," she adds.

Recent findings on the health effects of fiber show it may play a role in:

Cancer. Epidemiologic studies have consistently noted an association between low total fat and high fiber intakes and reduced incidence of colon cancer. A 1992 study by researchers at Harvard Medical School found that men who consumed 12 grams of fiber a day were twice as likely to develop precancerous colon changes as men whose daily fiber intake was about 30 grams. The exact mechanism for reducing the risk is not known, but scientists theorize that insoluble fiber adds bulk to stool, which in turn dilutes carcinogens and speeds their transit through the lower intestines and out of the body.

The evidence that a high-fiber diet can protect against breast cancer is equivocal. Researchers analyzing data from the Nurses' Health Study, which tracked 89,494 women for eight years, concluded in 1992 that fiber intake has no influence on breast cancer risk in middle-aged women. Previously, a review and analysis of 12 studies found a link between high fiber intake and reduced risk.

In the early stages, some breast tumors are stimulated by excess amounts of estrogen circulating in the bloodstream. Some scientists believe that fiber may hamper the growth of such tumors by binding with estrogen in the intestine. This prevents the excess estrogen from being reabsorbed into the bloodstream.

Digestive Disorders. Because insoluble fiber aids digestion and adds bulk to stool, it hastens passage of fecal material through the gut, thus helping to prevent or alleviate constipation. Fiber also may help reduce the risk of diverticulosis, a condition in which small pouches form in the colon wall (usually from the pressure of straining during bowel movements). People who already have diverticulosis often find that increased fiber consumption can alleviate symptoms, which include constipation and/or diarrhea, abdominal pain, flatulence, and mucus or blood in the stool.

Diabetes. As with cholesterol, soluble fiber traps carbohydrates to slow their digestion and absorption. In theory, this may help prevent wide swings in blood sugar level throughout the day. Additionally, a new study from the Harvard School of Public Health, published in the February 12, 1997 issue of the *Journal of the American Medical Association*, suggests that a high-sugar, low-fiber diet more than doubles women's risk of Type II (non-insulin-dependent) diabetes. In the study, cereal fiber was associated with a 28 percent decreased risk, with fiber from fruits and vegetables having no effect. In comparison, cola beverages, white bread, white rice, and french fries increased the risk.

Heart Disease. Clinical studies show that a heart-healthy diet (low in saturated fat and cholesterol, and high in fruits, vegetables and grain products that contain soluble fiber) can lower blood cholesterol. In these studies, cholesterol levels dropped between 0.5 percent and 2 percent for every gram of soluble fiber eaten per day.

As it passes through the gastrointestinal tract, soluble fiber binds to dietary cholesterol, helping the body to eliminate it. This reduces blood cholesterol levels, which, in turn, reduces cholesterol deposits on arterial walls that eventually choke off the vessel. There also is some evidence that soluble fiber can slow the liver's manufacture of cholesterol, as well as alter low-density lipoprotein (LDL) particles to make them larger and less dense. Researchers believe that small, dense LDL particles pose a bigger health threat.

Recent findings from two long-term large-scale studies of men suggest that high fiber intake can significantly lower the risk of heart attack. Men who ate the most fiber-rich foods (35 grams a day, on average) suffered one-third fewer heart attacks than those who had the lowest fiber intake (15 grams a day), according to a Finnish study of 21,903 male smokers aged 50 to 69, published in the December 1996 issue of Circulation. Earlier in the year, findings from an ongoing U.S. study of 43,757 male health professionals (some of whom were sedentary, overweight or smokers) suggest that those who ate more than 25 grams of fiber per day had a 36 percent lower risk of developing heart disease than those who consumed less than 15 grams daily. In the Finnish study, each 10 grams of fiber added to the diet decreased the risk of dying from heart disease by 17 percent; in the U.S. study, risk was decreased by 29 percent.

These results indicate that high-fiber diets may help blunt the effects of smoking and other risk factors for heart disease.

Obesity. Because insoluble fiber is indigestible and passes through the body virtually intact, it provides few calories. And since the digestive tract can handle only so much bulk at a time, fiber-rich foods are more filling than other foods—so people tend to eat less. Insoluble fiber also may hamper the absorption of calorie-dense dietary fat. So, reaching for an apple instead of a bag of chips is a smart choice for someone trying to lose weight.

But be leery of using fiber supplements for weight loss. In August 1991, FDA banned methylcellulose, along with 110 other ingredients, in over-the-counter diet aids because there was no evidence these ingredients were safe and effective. The agency also recalled one product that contained guar gum after receiving reports of gastric or esophageal obstructions. The manufacturer had claimed the product promoted a feeling of fullness when it expanded in the stomach.

An Apple a Day and More

Recent research suggests that as much as 35 grams of fiber a day is needed to help reduce the risk of chronic disease, including heart disease. A fiber supplement can help make up the shortfall, but should not be a substitute for fiber-rich foods. "Foods that are high in fiber also contain nutrients that may help reduce the risk of chronic disease," Saltsman notes. In addition, eating a variety of such foods provides several types of fiber, whereas some fiber supplements contain only a single type of fiber, such as methylcellulose or psyllium.

Slow Going

A word of caution: When increasing the fiber content of your diet, it's best to take it slow. Add just a few grams at a time to allow the intestinal tract to adjust; otherwise, abdominal cramps, gas, bloating, and diarrhea or constipation may result. Other ways to help minimize these effects:

- Drink at least 2 liters (8 cups) of fluid daily.
- Don't cook dried beans in the same water you soaked them in.
- Use enzyme products, such as Beano or Say Yes To Beans, that help digest fiber.

To Fit More Fiber into Your Day

- **Read food labels.** The labels of almost all foods will tell you the amount of dietary fiber in each serving, as well as the Percent Daily Value (DV) based on a 2,000-calorie diet. For instance, if a half cup serving of a food provides 10 grams of dietary fiber, one serving provides 40 percent of the recommended DV. The food label can state that a product is "a good source" of fiber if it contributes 10 percent of the DV—2.5 grams of fiber per serving. The package can claim "high in," "rich in" or "excellent source of" fiber if the product provides 20 percent of the DV—5 grams per serving.

- **Use the U.S. Department of Agriculture's food pyramid as a guide.** If you eat 2 to 4 servings of fruit, 3 to 5 servings of vegetables, and 6 to 11 servings of cereal and grain foods, as recommended by the pyramid, you should have no trouble getting 25 to 30 grams of fiber a day.

- **Start the day with a whole-grain cereal that contains at least 5 grams of fiber per serving.** Top with wheat germ, raisins, bananas, or berries, all of which are good sources of fiber.

- **When appropriate, eat vegetables raw.** Cooking vegetables may reduce fiber content by breaking down some fiber into its carbohydrate components. When you do cook vegetables, microwave or steam only until they are al dente—tender, but still firm to the bite.

- **Avoid peeling fruits and vegetables; eating the skin and membranes ensures that you get every bit of fiber.** But rinse with warm water to remove surface dirt and bacteria before eating. Also, keep in mind that whole fruits and vegetables contain more fiber than juice, which lacks the skin and membranes.

- **Eat liberal amounts of foods that contain unprocessed grains in your diet:** whole-wheat products such as bulgur, couscous or kasha and whole-grain breads, cereals and pasta.

- **Add beans to soups, stews and salads.** A couple of times a week, substitute legume-based dishes (such as lentil soup, bean burritos, or rice and beans) for those made with meat.

- **Keep fresh and dried fruit on hand for snacks.**

"So many foods contain fiber that it's really not that hard to get your intake up where it should be," Saltsman says.

—by Ruth Papazian

Ruth Papazian is a writer in Bronx, N.Y., specializing in health and safety issues.

Chapter 8

Does Dietary Fat Still Matter?

True or false: The less fat you eat, the better. Given the messages about fat broadcast by nutritionists and health organizations—and most strongly by low-fat advocates such as Dr. Dean Ornish—you probably said "true" without even thinking. For the past 20 years, Americans have been told to reduce their dietary fat intake to 30%, 20%, or even 10% of their total calories to help prevent coronary heart disease (CHD) and other disorders. And they have moved steadily toward those goals.

Today, fat intake averages 33% of daily calories, down from about 40% in the 1960s. That reduction in fat consumption is thought to be a major reason why the rate of CHD has declined by about 30% over the past 25 years. So, for many, it was quite a shock when a study published in the *Journal of the American Medical Association (JAMA)* found that men who ate the most fat were the least likely to suffer a stroke. A cluster of other recent studies also now suggests that the role fat plays in a healthy diet is far from settled.

The complexity of fat's effect on overall health is bound to lead to some confusion about just what to eat. Each of the several types of fat (see below) has a different impact on your risk of developing diseases, such as CHD and possibly cancer. Saturated and trans fats, the most harmful types, raise blood cholesterol levels, which can lead

Reprinted with permission from *The Johns Hopkins Medical Letter Health After 50*, © MedLetter Associates, 1998. To order a one-year subscription, call 800-829-9170.

to narrowed arteries and possibly a heart attack. Unsaturated fat does not raise blood cholesterol.

But nutrition experts and health organizations—such as the American Heart Association, the American Cancer Society, the National Heart, Lung, and Blood Institute—have recommended limiting all types of fat, so that fat makes up no more than 30% of daily calories. The recommendation's primary purpose is to achieve a low intake of saturated fat. But it's also based on some research that shows that reducing total fat helps prevent cancer and obesity. When it comes to overall health, however, what the new studies indicate is that the type of fat you eat is probably more important than the total amount of fat.

Types of Fat

Saturated fat. Solid at room temperature, saturated fat is found predominantly in beef, butter, whole milk dairy products, and three vegetable oils (coconut, palm, and palm kernel),. It raises blood cholesterol levels and may contribute to certain types of cancer.

Trans fat. Formed when food manufacturers add hydrogen to unsaturated fatty acids to make the fat firmer and less likely to spoil, trans fat behaves like saturated fat in the body. It is found in packaged products—cookies, cakes, crackers, frozen dinners, some breakfast, cereals—as well as in stick margarine and some fried fast foods. To spot foods that contain trans fat, look for "Partially hydrogenated" oils on the ingredients list of packaged products.

Polyunsaturated fat. Polyunsaturated fat is found in vegetable oils, fish, walnuts, and other nuts. The form of polyunsaturated fat in fish not only lowers cholesterol, but may have other cardioprotective properties.

Monounsaturated fat. Found primarily in olive and canola oils, peanuts, almonds, and avocados, this type of fat tends to lower blood cholesterol levels. Because it is less susceptible to damage from oxygen than polyunsaturated fat, monounsaturated fat should make up the majority of fat in your diet.

Fat and Your Heart

Many people experience a significant decline in blood cholesterol levels when they reduce their total dietary fat to 30% of calories or less. But research is showing that this blanket approach to fat may not be necessary—and that a very low total fat intake may sometimes even be harmful. The reason a low-fat diet translates into a better cholesterol profile is that eating less fat overall means you also cut down on saturated fat. But if you trim the saturated fat from your diet, you may not have to worry as much about the other types, as the following studies demonstrate.

Dietary Alternatives Study. The Dietary Alternatives Study looked at the impact of varying intakes of dietary fat on blood lipid levels in 444 men with high LDL ("bad") cholesterol levels. Not unexpectedly, men who lowered their fat intake to 26% reduced their LDL cholesterol levels by 13%.

But these levels didn't fall further in men who ate even less fat. In fact, they had an undesirable cholesterol response: Those who got only 18 to 22% of their calories from fat experienced moderate declines in HDL ("good") cholesterol and a 39% increase in triglyceride levels. Both changes increase the risk for CHD.

Nurses' Health Study. The Nurses' Health Study, which involved over 80,000 women, confirmed the importance of cutting back on saturated and trans fats, but found that total fat intake did not influence CHD risk. As long as saturated and trans fat intake was low, women who got as much as 46% of their calories from fat were no more likely to develop CHD than women who ate less fat.

This study also pointed to a seemingly paradoxical increase in CHD risk if carbohydrates are substituted for unsaturated fat, as is often advised. For example, replacing 5% of saturated fat calories with an equivalent amount of carbohydrate calories reduced CHD risk by about 10%. In contrast, replacing 5% of calories from monounsaturated or polyunsaturated fat with carbohydrates resulted in 20% and 60% increases in CHD risk, respectively. Replacing trans fat with unsaturated fat was also associated with a reduced chance of developing CHD.

The researchers concluded that replacing saturated and trans fats with unsaturated fat improves blood cholesterol levels: LDL cholesterol levels decline, while HDL cholesterol levels increase or at least remain the same. When carbohydrates are substituted for unsaturated fat, however, HDL as well as LDL cholesterol levels drop, and blood triglycerides may increase.

JAMA Study. A more surprising finding came from the *JAMA* study of stroke. Not only did it find that total fat intake did not matter when it came to stroke risk in men, but that a high intake of saturated fat was even protective.

"This study has several methodological problems," says Dr. Simeon Margolis, medical editor of *Health After 50*. "The most important is that the conclusions were based on what the subjects said they ate in a single 24-hour period at the start of the study. No further dietary information was collected, and it's certainly possible that the men changed their diets over the 20-year follow-up period."

If the findings of the *JAMA* study prove to be valid, the results also showed that monounsaturated fat is equally protective against stroke. For these reasons, the researchers still recommend limiting saturated fat intake. (In addition, although some studies have shown that elevated cholesterol levels are not a major risk factor for stroke, drug treatment to reduce cholesterol levels has significantly lowered the number of strokes, as well as heart attacks, in other studies.)

Fat and Cancer

Despite the evidence that limiting saturated and trans fats is what really counts for preventing CHD, experts are reluctant to tell people that the total amount of fat you eat does not matter, even if most of it is unsaturated. That's because there is some debate about the effect of dietary fats on cancer risk. In addition, a diet high in fat is thought to contribute to obesity, which in turn is associated with diabetes, CHD, and other disorders. However, accumulating evidence implicates saturated fat, but not other types of fat, in the development of cancer, and also demonstrates that a low-fat diet does not necessarily promote weight loss or prevent weight gain.

A combination of animal and human studies had suggested that a high intake of fat, no matter what the type, was associated with an increased risk of colon, prostate, and breast cancers. However, further analysis shows that this is probably not the case. For example, a study from Italy published in February [1998] found that saturated fat increased colon cancer risk, but there was no significant effect, good or bad, from unsaturated fat.

Nor has it been confirmed that a high total fat intake boosts the risk of breast cancer. In fact, a comprehensive 1996 review of studies examining the connection between breast cancer and diet concluded that there is no reduction in breast cancer risk among women following a low-fat diet, even when fat intake is very low (about 20% of calories). A more recent British study comparing 200 women with newly diagnosed breast cancer to 1,357 women without the disease also found no connection between the amount of dietary fat and the chances of developing the disease.

More surprisingly, a study from the *Annals of Internal Medicine* hints at a possible protective effect from monounsaturated fat. In this study, women who ate more monounsaturated fat were less likely to develop breast cancer than women who ate little monounsaturated fat. While this finding needs to be confirmed by further research, it seems safe to say that the amount of total fat in the diet does not increase breast cancer risk.

Fat and Weight Control

A low-fat diet is often recommended for people trying to control their weight because all types of fat have twice as many calories as carbohydrates or protein (9 vs. 4 per gram). Therefore, you cut more calories by eliminating small amounts of fatty foods from your diet than by eating fewer carbohydrates or less protein.

Still, the ultimate determinants of weight are the total number of calories consumed and the total expended by metabolism, daily activity, and exercise. Someone who eats little fat, but overeats low-fat foods, may fail to lose weight or may even gain weight. This is because many low-fat foods—especially low-fat snacks and desserts—still contain a significant number of calories. For example, three regular Oreo cookies contain 160 calories and 7 grams of fat. Reduced-fat Oreos contain half the fat (3.5 grams), but still have 130 calories—not much of a savings over the regular variety.

The Bottom Line

In general, the results of these studies represent good news for people who have been squeezing lemon juice over salads but would rather use oil, and for those who've reluctantly passed up the peanuts at a ball game. Even though these are high-fat foods, most of their fat is unsaturated. "Total fat probably does not matter, if most of the fat is unsaturated and you're careful not to consume too many calories," says Dr. Margolis. "But if you eat a typical American diet, limiting total fat to 30% of calories is the easiest way to keep your saturated fat intake low," he says.

Because saturated fat should contribute no more than 10% of calories (no more than 7% if you have high total or LDL cholesterol levels or already have CHD), you still don't have the green light to eat more hamburgers, butter, and ice cream. It is also important to minimize your intake of stick margarine and packaged foods that contain partially hydrogenated oils, which are the main sources of trans fat.

The best advice may be to follow a Mediterranean-style diet. The main source of fat in this diet is olive oil, a predominantly monounsaturated fat. Vegetables, fruits, grains, and legumes are its staples, supplemented by yogurt, fish, nuts, and small amounts of cheese. Meat, especially red meat, is consumed infrequently, and butter is almost never used. Years ago, researchers noticed that people who lived in Mediterranean countries—Greece, Italy, and Spain, for example—had low rates of CHD and cancer despite a high total fat intake. In a 1995 study in Lyon, France, men and women who'd had a heart attack and were assigned to follow a Mediterranean diet reduced their risk of having another heart attack by 70%.

The Mediterranean Diet

Following a Mediterranean-style diet involves more than simply adding olive oil to foods. Follow these easy steps:

- Eat more bread, whole grains (barley and brown rice, for example), and whole-grain cereals.

- Eat several vegetables a day, and don't let a day pass without consuming at least one piece of fruit.

- Eat more fish.

- Cut back on red meet (beef, pork, and lamb). Consider eating poultry instead. When you eat red meat, choose lean cuts and eat small portions (3 to ounces cooked).

- Incorporate legumes, such as chick-peas, kidney beans, and navy beans, into your diet several times a week. Canned beans are just as nutritious as dried ones.

- Skip the butter and cream. Use olive oil or canola oil instead.

- Eat nuts several times a week.

- Make dairy products a regular part of your daily meals, but choose low-fat versions. Eat full-fat cheeses in small portions.

- Reduce your, consumption of packaged products made with partially hydrogenated oils.

Chapter 9

The New Food Label

Grocery store aisles have become avenues to greater nutritional knowledge.

The new food label makes it possible. Under new regulations from the Food and Drug Administration of the Department of Health and Human Services and the Food Safety and Inspection Service of the U.S. Department of Agriculture, the food label offers more complete, useful and accurate nutrition information than ever before.

The purpose of the food label reform was simple: to clear up confusion that has prevailed on supermarket shelves for years, to help consumers choose more healthful diets, and to offer an incentive to food companies to improve the nutritional qualities of their products.

Among key features are:

- nutrition labeling for almost all foods. Consumers now can learn about the nutritional qualities of almost all of the products they buy.

- a new, distinctive, easy-to-read format that enables consumers to more quickly find the label and the information they need to make healthful food choices.

- information on the amount per serving of saturated fat, cholesterol, dietary fiber, and other nutrients that are of major health concern to today's consumers.

Food and Drug Administration, Publication No. BG 95-12, May 1995. Source: Excerpted from FDA flyer, 1994: The New Food Label: What Consumers Want to Know. Updated: November 1996, Office of Food Labeling.

- nutrient reference values, expressed as % Daily Values, that help consumers see how a food fits into an overall daily diet.

- uniform definitions for terms that describe a food's nutrient content—such as "light," "low-fat," and "high-fiber"—to ensure that such terms mean the same for any product on which they appear. These descriptors are particularly helpful for consumers trying to moderate their intake of calories or fat and other nutrients, or for those trying to increase their intake of certain nutrients, such as fiber.

- claims about the relationship between a nutrient or food and a disease or health-related condition, such as calcium and osteoporosis, and fat and cancer. These are helpful for people who are concerned about eating foods that may help keep them healthier longer.

- standardized serving sizes that make nutritional comparisons of similar products easier.

- declaration of total percentage of juice in juice drinks. This enables consumers to know exactly how much juice is in a product.

- voluntary nutrition information for many raw foods.

Nutritional Labeling and Education Act (NLEA)

These and other changes are part of final rules published in the Federal Register in 1992 and 1993. FDA's rules implement the provisions of the Nutrition Labeling and Education Act of 1990 (NLEA), which, among other things, requires nutrition labeling for most foods (except meat and poultry) and authorizes the use of nutrient content claims and appropriate FDA-approved health claims.

Meat and poultry products regulated by USDA are not covered by NLEA. However, USDA's regulations closely parallel FDA's rules, summarized here.

Nutrition Labeling—Applicable Foods

The regulations, most of which went into effect in 1994, call for nutrition labeling for most foods. In addition, they set up voluntary programs for nutrition information for many raw foods: the 20 most frequently eaten raw fruits, vegetables and fish each, under FDA's voluntary point-of-purchase nutrition information program, and the 45 best-selling cuts of meat, under USDA's program.

Although voluntary, FDA's program for raw produce and fish carries a strong incentive for retailers to participate. The program will remain voluntary only if at least 60 percent of a nationwide sample of retailers continue to provide the necessary information. (In a 1994 survey, FDA found that more than 70 percent of U.S. food stores were complying.

Nutrition information also will be provided for some restaurant foods. The current regulations require nutrition information for foods about which health or nutrient-content claims are made on restaurant signs or placards. In June 1993, FDA proposed similar requirements for restaurant menu items with such claims. Under that proposal, restaurants would have to provide a "reasonable basis" for making claims. They would be given some flexibility in demonstrating that reasonable basis. For example, they could rely on recipes endorsed by medical or dietary groups.

Nutrition Labeling—Exemptions

Under NLEA, some foods are exempt from nutrition labeling. These include:

- food served for immediate consumption, such as that served in hospital cafeterias and airplanes, and that sold by food service vendors—for example, mall cookie counters, sidewalk vendors, and vending machines.

- ready-to-eat food that is not for immediate consumption but is prepared primarily on site—for example, bakery, deli, and candy store items.

- food shipped in bulk, as long as it is not for sale in that form to consumers.

- medical foods, such as those used to address the nutritional needs of patients with certain diseases.

- plain coffee and tea, some spices, and other foods that contain no significant amounts of any nutrients.

Food produced by small businesses also is exempt, under 1993 amendments to NLEA. The NLEA amendments provide for a system in which exemptions are based on the number of people a company employs and the number of units within a product line it makes yearly.

Under this system, the allowances for each factor are gradually lowered. Between May 9, 1995, and May 8, 1996, a food is exempt from nutrition labeling if the company whose name appears on the label employs fewer than 300 full-time equivalent employees and makes fewer than 400,000 units of the product yearly. After May 1997, only businesses with fewer than 100 full-time equivalent employees producing fewer than 100,000 units within a product line for U.S. distribution can qualify for an exemption.

Almost all companies seeking an exemption will have to notify FDA that they meet the criteria. Those that do not have to notify FDA are U.S. firms with fewer than 10 employees making fewer than 10,000 units of a food in a year.

Although these foods are exempt, they are free to carry nutrition information, when appropriate—as long as it complies with the new regulations. Also, they will lose their exemption if their labels carry a nutrient content or health claim or any other nutrition information.

Nutrition information about game meats—such as deer, bison, rabbit, quail, wild turkey, and ostrich—is not required on individual packages. Instead, it can be given on counter cards, signs, or other point-of-purchase materials. Because few nutrient data exist for these foods, FDA believes that allowing this option will enable game meat producers to give first priority to collecting appropriate data and make it easier for them to update the information as it becomes available.

Nutrition Panel Title

The new food label features a revamped nutrition panel. It has a new title, "Nutrition Facts," which replaced "Nutrition Information Per Serving." The new title signals that the product has been labeled according to the new regulations. Also, for the first time, there are requirements on type size, style, spacing, and contrast to ensure a more distinctive, easy-to-read label.

Serving Sizes

The serving size remains the basis for reporting each food's nutrient content. However, unlike in the past, when the serving size was up to the discretion of the food manufacturer, serving sizes now are more uniform and reflect the amounts people actually eat. They also must be expressed in both common household and metric measures.

FDA allows as common household measures: the cup, tablespoon, teaspoon, piece, slice, fraction (such as "¼ pizza"), and common household containers used to package food products (such as a jar or tray). Ounces may be used, but only if a common household unit is not applicable and an appropriate visual unit is given—for example, 1 oz (28 g/about ½ pickle).

Grams (g) and milliliters (mL) are the metric units that are used in serving size statements.

NLEA defines serving size as the amount of food customarily eaten at one time. The serving sizes that appear on food labels are based on FDA-established lists of "Reference Amounts Customarily Consumed Per Eating Occasion."

These reference amounts, which are part of the regulations, are broken down into 139 FDA-regulated food product categories, including 11 groups of foods specially formulated or processed for infants or children under 4. They list the amounts of food customarily consumed per eating occasion for each category, based primarily on national food consumption surveys. FDA's list also gives the suggested label statement for serving size declaration. For example, the category "breads (excluding sweet quick type), rolls" has a reference amount of 50 g, and the appropriate label statement for sliced bread or rolls is "piece(s) (g)" or, for unsliced bread, "2 oz (56 g/inch slice)."

The serving size of products that come in discrete units, such as cookies, candy bars, and sliced products, is the number of whole units that most closely approximates the reference amount. Cookies are an example. Under the "bakery products" category, cookies have a reference amount of 30 g. The household measure closest to that amount is the number of cookies that comes closest to weighing 30 g. Thus, the serving size on the label of a package of cookies in which each cookie weighs 13 g would read "2 cookies (26 g)."

If one unit weighs more than 50 percent but less than 200 percent of the reference amount, the serving size is one unit. For example, the reference amount for bread is 50 g; therefore, the label of a loaf of bread in which each slice weighs more than 25 g would state a serving size of one slice.

Certain rules apply to food products that are packaged and sold individually. If such an individual package is less than 200 percent of the applicable reference amount, the item qualifies as one serving. Thus, a 360 mL (12 fluid ounce) can of soda is one serving, since the reference amount for carbonated beverages is 240 mL (8 ounces). However, if the product has a reference amount of 100 g or 100 mL or more and the package contains more than 150 percent but less than 200 percent of the reference amount, manufacturers have the option of deciding whether the product can be one or two servings.

An example is a 15 ounce (420 g) can of soup. The serving size reference amount for soup is 245 g. Therefore, the manufacturer has the option to declare the can of soup as one or two servings.

Nutrition Information

There is a new set of dietary components on the nutrition panel. The mandatory (boldface) and voluntary components and the order in which they must appear are:

- **total calories**
- **calories from fat**
- calories from saturated fat
- **total fat**
- **saturated fat**
- polyunsaturated fat
- monounsaturated fat
- **cholesterol**
- **sodium**
- potassium
- **total carbohydrate**
- **dietary fiber**
- soluble fiber
- insoluble fiber
- **sugars**
- sugar alcohol (for example, the sugar substitutes xylitol, mannitol and sorbitol)
- other carbohydrate (the difference between total carbohydrate and the sum of dietary fiber, sugars, and sugar alcohol if declared)
- **protein**
- **vitamin A**
- percent of vitamin A present as beta-carotene
- **vitamin C**
- **calcium**
- **iron**
- other essential vitamins and minerals

If a claim is made about any of the optional components, or if a food is fortified or enriched with any of them, nutrition information for these components becomes mandatory.

These mandatory and voluntary components are the only ones allowed on the nutrition panel. The listing of single amino acids, maltodextrin, calories from polyunsaturated fat, and calories from carbohydrates, for example, may not appear as part of the Nutrition Facts on the label.

The required nutrients were selected because they address today's health concerns. The order in which they must appear reflects the priority of current dietary recommendations.

Thiamin, riboflavin and niacin are no longer required in nutrition labeling because deficiencies of each are no longer considered of public health significance. However, they may be listed voluntarily.

Nutrition Panel Format

The format for declaring nutrient content per serving also has been revised. Now, all nutrients must be declared as percentages of the Daily Values—the new label reference values. The amount, in grams or milligrams, of macronutrients (such as fat, cholesterol, sodium, carbohydrates, and protein) still must be listed to the immediate right of each of the names of each of these nutrients. But, for the first time, a column headed "% Daily Value" appears.

Requiring nutrients to be declared as a percentage of the Daily Values is intended to prevent misinterpretations that arise with quantitative values. For example, a food with 140 milligrams (mg) of sodium could be mistaken for a high-sodium food because 140 is a relatively large number. In actuality, however, that amount represents less than 6 percent of the Daily Value for sodium, which is 2,400 mg.

On the other hand, a food with 5 g of saturated fat could be construed as being low in that nutrient. In fact, that food would provide one-fourth the total Daily Value because 20 g is the Daily Value for saturated fat based on a 2,000-calorie diet.

Nutrition Panel Footnote

The % Daily Value listing carries a footnote saying that the percentages are based on a 2,000-calorie diet. Some nutrition labels—at least those on larger packages—have these additional footnotes:

- a sentence noting that a person's individual nutrient goals are based on his or her calorie needs.
- lists of the daily values for selected nutrients for a 2,000- and a 2,500-calorie diet.

An optional footnote for packages of any size is the number of calories per gram of fat (9), and carbohydrate and protein (4).

Format Modifications

In limited circumstances, variations in the format of the nutrition panel are allowed. Some are mandatory. For example, the labels of foods for children under 2 (except infant formula, which has special labeling rules under the Infant Formula Act of 1980) may not carry information about saturated fat, polyunsaturated fat, monounsaturated fat, cholesterol, calories from fat, or calories from saturated fat.

The reason is to prevent parents from wrongly assuming that infants and toddlers should restrict their fat intake, when, in fact, they should not. Fat is important during these years to ensure adequate growth and development.

The labels of foods for children under 4 may not include the % Daily Values for total fat, saturated fat, cholesterol, sodium, potassium, total carbohydrate, and dietary fiber. They may carry % Daily Values for protein, vitamins, and minerals, however. These nutrients are the only ones for which FDA has set Daily Values for this age group.

Thus, the top portion of the "Nutrition Facts" panels of foods for children under 4 will consist of two columns. The nutrients' names will be listed on the left and their quantitative amounts will be on the right. The bottom portion will provide the % Daily Values for protein, vitamins, and minerals. Only the calorie conversion information may be given as a footnote.

Some foods qualify for a simplified label format. This format is allowed when the food contains insignificant amounts of seven or more of the mandatory nutrients and total calories. "Insignificant" means that a declaration of zero could be made in nutrition labeling, or, for total carbohydrate, dietary fiber, and protein, the declaration states "less than 1 g."

For foods for children under 2, the simplified format may be used if the product contains insignificant amounts of six or more of the following: calories, total fat, sodium, total carbohydrate, dietary fiber, sugars, protein, vitamins A and C, calcium, and iron.

If the simplified format is used, information on total calories, total fat, total carbohydrate, protein, and sodium—even if they are present in insignificant amounts—must be listed. Other nutrients, along with calories from fat, must be shown if they are present in more than insignificant amounts. Nutrients added to the food must be listed, too.

Some format exceptions exist for small and medium-size packages. Packages with less than 12 square inches of available labeling space (about the size of a package of chewing gum) do not have to carry nutrition information unless a nutrient content or health claim is made for the product. However, they must provide an address or telephone number for consumers to obtain the required nutrition information.

If manufacturers wish to provide nutrition information on these packages voluntarily, they have several options: (1) present the information in a smaller type size than that required for larger packages, or (2) present the information in a tabular or linear (string) format.

The tabular and linear formats also may be used on packages that have less than 40 square inches available for labeling and insufficient space for the full vertical format.

Other options for packages with less than 40 square inches of label space are:

- abbreviating names of dietary components
- omitting all footnotes, except for the statement that % Daily Values are based on a 2,000-calorie diet
- placing nutrition information on other panels readily seen by consumers.

A select group of packages with more than 40 square inches of labeling space is allowed a format exception, too. These are packages with insufficient vertical space (about 3 inches) to accommodate the required information. Some examples are bread bags, pie boxes, and bags of frozen vegetables. On these packages, the "Nutrition Facts" panel may appear horizontally, with footnote information appearing to the far right.

For larger packages in which there is not sufficient space on the principal display panel or the information panel to the right, FDA allows nutrition information to appear on any label panel that is readily seen by consumers. This intent lessens the chances of overcrowding of information and encourages manufacturers to provide the greatest amount of nutrition information possible.

For products that require additional preparation before eating, such as dry cake mixes and dry pasta dinners, or that are usually eaten with one or more additional foods, such as breakfast cereals with milk, FDA encourages manufacturers to provide voluntarily a second column of nutrition information. This is known as dual declaration.

With this variation, the first column, which is mandatory, contains nutrition information for the food as purchased. The second gives information about the food as prepared and eaten.

Still another variation is the aggregate display. This is allowed on labels of variety-pack food items, such as ready-to-eat cereals and assorted flavors of individual ice cream cups. With this display, the quantitative amount and % Daily Value for each nutrient are listed in separate columns under the name of each food.

Daily Values—DRVs

The new label reference value, Daily Value, comprises two sets of dietary standards: Daily Reference Values (DRVs) and Reference Daily Intakes (RDIs). Only the Daily Value term appears on the label, though, to make label reading less confusing.

DRVs have been established for macronutrients that are sources of energy: fat, carbohydrate (including fiber), and protein; and for cholesterol, sodium and potassium, which do not contribute calories.

DRVs for the energy-producing nutrients are based on the number of calories consumed per day. A daily intake of 2,000 calories has been established as the reference. This level was chosen, in part, because it approximates the caloric requirements for postmenopausal women. This group has the highest risk for excessive intake of calories and fat.

DRVs for the energy-producing nutrients are calculated as follows:

- fat based on 30 percent of calories
- saturated fat based on 10 percent of calories
- carbohydrate based on 60 percent of calories
- protein based on 10 percent of calories. (The DRV for protein applies only to adults and children over 4. RDIs for protein for special groups have been established.)
- fiber based on 11.5 g of fiber per 1,000 calories.

Because of current public health recommendations, DRVs for some nutrients represent the uppermost limit that is considered desirable. The DRVs for fats and sodium are:

- total fat: less than 65 g
- saturated fat: less than 20 g
- cholesterol: less than 300 mg
- sodium: less than 2,400 mg

Daily Values—RDIs

The RDI replaces the term "U.S. RDA," which was introduced in 1973 as a label reference value for vitamins, minerals and protein in voluntary nutrition labeling. The name change was sought because of confusion that existed over "U.S. RDAs," the values determined by FDA and used on food labels, and "RDAs" (Recommended Dietary Allowances), the values determined by the National Academy of Sciences for various population groups and used by FDA to figure the U.S. RDAs.

However, the values for the new RDIs remain the same as the old U.S. RDAs for the time being.

Nutrient Content Descriptors

The regulations also spell out what terms may be used to describe the level of a nutrient in a food and how they can be used. These are the core terms:

- **Free.** This term means that a product contains no amount of, or only trivial or "physiologically inconsequential" amounts of, one or more of these components: fat, saturated fat, cholesterol, sodium, sugars, and calories. For example, "calorie-free" means fewer than 5 calories per serving and "sugar-free" and "fat-free" both mean less than 0.5 g per serving. Synonyms for "free" include "without," "no" and "zero."

- **Low.** This term can be used on foods that can be eaten frequently without exceeding dietary guidelines for one or more of these components: fat, saturated fat, cholesterol, sodium, and calories. Thus, descriptors are defined as follows:
  - *low-fat:* 3 g or less per serving
  - *low-saturated fat:* 1 g or less per serving
  - *low-sodium:* 140 mg or less per serving
  - *very low sodium:* 35 mg or less per serving
  - *low-cholesterol:* 20 mg or less and 2 g or less of saturated fat per serving
  - *low-calorie:* 40 calories or less per serving.

  Synonyms for low include "little," "few," and "low source of."

- **Lean and extra lean.** These terms can be used to describe the fat content of meat, poultry, seafood, and game meats.
  - *lean:* less than 10 g fat, 4.5 g or less saturated fat, and less than 95 mg cholesterol per serving and per 100 g.

- *extra lean:* less than 5 g fat, less than 2 g saturated fat, and less than 95 mg cholesterol per serving and per 100 g.

- **High.** This term can be used if the food contains 20 percent or more of the Daily Value for a particular nutrient in a serving.

- **Good source.** This term means that one serving of a food contains 10 to 19 percent of the Daily Value for a particular nutrient.

- **Reduced.** This term means that a nutritionally altered product contains at least 25 percent less of a nutrient or of calories than the regular, or reference, product. However, a reduced claim can't be made on a product if its reference food already meets the requirement for a "low" claim.

- **Less.** This term means that a food, whether altered or not, contains 25 percent less of a nutrient or of calories than the reference food. For example, pretzels that have 25 percent less fat than potato chips could carry a "less" claim. "Fewer" is an acceptable synonym.

- **Light.** This descriptor can mean two things:

  - *First,* that a nutritionally altered product contains one-third fewer calories or half the fat of the reference food. If the food derives 50 percent or more of its calories from fat, the reduction must be 50 percent of the fat.

  - *Second,* that the sodium content of a low-calorie, low-fat food has been reduced by 50 percent. In addition, "light in sodium" may be used on food in which the sodium content has been reduced by at least 50 percent.

  The term "light" still can be used to describe such properties as texture and color, as long as the label explains the intent—for example, "light brown sugar" and "light and fluffy."

- **More.** This term means that a serving of food, whether altered or not, contains a nutrient that is at least 10 percent of the Daily Value more than the reference food. The 10 percent of Daily Value also applies to "fortified," "enriched" and "added" claims, but in those cases, the food must be altered.

Alternative spelling of these descriptive terms and their synonyms are allowed—for example, "hi" and "lo"—as long as the alternatives are not misleading.

Other Definitions

The regulations also address other claims. Among them:

- **Percent fat free:** A product bearing this claim must be a low-fat or a fat-free product. In addition, the claim must accurately reflect the amount of fat present in 100 g of the food. Thus, if a food contains 2.5 g fat per 50 g, the claim must be "95 percent fat free."

- **Implied:** These types of claims are prohibited when they wrongfully imply that a food contains or does not contain a meaningful level of a nutrient. For example, a product claiming to be made with an ingredient known to be a source of fiber (such as "made with oat bran") is not allowed unless the product contains enough of that ingredient (for example, oat bran) to meet the definition for "good source" of fiber. As another example, a claim that a product contains "no tropical oils" is allowed—but only on foods that are "low" in saturated fat because consumers have come to equate tropical oils with high saturated fat.

- **Meals and main dishes:** Claims that a meal or main dish is "free" of a nutrient, such as sodium or cholesterol, must meet the same requirements as those for individual foods. Other claims can be used under special circumstances. For example, "low-calorie" means the meal or main dish contains 120 calories or less per 100 g. "Low-sodium" means the food has 140 mg or less per 100 g. "Low-cholesterol" means the food contains 20 mg cholesterol or less per 100 g and no more than 2 g saturated fat. "Light" means the meal or main dish is low-fat or low-calorie.

- **Standardized foods:** Any nutrient content claim, such as "reduced fat," "low calorie," and "light," may be used in conjunction with a standardized term if the new product has been specifically formulated to meet FDA's criteria for that claim, if the product is not nutritionally inferior to the traditional standardized food, and the new product complies with certain compositional requirements set by FDA. A new product bearing a claim also must have performance characteristics similar to the referenced traditional standardized food. If the product doesn't, and the differences materially limit the product's use, its label must state the differences (for example, not recommended for baking) to inform consumers.

- **Healthy:** A "healthy" food must be low in fat and saturated fat and contain limited amounts of cholesterol and sodium. In addition, if it's a single-item food, it must provide at least 10 percent of one or more of vitamins A or C, iron, calcium, protein, or fiber. If it's a meal-type product, such as frozen entrees and multi-course frozen dinners, it must provide 10 percent of two or three of these vitamins or minerals or of protein or fiber, in addition to meeting the other criteria.

Limits on sodium will be phased in. By January 1996, FDA-regulated individual foods labeled "healthy" must provide no more than 480 mg of sodium per serving. After Jan. 1, 1998, the sodium limit for FDA-regulated foods will drop to 360 mg per serving for individual foods and 480 mg per serving for meal-type products that carry the "healthy" claims. Effective dates for the sodium phase-in for USDA-regulated products are November 1995 and November 1997. The sodium limits match FDA's.

"Fresh"

Although not mandated by NLEA, FDA has issued a regulation for the term "fresh." The agency took this step because of concern over the term's possible misuse on some food labels.

The regulation defines the term "fresh" when it is used to suggest that a food is raw or unprocessed. In this context, "fresh" can be used only on a food that is raw, has never been frozen or heated, and contains no preservatives. (Irradiation at low levels is allowed.) "Fresh frozen," "frozen fresh," and "freshly frozen" can be used for foods that are quickly frozen while still fresh. Blanching (brief scalding before freezing to prevent nutrient breakdown) is allowed.

Other uses of the term "fresh," such as in "fresh milk" or "freshly baked bread," are not affected.

Baby Foods

FDA is not allowing broad use of nutrient claims on infant and toddler foods. However, the agency may propose later claims specifically for these foods. The terms "unsweetened" and "unsalted" are allowed on these foods, however, because they relate to taste and not nutrient content.

Health Claims

Claims for eight relationships between a nutrient or a food and the risk of a disease or health-related condition are now allowed. They can be made in several ways: through third-party references, such as the National Cancer Institute; statements; symbols, such as a heart; and vignettes or descriptions. Whatever the case, the claim must meet the requirements for authorized health claims; for example, they cannot state the degree of risk reduction and can only use "may" or "might" in discussing the nutrient or food-disease relationship. And they must state that other factors play a role in that disease.

The claims also must be phrased so that consumers can understand the relationship between the nutrient and the disease and the nutrient's importance in relationship to a daily diet.

An example of an appropriate claim is: "While many factors affect heart disease, diets low in saturated fat and cholesterol may reduce the risk of this disease."

The allowed nutrient-disease relationship claims and rules for their use are:

- **Calcium and osteoporosis:** To carry this claim, a food must contain 20 percent or more of the Daily Value for calcium (200 mg) per serving, have a calcium content that equals or exceeds the food's content of phosphorus, and contain a form of calcium that can be readily absorbed and used by the body. The claim must name the target group most in need of adequate calcium intakes (that is, teens and young adult white and Asian women) and state the need for exercise and a healthy diet. A product that contains 40 percent or more of the Daily Value for calcium must state on the label that a total dietary intake greater than 200 percent of the Daily Value for calcium (that is, 2,000 mg or more) has no further known benefit.

- **Fat and cancer:** To carry this claim, a food must meet the descriptor requirements for "low-fat" or, if fish and game meats, for "extra lean."

- **Saturated fat and cholesterol and coronary heart disease (CHD):** This claim may be used if the food meets the definitions for the descriptors "low saturated fat," "low-cholesterol," and "low-fat," or, if fish and game meats, for "extra lean." It may mention the link between reduced risk of CHD and lower saturated fat and cholesterol intakes to lower blood cholesterol levels.

- **Fiber-containing grain products, fruits and vegetables and cancer:** To carry this claim, a food must be or must contain a grain product, fruit or vegetable and meet the descriptor requirements for "low-fat," and, without fortification, be a "good source" of dietary fiber.

- **Fruits, vegetables, and grain products that contain fiber and risk of CHD:** To carry this claim, a food must be or must contain fruits, vegetables, and grain products. It also must meet the descriptor requirements for "low saturated fat," "low-cholesterol," and "low-fat" and contain, without fortification, at least 0.6 g soluble fiber per serving.

- **Sodium and hypertension (high blood pressure):** To carry this claim, a food must meet the descriptor requirements for "low-sodium."

- **Fruits and vegetables and cancer:** This claim may be made for fruits and vegetables that meet the descriptor requirements for "low-fat" and that, without fortification, for "good source" of at least one of the following: dietary fiber or vitamins A or C. This claim relates diets low in fat and rich in fruits and vegetables (and thus vitamins A and C and dietary fiber) to reduced cancer risk. FDA authorized this claim in place of an antioxidant vitamin and cancer claim.

- **Folic acid and neural tube defects:** On January 4, 1994, FDA authorized the use of a health claim about the relationship between folic acid and the risk of neural tube birth defects for dietary supplements and for foods in conventional food form that are naturally high in folic acid. (In 1992, the U.S. Public Health Service had recommended that all women of childbearing age consume 0.4 mg folic acid daily to reduce their risk of giving birth to a child affected with a neural tube defect.) FDA plans to issue a final rule to allow the folic acid-neural tube defect claim for fortified foods, too.

Ingredient Labeling

The list of ingredients has undergone some changes, too. Chief among them is a requirement for full ingredient labeling on "standardized foods," which previously were exempt. Ingredient declaration is now required on all foods that have more than one ingredient.

Also, the ingredient list includes, when appropriate:

- FDA-certified color additives, such as FD&C Blue No. 1, by name.
- sources of protein hydrolysates, which are used in many foods as flavors and flavor enhancers.
- declaration of caseinate as a milk derivative in the ingredient list of foods that claim to be non-dairy, such as coffee whiteners.

The main reason for these new requirements is that some people may be allergic to such additives and now may be better able to avoid them.

As required by NLEA, beverages that claim to contain juice now must declare the total percentage of juice on the information panel. In addition, FDA's regulation establishes criteria for naming juice beverages. For example, when the label of a multi-juice beverage states one or more—but not all—of the juices present, and the predominantly named juice is present in minor amounts, the product's name must state that the beverage is flavored with that juice or declare the amount of the juice in a 5 percent range—for example, "raspberry-flavored juice blend" or "juice blend, 2 to 7 percent raspberry juice."

Economic Impact

It is estimated that the new food label will cost FDA-regulated food processors between $1.4 billion and $2.3 billion over the next 20 years. The benefits to public health—measured in monetary terms—are estimated to well exceed the costs. Potential benefits include decreased rates of coronary heart disease, cancer, osteoporosis, obesity, high blood pressure, and allergic reactions to food.

How Should I Use the % Daily Value (% DV) Column on the Food Label?

By using the % Daily Values, you can easily determine whether a food contributes a lot or a little of a particular nutrient. And you can compare different foods with no need to do any calculations. A high percentage means the food contains a lot of a nutrient and a low percentage means it contains a little.

Look to see whether the nutrients most of us need more of (such as total carbohydrate, dietary fiber, and certain vitamins and minerals) have high percentages. Look to see whether the nutrients most of us need to limit (such as fat, saturated fat, cholesterol, and—for some people—sodium) have low percentages.

The goal is to choose foods that together give you close to 100 percent of each nutrient for a day, or average about 100 percent a day over a few days, depending on the nutrient.

For example, if your goal is 2,000 calories, your total fat intake would be no more than 65 grams, the upper limit recommended for a 2,000 calorie daily diet. If the food you're preparing has 16 grams for fat per serving and shows the % Daily Value for total fat per serving at 25 percent, then you know that all the other foods you eat that day should total 75 percent or less of the Daily Value for total fat (or 49 grams of fat).

You can use the % Daily Value column to easily compare one product to another. If you want to lower the fat in your diet, you can compare products and select the ones with the lower %. You can also use the % Daily Value to make dietary trade-offs with other foods throughout the day. This means you don't have to deprive yourself of a favorite food that might be high in fat, if you watch what else you eat the rest of the day.

Obtaining Regulations and Related Information

Reprints of Federal Register documents on FDA's food labeling rules can be ordered by calling the National Technical Information Service at (703) 487-4650. Ask for #PB-93-139905. The cost is $91.

The January 6 document also can be downloaded from the National Agricultural Library's electronic bulletin board, Agricultural Library Forum (ALF). The electronic bulletin board can be accessed 24 hours a day, seven days a week. The telephone numbers are (301) 504-6510, (301) 504-5111, (301) 504-5496, and (301) 504-5497. For assistance, call the FDA/USDA Food Labeling Education Information Center at (301) 504-5719.

The January and April 1993 documents also are included in the April 1, 1993, edition of the Code of Federal Regulations, which is available from the Government Printing Office (Title 21, Parts 100-169) for $21. This may be ordered by calling (202) 512-1800.

Chapter 10

New Labels for Fat-Reduced Milk Products

Milk, that all-American food, is taking on some all-American names—like "fat free," "reduced fat" and "light."

Starting January 1, 1998, the labeling of fat-reduced milk products will have to follow the same requirements the Food and Drug Administration established almost five years ago for the labeling of just about every other food reduced in fat. From now on:

- 2 percent milk will become known, for example, as "reduced fat" or "less fat" instead of "low fat"

- 1 percent milk will remain "low fat" or become, for example, "little fat"

- skim will retain its name or be called, for example, fat-free, zero-fat, or no-fat milk.

Also, the regulations that implement the labeling changes give dairy processors more leeway to devise new formulations. As a result, consumers may see a broader range of milk and other dairy products, including "light" milk with at least 50 percent less fat than whole, or full-fat, milk and other reformulated milks with reduced fat contents but greater consumer appeal.

"I expect that there are going to be many more milk products for consumers to choose from" says Michelle Smith, a food technologist in FDA's Office of Food Labeling. "This is positive for milk consumption

"Skimming the Milk Label," *FDA Consumer*, January-February 1998.

in general, and it's likely that consumers will be able to find a lower fat milk product that they like."

FDA issued a final rule in November 1996 that revoked the standards of identity—the prescribed recipes that manufacturers of a particular food must follow—for many fat-reduced milk and other dairy products. This allowed the agency to bring milk labeling in line with existing labeling requirements for nutrient content claims, such as "fat free," "low fat," "high protein," and others.

Lower fat milk products will still need to be nutritionally equivalent to full-fat milk and provide at least the same amounts of the fat-soluble vitamins A and D as full-fat milk. Vitamins A and D are lost when milk fat is reduced or removed.

"[Milk] is just as nutritional as before," says LeGrande "Shot" Hudson, dairy plant manager for the Landover, Md.–based Giant Food Inc. "[The milk industry] just changed the name[s] a little."

Joint Effort

FDA's final rule was prompted in part by a petition filed jointly by the Milk Industry Foundation and the Center for Science in the Public Interest (CSPI), a consumer advocacy group, and a separate petition filed by the American Dairy Products Institute. The petitions

Table 10.1. Milk's New Names

Old Name	Possible New Names	Total Fat (per 240 mL; 1cup)		Calories per 240 mL
		Grams	%Daily Value	
Milk	Milk	8.0g	12%	150
Low- fat 2 percent milk	Reduced-fat or less-fat milk	4.7g	7%	122
Not on the Market	Light milk	4 g or less	6% or less	116 or less
Low-fat 1 percent milk	Low-fat milk	2.6g	4%	102
Skim milk	Fat-free, skim, zero-fat, no-fat or non-fat milk	less than 0.5g	0%	80

asked FDA to lift the labeling exemption provided for in the Nutrition Labeling and Education Act of 1990 for lower fat dairy products.

FDA agreed to revoke the standards of identity for low-fat milk and 11 other lower fat dairy products, including low-fat cottage cheese, sweetened condensed skimmed milk, sour half-and-half, evaporated skimmed milk, and low-fat dry milk. These products are now bound by the "general standard" for nutritionally modified standardized foods. This means the nutrients that lower fat milk products provide, other than fat, must be at least equal to full-fat milk before vitamins A and D are added.

FDA also agreed to allow manufacturers to use "skim" as a synonym for "fat free" in the labeling of dairy products because, the agency concluded, most consumers realize that skim milk means no fat.

The changes do not affect lower fat yogurt products. FDA decided to keep the standards of identity for the time being to further consider manufacturers' concerns about fortifying yogurt with vitamin A, a nutrient found in full-fat yogurt.

FDA, along with the milk industry and nutrition educators, believes the label changes will give consumers more accurate, useful information about milk. Because claims on milk labels will be consistent with claims on other foods, consumers will know, for example, that "low-fat" milk (formerly known as 1 percent milk) will be similar in fat content to "low-fat" cookies. (Both can provide no more than 3 grams of fat per serving. The serving size for each is listed on their label's Nutrition Facts panel.)

The improved accuracy of milk labeling is particularly important for skim milk, experts say, because "skim" carries a negative connotation for many consumers. "They think it is skimmed of all its good nutrients," says Brad Legreid, executive director of the Wisconsin Dairy Products Association. "That it's flat and tasteless. But that's not it at all."

Or, they view it in the same negative light as dry powdered milk, says Margo Wootan, a senior scientist with CSPI. She coordinates the group's public health campaign to encourage consumers to use milk that provides 4 percent or less of the Daily Value for fat—that is, low-fat or skim milk. She prefers the term "fat-free" to describe skim milk because she says: "It is more recognizable to the public. And "fat-free" better describes the benefits of skim milk."

Dietary Significance

The goal of the labeling changes, as many nutrition experts see it, is to help consumers select milk products that can help them lower their fat and saturated fat intakes to recommended levels. The Dietary Guidelines for Americans recommends limiting fat to no more than 30 percent of calories and saturated fat to less than 10 percent of calories. There is substantial scientific evidence to show that low fat intakes may help reduce the risk of some cancers, and diets low in saturated fat and cholesterol may reduce the risk of heart disease.

Switching from higher fat to lower fat milk products can have a particularly significant impact on lowering fat and saturated fat intakes because milk plays such an important role in the American diet, CSPI's Wootan says. She says that milk is a major contributor of saturated fat to the American adult's diet. Only cheese and beef contribute more.

Considering that 240 milliliters (one cup) of full-fat milk provides 26 percent of the Daily Value for saturated fat, while fat-free milk provides none, switching from full-fat to fat-free milk can drop saturated fat intake considerably, she says.

"It's an easy way to lower fat intake," she says. "It doesn't take a lot of time. No preparation skills are needed. It takes only five seconds at the dairy case to move your hand to the fat-free [skim] or low-fat [formerly 1 percent] milk. It's a good first step towards healthy eating."

Wootan believes that the revised milk labeling will make especially clear to consumers the difference between reduced-fat (formerly 2 percent low-fat milk) and low-fat (1 percent low-fat milk). "A lot of people use 2 percent milk thinking it is the same as 1 percent," she says, because the previous labels referred to both as "low fat." However, reduced-fat milk provides almost twice the amount of fat and saturated fat as low-fat milk.

The new labels will "show a difference," she says, "and, [I think,] more people will go to drinking 1 percent or skim milk."

New Names in the Dairy Case

But first, they'll need to get used to milk's new names. Joan Taylor, consumer affairs manager for Schnuck Markets Inc., of St. Louis, recalls the confusion that arose when manufacturers began relabeling ice milk as "low-fat" ice cream in 1994, under another FDA rule. The company received a number of calls from shoppers wanting to know why they had stopped selling ice milk, she says. "We hadn't," she says. "We only changed the name."

Some groceries and milk processors plan to educate consumers about the label changes. Schnuck Markets, for example, was planning at press time to post signs at their stores' dairy cases explaining what the new names mean. And its dairy plant planned to label, at least at first, lower fat milk with both the new name, followed by its former name or the milk's fat content. An example might be "reduced-fat milk, contains 2 percent milk fat."

Efforts such as these should help consumers catch on quickly to the new names, but nutrition and industry experts hope the new labels' potential benefits will be longer lasting.

"This is not just a cosmetic change," CSPI's Wootan says. "This is an important strategy to healthier eating."

Raising Milk Consumption

While the new labels may promote greater consumption of the lower fat milk products, some nutrition experts—and industry members in particular—hope the changes will increase milk consumption overall.

LeGrande "Shot" Hudson, dairy plant manager for Giant Food Inc., in Landover, Md., notes that the industry already has taken steps to entice consumers, especially teens and young adults, to drink more milk. It's undertaken major advertising campaigns and, in an effort to make milk more palatable to people who dislike the taste of plain milk, has begun marketing novel flavored products, such as banana, blueberry, raspberry, strawberry, and mocha milk products.

"We don't all wear the moustache," he says, alluding to the industry's current milk advertisements in which celebrities tout their preference for plain milk.

Michelle Smith, a food technologist in FDA's Office of Food Labeling, believes that milk processors will have even more flexibility to develop products with greater consumer appeal, now that the standards of identity for lower fat milks have been revoked. For example,

Table 10.2. Milk Sales Since 1976 (in billion pounds)

Type of Milk	1976	1986	1996
Full fat	35.2	26.4	18.8
Reduced-fat (2%)	12.4	21.2	24.2
Fat-free (skim)	2.5	3.2	8.9

processors will be able to add fat substitutes, stabilizers or thickeners to give lower fat milks a creamier texture and better sensation in the mouth or coloring to make the products whiter. When added, these ingredients must be listed on the label.

"There are many ways to modify a food," she says. "So, if you come across a reduced-fat product, and you want to know how they did it, look at the ingredient list."

With greater product development comes greater product choices for consumers, she says, and that will allow consumers to make better, lower fat choices that they can enjoy.

—by Paula Kurtzweil

Paula Kurtzweil is a member of FDA's public affairs staff.

Chapter 11

Are Restaurants' Nutrition Claims Accurate?

Remember the dieter's plate? For many years, it was the only menu item that really catered to the health conscious among us. It usually came with cottage cheese, several pieces of fruit, and a few crackers neatly arranged atop a lettuce leaf. If you looked carefully, you could usually spot it on the menu between other such fine restaurant fare as gelatin cubes and fruit cocktail in syrup.

These days, restaurants have a lot more to offer consumers concerned about calories and cholesterol, fat, and other nutrients that may help reduce their risk of certain diseases. Menus now may carry items ranging from low-fat, low-calorie tostados to full-course meals featuring seafood or chicken dishes that are low in sodium and fat and high in fiber and vitamins A and C. And restaurants boast about their nutritionally modified dishes with symbols, such as a big red heart signifying that the dish fits in with a diet that is consistent with general dietary recommendations or with claims such as "low fat," "light," or "heart healthy."

But the question is: Are these claims accurate and can they be trusted?

Regulations from the Food and Drug Administration effective May 2 are designed to ensure that the answer is "yes." The regulations, published in the August 2, 1996, *Federal Register*, apply the Nutrition Labeling and Education Act (NLEA) of 1990 to restaurant menu items that carry a claim about the food's nutritional content or health benefits.

"Today's Special: Nutrition Information," *FDA Consumer*, May-June1997.

91

Under NLEA, FDA established regulations mandating specific nutrition information on the labels of most store-bought products and set up criteria under which nutrient and health claims can be used in food labeling. Claims like these that appear on signs or placards in most restaurants have been covered by the requirements of the food labeling regulations since 1994.

The new menu regulations affect all eating establishments— whether a small-town corner tavern or a big-city four-star restaurant, a grocery store deli or a deli that delivers. All will have to follow requirements for nutrition and health claims for menu items that bear a claim and give customers the appropriate nutrition information for these items when requested.

"The idea is for the claims to mean the same thing wherever they show up—on food labels in the store or on menus in a restaurant," said Michelle Smith, a food technologist in FDA's Office of Food Labeling.

Eating Out in the 1990s

According to Smith, nutrition and health claims on menus can help people better understand the role of diet in health and choose restaurant foods that contribute to a healthy diet.

This is important, considering that more and more Americans are eating their meals outside the home. According to the National Restaurant Association, Americans spent 44 percent of their food dollars outside the home in 1996, up from 25 percent in 1955.

According to the association's report, *Tableservice Restaurant Trends—1995*, more than half of consumers 35 and older and 2 out of 5 consumers 18 to 34 look for lower fat menu options when eating out. Also, restaurateurs report that their customers are increasingly requesting meatless dishes.

The frequency with which eating establishments have been catering to these preferences by making claims about menu items is not well known. In its final rule on claims for restaurant foods, FDA cited information from the National Restaurant Association's annual menu contest, in which the group found that 89 percent of all printed menu entries had at least one nutritional or health claim. But it is not known how representative this number is for menu practices across the country.

In 1996, after a federal district court ordered FDA to include menu claims under food labeling regulations, Bruce Silverglade, legal director for the Center for Science in the Public Interest, said in a press statement: "For years, many restaurant menus have made misleading health and nutrition claims from 'low fat' claims for high-fat desserts to claims that foods flavored with Chinese herbs will lower blood pressure and improve vision. A restaurant menu should not be a work of fiction." (CSPI and another public advocacy group, Public Citizen, filed suit in 1993 against the government for excluding menu claims from the labeling regulations.)

There are indications that interest in healthier restaurant fare is growing. Heart Smart Restaurants, an Arizona-based company that helps restaurants, food processors, and vending companies develop and promote products suitable for nutrition and health claims, has seen a steady rise in the number of its restaurant clients since the early 1990s. Judy Peters, director of customer relations for the company, reports that the company's restaurant clients now number in the hundreds and offer from one to many Heart Smart dishes. The clients are located across the country and include both single restaurants and national chains, ranging from juice bars to steakhouses and ethnic restaurants.

Heart Smart is among a number of companies, health professionals, and other consultants that offer such services to restaurants, usually for a fee. Their services are not endorsed by FDA because, as a federal agency, FDA cannot endorse any particular third-party certification programs.

On a smaller scale, the health, fitness and nutrition program of Suburban Hospital in Bethesda, Maryland, a suburb of Washington, D.C., found considerable interest from area restaurateurs in its Heart Healthy Restaurant Program. This program, which helps chefs create and promote heart-healthy foods on their menus, signed up 20 fine-dining restaurants within a county-wide area in the first six months of its operation, according to Linda Dolan, a registered dietitian and director of Suburban's Well Works program. Many of the participating restaurants offer Italian and French cuisine.

Look to the Menu

FDA's regulations permit restaurants to promote their healthier menu fare using the following:

- Specific claims about a menu item's nutrient content: for example, low fat or high fiber. These are known as nutrient claims.

- Claims about the relationship between a nutrient or food and a disease or health condition: for example, a dish that is low in fat, saturated fat, and cholesterol might be able to carry a claim about how diets low in saturated fat and cholesterol may reduce the risk of heart disease. These are known as health claims, and they may initially appear on the menu in simple terms, such as "heart healthy." Further information about the claim should be available somewhere on the menu or in other labeling—for example, with the accompanying nutrition information that must be provided on request.

Consumers can use these claims to spot foods that may be more healthful for them. They also can look for statements giving what FDA considers general dietary guidance. For example, the salad section may start with the message "Eating five fruits and vegetables a day is an important part of a healthy diet." This statement would refer to the National Cancer Institute's recommendation that Americans eat more fruits and vegetables to help reduce their risk of cancer and heart disease.

Restaurants do not have to provide nutrition information about foods that do not bear nutrient content or health claims or that are referred to in general dietary guidance messages. However, restaurateurs need to be careful that the general guidance they provide on the menu doesn't turn into a claim, such as "Fruits and vegetables can help reduce the risk of cancer." This, then, would require the item to meet FDA's nutrition information and claims' requirements.

Claims that promote a nutrient or health benefit must meet certain criteria established by FDA and the U.S. Department of Agriculture; for example, the food must provide a requisite amount of the nutrient or nutrients referred to in the claim. In addition, a menu item carrying a health claim must provide significant amounts of one or more of six key nutrients, such as vitamin C, iron or fiber, and cannot contain a food substance at a level that increases the risk of a disease or health condition. For example, a restaurant meal that contains 26 grams of fat (40 percent of the Daily Value for fat) or 960 milligrams of sodium (40 percent of the Daily Value for sodium) is disqualified from making a heart-healthy claim.

These same rules apply to claims used in the labeling of commercial food products. But the requirements for further information differ between restaurant and commercially manufactured foods.

To meet FDA's criteria, food manufacturers may choose to do chemical analyses to determine the nutritional value of their products. But the criteria for menu items are more flexible, and, under FDA's requirements, restaurants may back up their claims with any "reasonable" base, such as databases, cookbooks, or other secondhand sources that provide nutrition information.

Also, restaurants do not have to provide the standard nutrition information profile and more exacting nutrient content values required in the Nutrition Facts panel of packaged foods. Instead, restaurants can present the information in any format desired, and they have to provide only information about the nutrient or nutrients that the claim is referring to. They can say simply that the amount of the nutrient in question does not exceed the limit imposed by FDA—for example, "This low-fat restaurant dish provides no more than 5 grams of fat per serving."

"It should be accurate," FDA's Smith said, "but not necessarily precise."

Although nutrition information is not required to appear on the menu, it must be made available to consumers when they request it. Restaurants can present it in a printed format—such as a notebook— or by having the staff recite it.

FDA is granting restaurants more flexibility because they don't produce foods according to the more exacting standards that food manufacturers follow, Smith said. She notes that restaurants change their menus frequently and produce smaller quantities than commercial food operations. And restaurant products often vary, depending on the type of ingredients available.

"A commercial operation has more stability than a restaurant," she said. "It would be an unreasonable burden to require restaurants to follow the same labeling regulations for packaged foods."

Much of the enforcement of the menu claims' regulations will likely be provided by state and local public health departments. The reason, Smith said, is that state and local health departments have direct jurisdiction over restaurants, including monitoring their food safety and sanitation practices, and regularly visit them to ensure compliance with various federal and state laws. Also, she said, FDA doesn't have the resources.

Whether restaurants will continue to make claims on menus now that they will be more closely monitored remains to be seen. "We're not sure what the result will be," said Bob Harrington, vice president of technical services for the National Restaurant Association. "Our fear is that the rules are so complex and compliance so confusing that [restaurants] will quit giving claims at all."

Healthful Foods with Flair

But some restaurants that have added healthier menu choices highlighted with claims report that those dishes sell well. Barbara Hartman, head chef for Geppetto, an Italian restaurant in Bethesda,

Maryland, and a participant in Suburban Hospital's Heart Healthy Restaurant Program, said the restaurant's "Healthy Menu" items account for 5 to 10 percent of daily sales. The sandwiches—Tuna Sandwich Dijon, Grilled Vegetable Sub, and others—represent as much as 20 percent of all sandwich sales, she said.

"We've had an excellent response," she said. "Better than we thought we would have."

Although most of the customer feedback has been positive, she noted that customers sometimes complain about the blandness of the food. "There's no salt, no sugar, no oil added," she said. "So I coach the waiters to let customers know that the food may not be as tasty as what they're used to. Then they won't be taken aback by what they're getting."

Healthy menu choices aren't going to appeal to every customer, either. Heart Smart's Peters noted that one previous client, a restaurant that offered only healthy-type foods, went out of business because its selection was too narrow. "People need a choice," she said.

And not every dish is suitable for dietary modification. Some lose their palatability when the fat and sodium contents are reduced to low levels, Peters said, citing fettuccine Alfredo as a prime example. Dishes containing cheese or cream sauces are difficult to modify, dietitian Dolan noted. And chef Hartman said the poached salmon that used to be on her restaurant's Healthy Menu had to be removed because the salmon didn't fit the criteria for a "heart healthy" claim.

But there still are plenty of other dishes that can easily be used or reworked as more healthful food offerings. Among those cited by restaurant menu experts are grilled seafood, chicken, venison, and ostrich; spaghetti with turkey meatballs; several Mexican dishes; salads; and pasta dishes and other entrees traditionally made with wine or herb sauces. Geppetto, for example, offers a single-serving California Bambino Pizza with a whole-wheat crust, fat-reduced mozzarella cheese, tomato basil sauce, roasted garlic, fresh mushrooms, broccoli, and roasted peppers. It provides 506 calories, 10 grams of fat, and 24 milligrams of cholesterol.

Tasty, yet healthful. And, one might add, a far cry from its predecessor, the dieter's plate.

Claims Sure to Strike Menus

Nutrient Claims

Low sodium, Low fat, Low cholesterol: These claims mean the item contains low amounts of these nutrients.

Light: Means the item has fewer calories and less fat than the food to which it's being compared. (Restaurants may continue to use the term "light" for reasons other than as a nutrient content claim—for example, "lighter fare" to mean the dishes contain smaller portions. However, its meaning must be clarified on the menu.)

Healthy: Means the item is low in fat and saturated fat, has limited amounts of cholesterol and sodium, and provides significant amounts of one or more of the key nutrients vitamins A and C, iron, calcium, protein, or fiber.

Health Claims

Heart Healthy has two possible meanings:

1. The item is low in saturated fat, cholesterol, and fat and provides without fortification significant amounts of one or more of six key nutrients. This claim will indicate that a diet low in saturated fat and cholesterol may reduce the risk of heart disease.

2. The item is low in saturated fat, cholesterol, and fat, provides without fortification significant amounts of one or more of six key nutrients, and is a significant source of soluble fiber (found in fruits, vegetables and grain products). This claim will indicate that a diet low in saturated fat and cholesterol and rich in fruits, vegetables and grain products that contain some types of fiber (particularly soluble fiber) may reduce the risk of heart disease.

—by Paula Kurtzweil

Paula Kurtzweil is a member of FDA's public affairs staff.

Chapter 12

Clearing Up Common Misconceptions about Vegetarianism

You know vegetarianism has gone mainstream when you can buy a meatless burger at a Subway shop. But while the image of who might be a vegetarian has gone from a granola-munching hippie to your average Joe grabbing a meal at a fast-food outlet, myths about vegetarianism persist. Herewith, five of the most common ones—and the truths behind them.

Myth number 1: *Vegetarian, diets are automatically more healthful than diets that include animal foods.*

Fact: Vegetarian diets are often much lower in saturated fat and cholesterol and higher in fiber than non-vegetarian diets. And studies suggest that in general, vegetarians are less likely to suffer from chronic degenerative conditions that plague the American population: diabetes, high blood pressure heart disease, and obesity.

But just leaving out animal foods does not undo all the "wrongs" of the typical American diet. Consider that a lacto-ovo vegetarian, meaning one who eats dairy products and eggs, can pile on the saturated fat with full-fat dairy products like butter, cream, and cheese. Candy, chips, and other foods that fall under the vegetarian heading also tend to have a lot of fat—and calories—and relatively little in the way of nutrients.

© April 1998; Reprinted with permission, *Tufts University Health & Nutrition Letter*, 50 Broadway, 15th Floor, New York, NY 10004.

By the same token, healthful vegetarian diets have to be planned (just like the diets of meat eaters) according to the rules of nutrition science. Without sufficient knowledge of nutrient needs, going on a vegetarian diet because it seems "cool" or like the right thing to do could lead to serious vitamin and mineral deficiencies.

Myth number 2: *Vegetarians eat weird foods.*

Fact: Vegetarians often do eat items that are not part of traditional American meals: soybean-based products like tofu and tempeh and different types of beans, nuts, and seeds. Such foods are particularly important for vegetarians known as vegans, who eat no animal products whatsoever, dairy foods and eggs included. The soy items, beans, and nuts provide them with the calcium that others get from milk, yogurt, and cheese. Many of these items also contain iron—a good thing for all vegetarians because anyone who foregoes beef and poultry foregoes the major sources of iron in the American diet.

Still, in no way does eating a vegetarian diet have to mean giving up familiar fare, especially for lacto-ovo vegetarians. Eggplant parmesan; vegetable lasagna; split pea or lentil soup with a hunk of bread and a garden salad; meatless chili; stuffed peppers; pizza—all these fit into a vegetarian menu.

Myth number 3: *Vegetarians don't get enough protein.*

Fact: Even vegans, who go without all the protein in dairy foods and eggs, tend not to be deficient in protein. A 160-pound man needs about 60 grams of protein a day; a 125-pound woman, about 45 grams. But a cup and a half of pasta alone contains 11 grams. Add in a cup of broccoli and a half cup of tomato sauce, and the protein tally jumps to 19 grams. And that's just at dinner.

Related to the not-enough-protein myth is the myth that vegetarians have to eat certain foods at the same time to make their proteins "complete." Granted, unlike a meat or dairy product, any one plant food is "incomplete" on its own because it does not contain all the amino acids (protein building blocks) that the body is unable to synthesize by itself. Therefore, vegan diets must include various combinations of plant foods to ensure that the amino acids absent from one are provided by another.

But researchers now have some evidence that those combinations—beans with grains or cereals; cereals with leafy vegetables; peanuts with wheat, oats, corn or rice; soy with corn, wheat, or rye—

do not have to be eaten at the same time. An over-the-course of-the day approach appears fine.

From a practical standpoint, it doesn't matter either way. Rice and beans, peanut butter and jelly sandwiches, bread dipped into a bean-based soup—these and many other meals that people eat without thinking about protein needs meet the requirement.

Myth number 4: *Vegetarians are seriously deficient in iron, calcium, and other essential nutrients.*

Fact: There are five nutrients that present special concerns for vegetarians: iron, calcium, vitamin D, vitamin$_{12}$, and zinc. But that said, the rate of consumption, at least among lacto-ovo vegetarians, is similar to the calcium consumption of nonvegetarians.

To be sure, the iron in plant foods, known as nonheme iron, is not as well absorbed as the heme iron in animal foods. But vegetarians tend to take in more iron than nonvegetarians overall, which helps offset the absorption problem. Indeed, the vegan menu shown below has 29 milligrams of iron, more than twice as much as many Americans typically consume. What's more, the vitamin C contained in much of the produce that vegetarians eat aids iron absorption. See Table 12.1. for a listing of some iron-rich plant foods.

As for calcium, vegetarians who don't eat dairy products do have to try to get plenty of calcium from other sources. But there are more calcium-containing nondairy foods than most people are aware of. For example, a tablespoon of blackstrap molasses (mixed into, say, a bowl of oatmeal) contains 172 milligrams, as Table 12.2 shows.

Along with calcium, non-dairy-eating vegans need to make sure they get enough vitamin D—necessary for the proper absorption of calcium and found most abundantly in milk. Non-animal sources of D include sunlight (the nutrient is synthesized in the skin), fortified breakfast cereals, fortified soymilk, and multivitamin supplements.

One nutrient that presents a challenge for vegans and lacto-ovo vegetarians a like is vitamin B_{12}, long-term deficiencies of which could cause nerve damage. Many vegetarians rely on tempeh and miso for B_{12} and on certain vegetables, too. But much of the B_{12} in those foods is an inactive B_{12} analog, not the active vitamin found in animal foods.

Dairy products and eggs contain B_{12}, but research suggests that even lacto-ovo vegetarians have low levels of that nutrient. For that reason, all vegetarians should make a conscious effort to consume more B_{12}. Like vitamin D, it is found in fortified breakfast cereals, fortified soymilk, and multivitamin supplements.

Finally, vegetarians should try to take in more zinc, needed for protein synthesis, wound healing, and proper immunity. That's because zinc from plant foods is less available to the body than zinc from meat and poultry. The Recommended Dietary Allowance for zinc is 15 milligrams a day for men and 10 milligrams for women. Plant sources include grain products like corn and wheat germ, fortified cereals, beans, and soy-based foods like tofu. Zinc is also available in dairy foods.

Table 12.1. Iron Content of Plant Foods

For women of childbearing years, the Recommended Dietary Allowance for iron is 15 milligrams. For women who have reached menopause and for men, the RDA is 10 milligrams.

	Iron(*)†
½ cup raw tofu	7
1 tablespoon blackstrap molasses	4
½ cup lentils	3
2 tablespoons pumpkin seeds	3
½ cup garbanzo beans (chickpeas)	2
½ cup Swiss chard	2
5 dried apricots	1
2 tablespoons cashews	1
1 cup tomato juice	1
1 cup white rice	1
1 slice whole wheat bread	1

(*) Substances in coffee and tea called polyphenols can reduce the absorption of iron in plant foods by up to 76 percent. Those making a conscious effort to get enough iron should not drink coffee or tea for an hour and a half after they eat iron-containing foods. They should also eat some iron-rich foods with foods that contain vitamin C, which enhances iron absorption. Many breakfast cereals are also fortified with iron.

† For foods that require cooking, values are for cooked weight or volume.

Myth number 5: It would be better for the environment if we stopped killing animals for food.

Fact: Animals compete with humans for food and other resources, including space. Thus, if we were to stop using animals for food completely, humans would be in trouble.

Says Joan Dye Gussow, EdD, a professor emeritus of nutrition and education at Columbia University Teacher's College, "Some people have the idea that if we just freed the cattle and stopped eating beef,

Table 12.2. Calcium Content of Plant Foods

Men and women through age 50 should shoot for 1,000 milligrams of calcium a day; after age 50, 1,200 milligrams daily.

	Calcium†
1 cup fortified soymilk	250-300
1 cup calcium-fortified orange juice	300
½ cup raw tofu	100-250(**)
½ cup frozen collard greens	179
1 tablespoon blackstrap molasses	172
5 dried figs	135
1 cup frozen turnip greens	125
1 cup frozen kale	90
1 cup navy beans	64
2 tablespoons almonds	50
1 orange	50
½ cup frozen broccoli	47

†For foods that require cooking, values are for cooked weight or volume.

(**) Calcium content varies. Check labels.

the buffalo would return to the prairie; the foxes would come back; and we could grow crops where the cattle used to graze. But it's not that simple.

"One consequence would be that animals like deer would return to where the cattle were. And they'd eat the foods we planted for ourselves." In other words, at a certain point, it's "them or us" when it comes to animals.

To be sure, Dr. Gussow comments, "the way we do kill animals currently to produce food is an ecological horror." Small pens for cattle, hog confinement facilities, chicken "tenements"—all of these huge concentrations of animals and their waste pollute the soil, water, and air. And, of course, they make the animals' lives unnecessarily miserable.

Dr. Gussow says it would be much better for the planet to raise fewer animals for food in a much less concentrated manner—and consequently eat much less flesh food. But, she says, "the idea of taking no animals' lives for food does not allow for the continuance of human life or for the earth's ecosystems to be sustained."

Vegetarian for a Day

The following menu is for a vegan, who would eat no dairy foods or eggs. Lacto-ovo vegetarians, who include milk, yogurt, cheese, and eggs in their diets, would have an even easier time meeting nutrient requirements.

The one-day example here provides 1,850 calories. It also supplies 66 grams of protein, 29 grams of iron, 870 milligrams of calcium, and 10 milligrams of zinc—meeting or exceeding current recommendations for most of those minerals, which are traditionally thought of as animal-food nutrients. In addition, it contributes just 10 grams of saturated fat—a mere 5 percent of total calories.

Breakfast

1 cup Kellogg's Raisin Bran
1 cup soymilk
1 cup calcium-fortified orange juice

Mid-morning Snack

1 banana
1 tablespoon peanut butter

Lunch

1 cup split pea soup
2 slices whole wheat bread
Salad tossed with 1 tablespoon slivered almonds

Mid-afternoon Snack

2 tablespoons sunflower seeds

Dinner

1½ cups pasta
½ cup tomato sauce
1 cup broccoli mixed with ¼ cup tofu

Evening Snack

1 cup cut-up cantaloupe

Chapter 13

Are Food Cravings Related to Nutritional Needs?

You crave a steak or a burger, so you assume you must be low on iron. Or you often crave chocolate or other sweets and figure you have a sugar addiction. Some 97 percent of women and 68 percent of men experience food cravings, according to a survey conducted at Canada's McMaster University in Ontario. But despite the fact that cravings are so widespread, researchers are still hard-pressed for a scientific explanation as to why they arise, and what purpose they serve.

To gain some insight on food cravings, we turned to Marcia Levin Pelchat, PhD. Dr. Pelchat is a biological psychologist who specializes in the "hows" and "whys" of food choices at Philadelphia's Monell Chemical Senses Center—a world-renowned research institute founded to study taste, smell, and nutrition.

What's the difference between simply feeling like eating a food and having a food craving?

Dr. Pelchat: Cravings are difficult to define. There's really no objective way to measure them—we have to rely on what people tell us they're experiencing. At Monell, we tell people that a food craving is a very intense desire to eat a particular food, strong enough that you may go out of your way to get it. For example, I may like pizza, but that doesn't mean I'll go out in a rainstorm at midnight to get some.

We also know that food cravings are different from hunger. When you're hungry, any number of foods could be satisfying. But a craving is highly specific for one food or type of food. If it's pizza you really crave, eating spaghetti with tomato sauce and grated cheese may not do the trick.

Don't food cravings stem from nutrient deficiencies? In other words, if I crave meat, doesn't that mean my body needs iron?

Dr. Pelchat: The idea that food cravings somehow reflect the "wisdom of the body" is probably one of the most popular views around — but it's not one for which there's much proof.

Granted, there is some evidence that people who have a severe sodium deficiency may develop cravings for salt. There's a well-known medical report of a young boy who ate immense amounts of salt; it turned out he was deficient in sodium due to an adrenal gland disorder.

But when you look at the sodium intake of most people in the United States [which averages more than 3,200 milligrams a day], and compare it to what we actually need [about 500 milligrams a day], the two don't match up at all. It's very rare for people to have any kind of medically significant sodium deficiency, and yet it's fairly common for people to crave salty foods.

For other nutrients, the evidence gets even shakier. For instance, iron-deficiency anemia is frequently accompanied by cravings, but the cravings aren't necessarily for high-iron foods, like red meal One study that came out a few years ago showed that eating red clay is associated with iron-deficiency anemia, which might make you think that the people were somehow getting minerals from the clay. But it turns out that some red clays actually chelate, or trap, the iron coming from foods — making the craving for red clay the cause of the anemia rather than the result.

So then what might cause a food craving?

Dr. Pelchat: One hypothesis is that just the sights and smells around you — something like the aroma of baking bread — can trigger a food craving. Or, it might be what happens after you eat a craved food that makes you want it in the first place. There's a hypothesis, for example, that eating sweet foods causes the release of compounds in the brain that create a feeling similar to a runner's high.

Cravings could also be caused simply by a need for more variety in your diet, which in turn could ensure that you take in a wider array of essential nutrients. In one study, we asked people to consume nothing but vanilla Sustacal and water for 5 days. It was a very sweet-tasting, liquid, monotonous diet. When we asked the volunteers whether they craved certain foods during that time, they reported craving entrees like pizza and steak—foods with a different aroma, flavor, or texture—over sweet foods like ice cream or cookies.

Now in that case, it wasn't nutritional deficiency that had anything to do with their cravings, because the Sustacal diet was designed to be nutritionally complete. But that was unusual. Most monotonous diets, if followed long enough, could become nutritionally inadequate because they lack variety. So perhaps craving different foods simply ensures eating a more varied diet, which is more likely to contain all the essential nutrients than a diet that includes relatively few foods.

Are some people more susceptible to food cravings than others?

Dr. Pelchat: Women, both older and younger, seem to report cravings more often than men. But cravings do differ by age—that's a big one. Older people are less driven by cravings in general, and old men really report very few cravings. We don't know whether they simply don't have them or whether they just don't talk about that type of thing.

There are differences with time of day, too. Cravings tend to occur late in the day—in the late afternoon or evening. No one knows precisely why that is, although there are quite a few hypotheses out there: low blood sugar, the smell of dinner cooking, food commercials on television, to name a few.

Which foods do people crave most?

Dr. Pelchat: In the United States and Canada, where most of the research has been done, the most commonly craved food usually turns out to be chocolate candy. Pizza is a very close second. These are two highly palatable foods, very aromatic and big on flavor. People don't tend to crave things that they don't enjoy the flavor of.

Does the menstrual cycle affect women's cravings?

Dr. Pelchat: Yes. Hormonal state, particularly during pregnancy and certain parts of a woman's cycle, may have a strong influence on cravings. The association between cravings and the menstrual cycle, in particular, has been very well documented. What researchers have noticed is that, at least in some women, cravings increase in the perimenstrual period: that is, the few days before and after the onset of menses. It's not just premenstrual, which makes sense if you look at hormone levels. They are about the same 3 days before and 3 days after menses begin.

But it's an association, not a mechanism: we don't know how shifting hormone levels might cause cravings.

Are women's cravings any different from men's?

Dr. Pelchat: Most women report that their cravings are primarily for carbohydrates, mostly sweets, and especially chocolate. But it's a misconception that women crave only sweets and that men crave only meats and savory (spicy or aromatic) foods. That fits in with a lot of gender stereotypes. To some extent, we do see it when we collect data on cravings, but it depends on how you conduct the research study. Some methods are more open to bias than others.

In studies where people are given a questionnaire and asked to remember their cravings, a method which could be biased by knowing the male and female cultural stereotypes, you do see big gender differences. Females appear to crave sweets more than savory foods, and for males you see the opposite pattern. But—in studies where people simply record their cravings every day rather than respond to a survey, bias is less likely, and gender differences don't necessarily come through.

Why, then, do so many women crave chocolate?

Dr. Pelchat: There's one idea, although it's controversial, that premenstrual cravings for carbohydrates and chocolate are a sort of natural anti-depressant mechanism. It's called the serotonin hypothesis. The thinking is that women become depressed due to low levels of serotonin, a brain chemical, and develop carbohydrate cravings to provide the body with more. Serotonin levels rise when high-carbohydrate foods are eaten, and it supposedly produces a calming effect that improves mood.

But the serotonin hypothesis doesn't explain why chocolate would be more popular than other high-carbohydrate foods. Using this theory to explain premenstrual chocolate craving also neglects the fact that chocolate is high in fat. It may be that we just like chocolate for its sweet taste, aroma, and texture.

Do people on weight-loss diets get food cravings more often than others?

Dr. Pelchat: It's possible that cravings could be caused by a calorie deficit—eating less than you're used to. But in studies that have been done with people who are quite overweight and who have been on diets for a long time, it doesn't look like dieting produces a lot of cravings. Among more casual dieters—people who aren't quite as heavy and don't stick to their diets for long periods of time—there is some association between dieting and cravings.

So it seems like cravings are there at first and then fade. How does that work?

Dr. Pelchat: We don't know what the mechanism is yet. People may be most bothered by cravings when they first start a diet, which could be why people on diets for a long time stop having them. Or it could be that people who can follow a diet for a long time are following a sensible one with a wide variety of foods and not too much deprivation. Short-term dieters, on the other hand, may be following a plan that's too restrictive. Maybe it's monotonous, for instance, if the dieters are restricting themselves to eating only foods that they believe are healthy, or to those foods that are "allowed" on a particular diet. That could trigger cravings for the "missing" foods.

Dieters' food cravings could also just be an emotional response to the knowledge that they're "supposed" to be depriving themselves. Just knowing that something is forbidden may make people want it more. It's important to remember, though, that this is all speculation. There still aren't any studies out there to prove or dispel these theories.

How can someone best manage a craving? Ride it out—or just give in to it?

Dr. Pelchat: We don't know of a "magic bullet" that will stop a craving in its tracks. Some people try to substitute foods. For example, they'll have a glass of chocolate milk instead of a chocolate bar. But that doesn't work for everyone. Others try to exercise portion control. For example, going out for ice cream and ordering a dip or two rather than having a half-gallon talking to you in the freezer is a way to indulge yourself without going overboard.

Of course, for the average person—someone who's not on a medically restricted diet—it's not even clear that cravings are "bad" per se and need to be gotten around. For many people, in fact, just giving in to a craving when it strikes can keep it from getting out of hand.

Chapter 14

Alcohol and Nutrition

Nutrition is a process that serves two purposes: to provide energy and to maintain body structure and function. Food supplies energy and provides the building blocks needed to replace worn or damaged cells and the nutritional components needed for body function. Alcoholics often eat poorly, limiting their supply of essential nutrients and affecting both energy supply and structure maintenance. Furthermore, alcohol interferes with the nutritional process by affecting digestion, storage, utilization, and excretion of nutrients.[1]

Impairment of Nutrient Digestion and Utilization

Once ingested, food must be digested (broken down into small components) so it is available for energy and maintenance of body structure and function. Digestion begins in the mouth and continues in the stomach and intestines, with help from the pancreas. The nutrients from digested food are absorbed from the intestines into the blood and carried to the liver. The liver prepares nutrients either for immediate use or for storage and future use.

Alcohol inhibits the breakdown of nutrients into usable molecules by decreasing secretion of digestive enzymes from the pancreas.[2] Alcohol impairs nutrient absorption by damaging the cells lining the

Alcohol Alert, National Institute on Alcohol Abuse and Alcoholism (NIAAA), No. 22, PH 346, October 1993. Copies of the *Alcohol Alert* are available free of charge from the Scientific Communications Branch, Office of Scientific Affairs, NIAAA, 5600 Fishers Lane, Room 16C-14, Rockville, MD 20857. Telephone (301) 443-3860.

stomach and intestines and disabling transport of some nutrients into the blood.[3] In addition, nutritional deficiencies themselves may lead to further absorption problems. For example, folate deficiency alters the cells lining the small intestine, which in turn impairs absorption of water and nutrients including glucose, sodium, and additional folate.[3]

Even if nutrients are digested and absorbed, alcohol can prevent them from being fully utilized by altering their transport, storage, and excretion.[4] Decreased liver stores of vitamins such as vitamin A,[5] and increased excretion of nutrients such as fat, indicate impaired utilization of nutrients by alcoholics.[3]

Alcohol and Energy Supply

The three basic nutritional components found in food—carbohydrates, proteins, and fats—are used as energy after being converted to simpler products. Some alcoholics ingest as much as 50 percent of their total daily calories from alcohol, often neglecting important foods.[3,6]

Even when food intake is adequate, alcohol can impair the mechanisms by which the body controls blood glucose levels, resulting in either increased or decreased blood glucose (glucose is the body's principal sugar).[7] In nondiabetic alcoholics, increased blood sugar, or hyperglycemia—caused by impaired insulin secretion—is usually temporary and without consequence. Decreased blood sugar, or hypoglycemia, can cause serious injury even if this condition is short lived. Hypoglycemia can occur when a fasting or malnourished person consumes alcohol. When there is no food to supply energy, stored sugar is depleted, and the products of alcohol metabolism inhibit the formation of glucose from other compounds such as amino acids.[7] As a result, alcohol causes the brain and other body tissue to be deprived of glucose needed for energy and function.

Although alcohol is an energy source, how the body processes and uses the energy from alcohol is more complex than can be explained by a simple calorie conversion value.[8] For example, alcohol provides an average of 20 percent of the calories in the diet of the upper third of drinking Americans, and we might expect many drinkers who consume such amounts to be obese. Instead, national data indicate that, despite higher caloric intake, drinkers are no more obese than nondrinkers.[9,10] Also, when alcohol is substituted for carbohydrates, calorie for calorie, subjects tend to lose weight, indicating that they derive less energy from alcohol than from food (summarized in reference 8).

The mechanisms accounting for the apparent inefficiency in converting alcohol to energy are complex and incompletely understood,[11] but several mechanisms have been proposed. For example, chronic drinking triggers an inefficient system of alcohol metabolism, the microsomal ethanol-oxidizing system (MEOS).[1] Much of the energy from MEOS-driven alcohol metabolism is lost as heat rather than used to supply the body with energy.

Alcohol and the Maintenance of Cell Structure and Function

Structure

Because cells are made mostly of protein, an adequate protein diet is important for maintaining cell structure, especially if cells are being damaged. Research indicates that alcohol affects protein nutrition by causing impaired digestion of proteins to amino acids, impaired processing of amino acids by the small intestine and liver, impaired synthesis of proteins from amino acids, and impaired protein secretion by the liver.[3]

Function

Nutrients are essential for proper body function; proteins, vitamins, and minerals provide the tools that the body needs to perform properly. Alcohol can disrupt body function by causing nutrient deficiencies and by usurping the machinery needed to metabolize nutrients.

Vitamins. Vitamins are essential to maintaining growth and normal metabolism because they regulate many physiological processes. Chronic heavy drinking is associated with deficiencies in many vitamins because of decreased food ingestion and, in some cases, impaired absorption, metabolism, and utilization.[1,12] For example, alcohol inhibits fat absorption and thereby impairs absorption of the vitamins A, E, and D that are normally absorbed along with dietary fats.[12,13] Vitamin A deficiency can be associated with night blindness, and vitamin D deficiency is associated with softening of the bones.[6]

Vitamins A, C, D, E, K, and the B vitamins, also deficient in some alcoholics, are all involved in wound healing and cell maintenance.[14] In particular, because vitamin K is necessary for blood clotting, deficiencies of that vitamin can cause delayed clotting and result in excess bleeding. Deficiencies of other vitamins involved in brain function can cause severe neurological damage.

Minerals. Deficiencies of minerals such as calcium, magnesium, iron, and zinc are common in alcoholics, although alcohol itself does not seem to affect the absorption of these minerals.[15] Rather, deficiencies seem to occur secondary to other alcohol-related problems: decreased calcium absorption due to fat malabsorption; magnesium deficiency due to decreased intake, increased urinary excretion, vomiting, and diarrhea;[16] iron deficiency related to gastrointestinal bleeding;[3,15] and zinc malabsorption or losses related to other nutrient deficiencies.[17] Mineral deficiencies can cause a variety of medical consequences from calcium-related bone disease to zinc-related night blindness and skin lesions.

Alcohol, Malnutrition, and Medical Complications

Liver Disease

Although alcoholic liver damage is caused primarily by alcohol itself, poor nutrition may increase the risk of alcohol-related liver damage. For example, nutrients normally found in the liver, such as carotenoids, which are the major sources of vitamin A, and vitamin E compounds, are known to be affected by alcohol consumption.[18,19] Decreases in such nutrients may play some role in alcohol-related liver damage.

Pancreatitis

Research suggests that malnutrition may increase the risk of developing alcoholic pancreatitis,[20,21] but some research performed outside the United States links pancreatitis more closely with overeating.[21] Preliminary research suggests that alcohol's damaging effect on the pancreas may be exacerbated by a protein-deficient diet.[22]

Brain

Nutritional deficiencies can have severe and permanent effects on brain function. Specifically, thiamin deficiencies, often seen in alcoholics, can cause severe neurological problems such as impaired movement and memory loss seen in Wernicke/Korsakoff syndrome.[23]

Pregnancy

Alcohol has direct toxic effects on fetal development, causing alcohol-related birth defects, including fetal alcohol syndrome. Alcohol itself is toxic to the fetus, but accompanying nutritional deficiency can affect fetal development, perhaps compounding the risk of developmental damage.[24,25]

The nutritional needs during pregnancy are 10 to 30 percent greater than normal; food intake can increase by as much as 140 percent to cover the needs of both mother and fetus.[24] Not only can nutritional deficiencies of an alcoholic mother adversely affect the nutrition of the fetus, but alcohol itself can also restrict nutrition flow to the fetus.[24,25]

Nutritional Status of Alcoholics

Techniques for assessing nutritional status include taking body measurements such as weight, height, mass, and skin fold thickness to estimate fat reserves, and performing blood analysis to provide measurements of circulating proteins, vitamins, and minerals. These techniques tend to be imprecise, and for many nutrients, there is no clear "cut-off" point that would allow an accurate definition of deficiency.[4] As such, assessing the nutritional status of alcoholics is hindered by the limitations of the techniques. Dietary status may provide inferential information about the risk of developing nutritional deficiencies. Dietary status is assessed by taking patients' dietary histories and evaluating the amount and types of food they are eating.

A threshold dose above which alcohol begins to have detrimental effects on nutrition is difficult to determine. In general, moderate drinkers (two drinks or less per day) seem to be at little risk for nutritional deficiencies. Various medical disorders begin to appear at greater levels.

Research indicates that the majority of even the heaviest drinkers have few detectable nutritional deficiencies but that many alcoholics who are hospitalized for medical complications of alcoholism do experience severe malnutrition.[1,12] Because alcoholics tend to eat poorly—often eating less than the amounts of food necessary to provide sufficient carbohydrates, protein, fat, vitamins A and C, the B vitamins, and minerals such as calcium and iron[6,9,26]—a major concern is that alcohol's effects on the digestion of food and utilization of nutrients may shift a mildly malnourished person toward severe malnutrition.

A Commentary by NIAAA Director Enoch Gordis, M.D.

The combination of an adequate diet and abstention from alcohol is the best way to treat malnourished alcoholic patients. Nutritional supplements have been used to replace nutrients deficient in malnourished alcoholics in an attempt to improve their overall health. Dosages of nutritional supplements such as vitamin A that exceed normally prescribed levels may result in overdose.

Although various nutritional approaches have been touted as "cures" for alcoholism, there is little evidence to support such claims. However, renewed research attention to the nutritional aspects of alcohol leaves open the possibility that a role for nutritional therapy in alcoholism treatment may yet be defined.

References

1. Lieber, C.S. The influence of alcohol on nutritional status. *Nutrition Reviews* 46(7):241-254, 1988.

2. Korsten, M.A. Alcoholism and pancreatitis: Does nutrition play a role? *Alcohol Health & Research World* 13(3):232-237, 1989.

3. Feinman, L. Absorption and utilization of nutrients in alcoholism. *Alcohol Health & Research World* 13(3):207-210, 1989.

4. Thomson, A.D., and Pratt, O.E. Interaction of nutrients and alcohol: Absorption, transport, utilization, and metabolism. In: Watson, R.R., and Watzl, B., eds. *Nutrition and Alcohol.* Boca Raton, FL: CRC Press, 1992. pp. 75-99.

5. Sato, M., and Lieber, C.S. Hepatic vitamin A depletion after chronic ethanol consumption in baboons and rats. *Journal of Nutrition* 111:2015-2023, 1981.

6. Feinman, L., and Lieber, C.S. Nutrition: Medical problems of alcoholism. In: Lieber, C.S., ed. *Medical and Nutritional Complications of Alcoholism: Mechanisms in Management.* New York: Plenum Publishing Corp., 1992. pp. 515-530.

7. Patel, D.G. Effects of ethanol on carbohydrate metabolism and implications for the aging alcoholic. *Alcohol Health & Research World* 13(3):240-246, 1989.

8. U.S. Department of Health and Human Services. *The Surgeon General's Report on Nutrition and Health.* DHHS Pub. No. (PHS)88-50210. Washington, DC: Supt. of Docs., U.S. Govt. Print. Off., 1988.

9. Gruchow, H.W.; Sobocinski, K.A.; Barboriak, J.J.; and Scheller, J.G. Alcohol consumption, nutrient intake and relative body

weight among U.S. adults. *American Journal of Clinical Nutrition* 42(2):289-295, 1985.

10. Colditz, G.A.; Giovannucci, E.; Rimm, E.B.; Stampfer, M.J.; Rosner, B.; Speizer, F.E.; Gordis, E.; and Willett, W.C. Alcohol intake in relation to diet and obesity in women and men. *American Journal of Clinical Nutrition* 54(1):49-55, 1991.

11. World, M.J.; Ryle, P.R.; Pratt, O.E.; and Thomson, A.D. Alcohol and body weight. *Alcohol and Alcoholism* 19(1):1-6, 1984.

12. Lieber, C.S. Alcohol and nutrition: An overview. *Alcohol Health & Research World* 13(3):197-205, 1989.

13. Leo, M.A., and Lieber, C.S. Alcohol and vitamin A. *Alcohol Health & Research World* 13(3):250-254, 1989.

14. Tortora, G.J., and Anagnostakos, N.P., eds. *Principles of Anatomy and Physiology. 5th ed.* New York: Harper & Row Publishers, 1987.

15. Marsano, L., and McClain, C.J. Effects of alcohol on electrolytes and minerals. *Alcohol Health & Research World* 13(3):255-260, 1989.

16. Flink, E.B. Magnesium deficiency in alcoholism. *Alcoholism: Clinical and Experimental Research* 10(6):590-594, 1986.

17. McClain, C.J.; Antonow, D.R.; Cohen, D.A.; and Shedlofsky, S.I. Zinc metabolism in alcoholic liver disease. *Alcoholism: Clinical and Experimental Research* 10(6):582-589, 1986.

18. Leo, M.A.; Kim, C.-I.; Lowe, N.; and Lieber, C.S. Interaction of ethanol with *-carotene: Delayed blood clearance and enhanced hepatotoxicity. *Hepatology* 15(5):883-891, 1992.

19. Leo, M.A.; Rosman, A.S.; and Lieber, C.S. Differential depletion of carotenoids and tocopherol in liver disease. *Hepatology* 17(6):977-986, 1993.

20. Mezey, E.; Kolman, C.J.; Diehl, A.M.; Mitchell, M.C.; and Herlong, H.F. Alcohol and dietary intake in the development of chronic pancreatitis and liver disease in alcoholism. *American Journal of Clinical Nutrition* 48(1):148-151, 1988.

21. Korsten, M.A.; Pirola, R.C.; and Lieber, C.S. Alcohol and the pancreas. In: Lieber, C.S., ed. *Medical and Nutritional Complications of Alcoholism: Mechanisms in Management.* New York: Plenum Publishing Corp., 1992. pp. 341-358.

22. Korsten, M.A.; Wilson, J.S.; and Lieber, C.S. Interactive effects of dietary protein and ethanol on rat pancreas: Protein synthesis and enzyme secretion. *Gastroenterology* 99(1):229-236, 1990.

23. Victor, M. The effects of alcohol on the nervous system: Clinical features, pathogenesis, and treatment. In: Lieber, C.S., ed. *Medical and Nutritional Complications of Alcoholism: Mechanisms in Management.* New York: Plenum Publishing Corp., 1992. pp. 413-457.

24. Weinberg, J. Nutritional issues in perinatal alcohol exposure. *Neurobehavioral Toxicology and Teratology* 6(4):261-269, 1984.

25. Phillips, D.K.; Henderson, G.I.; and Schenker, S. Pathogenesis of fetal alcohol syndrome: Overview with emphasis on the possible role of nutrition. *Alcohol Health & Research World* 13(3):219-227, 1989.

26. Hillers, V.N., and Massey, L.K. Interrelationships of moderate and high alcohol consumption with diet and health status. *American Journal of Clinical Nutrition* 41(2):356-362, 1985.

Part Two

Nutrition Needs throughout Life

Chapter 15

Infant Formula: Second Best

A century ago, babies who couldn't be breast-fed usually didn't survive. Today, although breast-feeding is still the best nourishment for infants, infant formula is a close enough second that babies not only survive but thrive.

Commercially prepared formulas are regulated by the Food and Drug Administration.

The safety of commercially prepared formula is also ensured by the agency's nutrient requirements (see "Nutrient Requirements" below) and by strict quality control procedures that require manufacturers to analyze each batch of formula for required nutrients, to test samples for stability during the shelf life of the product, to code containers to identify the batch, and to make all records available to FDA investigators.

The composition of infant formula is similar to breast milk, but it isn't a perfect match, because the exact chemical makeup of breast milk is still unknown.

Human milk is very complex, and scientists are still trying to unravel and understand what makes it such a good source of nutrition for rapidly growing and developing infants. However, John C. Wallingford, Ph.D., an infant nutrition specialist with FDA's Center for Food Safety and Applied Nutrition, notes that "infant formula is increasingly close to breast milk."

"Infant Formula: Second Best but Good Enough," U.S. Food and Drug Administration (FDA), *FDA Consumer*, June 1996; and "Overview of Infant Formula," FDA Center for Food Safety and Applied Nutrition, August 1997.

More than half the calories in breast milk come from fat, and the same is true for today's infant formulas. This may be alarming to many American adults watching their intake of fat and cholesterol, especially when sources of saturated fats, such as coconut oil, are used in formulas. (In adults, high intakes of saturated fats tend to increase blood cholesterol levels more than other fats or oils.) But the low-fat diet recommended for adults doesn't apply to infants.

"Infants have a very high energy requirement, and they have a restricted volume of food that they can digest," says Wallingford. "The only way to get the energy density of a food up is to have a high amount of fat."

While greater knowledge about human milk has helped scientists improve infant formula, it has become "increasingly apparent that infant formula can never duplicate human milk," write John D. Benson, Ph.D, and Mark L. Masor, Ph.D., in the March 1994 issue of Endocrine Regulations. "Human milk contains living cells, hormones, active enzymes, immunoglobulins and compounds with unique structures that cannot be replicated in infant formula."

Benson and Masor, both of whom are pediatric nutrition researchers at infant formula manufacturer Abbott Laboratories, believe creating formula that duplicates human milk is impossible. "A better goal is to match the performance of the breastfed infant," they write. Performance is measured by the infant's growth, absorption of nutrients, gastrointestinal tolerance, and reactions in blood.

Wallingford agrees, explaining that while FDA's regulations on what goes into infant formula are to ensure there are enough nutrients, "that's just a starting point. What's really important is how infants thrive."

Cow's Milk or Soy?

Normal, full-term infants should get a conventional cow's-milk-based formula, says John N. Udall Jr., M.D., chief of nutrition and gastroenterology at Children's Hospital of New Orleans. However, adverse reactions to the protein in cow's milk formula or symptoms of lactose intolerance (lactose is the carbohydrate in cow's milk) may require switching to another type of formula, he says.

Symptoms that may indicate an adverse reaction to cow's milk protein include vomiting, diarrhea, abdominal pain, and rash. With lactose intolerance, the most common symptoms are excessive gas, abdominal distension and pain, and diarrhea. Since some of the symptoms overlap, a stool test may be necessary to determine the culprit.

Usually, lactose intolerance will produce acidic stools that contain glucose. If the protein is the problem, stools will be nonacidic and have flecks of blood.

The main alternative to cow's milk formula is soy formula. About 20 percent of the formula sold in the United States is soy. "Lactose intolerance is probably the biggest reason to switch to soy formula," says William J. Klish, M.D., chairman of the American Academy of Pediatrics Committee on Nutrition.

The carbohydrates in most soy formulas are sucrose and corn syrup, which are easily digested and absorbed by infants. However, soy is not as good a protein source as cow's milk. Also, babies don't absorb some minerals, such as calcium, as efficiently from soy formulas. Therefore, according to the American Academy of Pediatrics, "Healthy full-term infants should be given soy formula only when medically necessary."

For a child who can't tolerate cow's milk protein, Klish recommends the use of hydrolyzed-protein formula. Although hydrolyzed-protein formulas are made from cow's milk, the protein has been broken up into its component parts. Essentially, it's been predigested, which decreases the likelihood of an allergic reaction.

Iron

The infant formulas currently available in the United States are either "iron-fortified"—with approximately 12 milligrams of iron per liter—or "low iron"—with approximately 2 milligrams of iron per liter.

"There should not be a low-iron formula on the market for the average child because a low-iron formula is a nutritionally deficient formula," says Klish. "It doesn't provide enough iron to maintain proper blood cell counts or proper hemoglobin." (Hemoglobin is a blood protein that carries oxygen from the lungs to the tissues, and carbon dioxide from the tissues to the lungs.)

In addition, studies have shown that school children who had good iron status as infants because they were fed iron-fortified formula performed better on standardized developmental tests than children with poor iron status. However, Wallingford says that "FDA has permitted marketing of low-iron formulas because some pediatricians prefer to use them, with the caveat that the physician would be monitoring iron status and prescribing iron supplements when appropriate."

Why is there low-iron formula on the market? "In the past there have been a lot of symptoms that have been attributed to iron, including abdominal discomfort, constipation, diarrhea, colic, and irritability," says Klish. "Also there was some concern about too much iron interfering with the immune system. All of those concerns and questions have been laid to rest with appropriate studies."

Another reason for originally producing low-iron formulas was that human milk contains low amounts of iron—less than a milligram per liter. However, it is now understood that an infant absorbs virtually 100 percent of the iron from human milk, but considerably less from infant formula.

Researchers continue to try to determine the best amount of iron for infant formula. While low-iron formulas don't supply enough iron, the best amount of iron for formulas has not been established. "We did not have much data at the time the regulations were written for different intake levels of iron," says Wallingford. He explains that the current amounts give good developmental results, "but, based on European experience, half [of the high level] is probably good enough to do the same thing." Currently, the Federation of American Societies for Experimental Biology is evaluating what the best levels may be and will make recommendations to FDA on what levels of iron to require in formulas. The study is also reviewing the level of all other nutrients in infant formula, as well as the need for nutrients not currently included.

Cooking Lessons

Both milk and soy formulas are available in powder, liquid concentrate, or ready-to-feed forms. The choice should depend on whatever the parents find convenient and can afford.

Whatever form is chosen, proper preparation and refrigeration are essential. Opened cans of ready-to-feed and liquid concentrate must be refrigerated and used within the time specified on the can. Once the powder is mixed with water, it should also be refrigerated if it is not used right away. The exact amounts of water recommended on the label must be used. Under-diluted formula can cause problems for the infant's organs and digestive system. Over-diluted formula will not provide adequate nutrition, and the baby may fail to thrive and grow.

Until recently, the American Academy of Pediatrics felt that municipal water supplies were safe enough without boiling the water before mixing with the formula. But because of the contamination of Milwaukee's water with the parasite *Cryptosporidium* in 1993, "the whole business of boiling water has come up again," says Klish. "The academy is now again recommending boiling water for infant formulas."

Klish advises heating the water until it reaches a rolling boil, continue to boil for one to two minutes, and then let it cool. "That should take care of all the bacteria and parasites that might be in the water," he explains.

The American Academy of Pediatrics does not have any recommendations about bottled water. Klish says bottled water is fine, but it still needs to be boiled. "There's no reason to think that bottled water is any safer than city water," he says.

Bottled water must meet specific FDA quality standards for contaminants. These are set in response to requirements that the Environmental Protection Agency has established for tap water.

A new regulation published in the November 13, 1995, *Federal Register* sets standard definitions for different types of bottled waters, helping resolve possible confusion about what different terms mean.

The regulation also requires accurate labeling of bottled waters marketed for infants. If a product is labeled "sterile," it must be processed to meet FDA's requirements for commercial sterility. Otherwise, the labeling must indicate that it is not sterile and should be used as directed by a physician or according to infant formula preparation instructions.

What about sterilizing the bottles and nipples? "Dishwashers tend to sterilize bottles and nipples fairly well," says Klish. They can also be sterilized by placing in a pan of boiling water for five minutes.

Warming the formula before feeding isn't necessary for proper nutrition, but most infants prefer the formula at least at room temperature. The best way to warm a bottle of formula is by placing the bottle in a pot of water and heating the pot on the stove.

Don't Try This at Home

Homemade formulas should not be used, says Nick Duy, a consumer safety officer in FDA's Office of Special Nutritionals. Homemade formulas based on cows' milk don't meet all of an infant's nutritional needs, and cow's milk protein that has not been cooked or processed is difficult for an infant to digest. In addition, the high protein and electrolyte (salt) content of cow's milk may put a strain on an infant's immature kidneys. Substituting evaporated milk for whole milk may make the homemade formula easier to digest because of the effect of processing on the protein, but the formula is still nutritionally inadequate and still may stress the kidneys.

Today's infant formula is a very controlled, high-tech product that can't be duplicated at home, says Udall.

Nutrient Requirements

FDA regulations specify minimum and, in some cases, maximum nutrient level requirements for infant formulas, based on recommendations by the American Academy of Pediatrics Committee on Nutrition. The following must be included in all formulas:

- protein
- fat
- linoleic acid
- vitamin A
- vitamin D
- vitamin E
- vitamin K
- thiamin (vitamin B_1)
- riboflavin (vitamin B_2)
- vitamin B_6
- vitamin B_{12}
- niacin
- folic acid

- pantothenic acid
- vitamin C
- calcium
- phosphorus
- magnesium
- iron
- zinc
- manganese
- copper
- iodine
- sodium
- potassium
- chloride

In addition, formulas not made with cow's milk must include biotin, choline and inositol.

Counterfeit Formulas

In February 1995, FDA special agents arrested a suspect in Southern California in a scheme to distribute infant formula in counterfeit packaging. The agency also seized 17,236 kilograms (38,000 pounds) of powdered formula at the suspect's counterfeit manufacturing operations in Southern California and 6,366 0.45-kilogram (1-pound) cans from retail and wholesale outlets.

The scheme involved the purchase of bulk infant formula labeled "for export only" from a legitimate manufacturer. The bulk formula was then packaged in the 1-pound cans that looked like Similac, an authentic formula made by Ross Products Division of Abbott Laboratories, Columbus, Ohio.

The agency did not receive any reports of illness attributable to the counterfeit formula.

The California counterfeit scheme has been completely suppressed, but it is just part of a diversion market in numerous products. One of FDA's concerns is the conditions the formula is subjected to during the illegal manufacturing operations.

Production records like those normally kept by legitimate manufacturers don't exist, explains Jim Dahl, assistant director of FDA's Office of Criminal Investigations. "How it was transported, what temperature conditions, what sanitary conditions, how cans were treated, how long they were held in those conditions, all of that is unknown," he says.

To protect their babies, parents need to be on the lookout for any changes in formula color, smell or taste, Dahl says. He also advises parents and retailers to:

- make sure lot numbers and expiration dates on both the can and the cardboard case are the same
- check containers for damage
- call the manufacturer's toll-free number with any concerns or questions.

Whole Milk for First Birthday

There's nothing like a cold glass of milk with a slice of birthday cake. That works out great for babies because, in general, parents should stop the formula and introduce milk around the time of a baby's first birthday.

The milk, however, should be whole milk. Low-fat and skim milk do not have enough fat and calories to supply the nutritional needs of a 1-year-old, explains John Udall, chief of nutrition and gastroenterology at Children's Hospital of New Orleans. At that age, "the child is growing so quickly, and the fat is so important for brain and central nervous system development," he says. "The recommendation that our daily intake of fat should compose less than 30 percent of our caloric intake does not apply to children under 2 years of age."

New on the market are special toddler formulas that claim to be better than milk. The formulas are good nutritionally, says Udall, but they're not necessary. "A well-balanced diet with milk and juices would be just as good in a healthy, normally active, normally growing child," says Udall.

William Klish, chairman of the American Academy of Pediatrics Committee on Nutrition, says that if a child needs to take a vitamin supplement, the toddler formula, fortified with a full range of vitamins and minerals, including iron, can serve that purpose. In addition, the toddler formulas don't need refrigeration, making them a convenient choice for snacks away from home.

— by Isadora B. Stehlin

Isadora B. Stehlin is a member of FDA's public affairs staff.

Additional Questions and Answers about Infant Formulas

What Is an Infant Formula?

Infant formulas are liquids or reconstituted powders fed to infants and young children. They serve as substitutes for human milk. Infant formulas have a special role to play in the diets of infants because they are often the only source of nutrients for infants. For this reason, the composition of commercial formulas is carefully controlled and FDA requires that these products meet very strict standards.

How Does FDA Regulate Infant Formulas?

The safety and nutritional quality of infant formulas are ensured by requiring that manufacturers follow specific procedures in manufacturing infant formulas. In fact, there is a law — known as the Infant Formula Act — which gives FDA special authority to create and enforce standards for commercial infant formulas. Manufactures must analyze each batch of formula to check nutrient levels and make safety checks. They must then test samples to make sure the product remains in good condition while it is on the market shelf. Infant formulas must also have codes on their containers to identify each batch and manufacturers must keep very detailed records of production and analysis.

How Do I Report a Problem or Illness Caused by an Infant Formula?

If a consumer has a general complaint or concern about a food product including an infant formula, FDA is the appropriate agency to contact. These problems, complaints, or injuries can be reported in writing or by telephone.

If you think your infant has suffered a serious harmful effect or illness from an infant formula, your health care provider can report this by calling FDA's MedWatch hotline at 1-800-FDA-1088 or by using the website www.fda.gov/medwatch/report/hcp.htm. The MedWatch program allows health care providers to report problems possibly caused by FDA-regulated products such as drugs, medical devices, medical foods and dietary supplements. The identity of the patient is kept confidential.

Consumers may also report an adverse event or illness they believe to be related to the use of an infant formula by calling FDA at

1-800-FDA-1088 or using the website www.fda.gov/medwatch/report/ consumer/consumer.htm. FDA would like to know when a product causes a problem even if you are unsure the product caused the problem or even if you and the baby do not visit a doctor or clinic.

Are there Approved Recipes for Homemade Infant Formulas?

FDA regulates commercially available infant formulas, which are in liquid and powder forms, but does not regulate recipes for homemade formulas. Great care must be given to the decision to make infant formulas at home, and safety should be of prime concern. The potential problems associated with errors in selecting and combining the ingredients for the formula are very serious and range from severe nutritional imbalances to unsafe products that can harm infants. Because of these potentially very serious health concerns, FDA does not recommend that consumers make infant formulas at home.

Product that Consumers Have inquired About: Recipe for Homemade Formula Developed by a Naturopath

Recently FDA has become aware of a homemade infant formula recipe which is attributed to a naturopath at a company that makes nutritional supplements. It has been distributed to at least one Down's Syndrome support group. The recipe includes the ingredients flaxseed oil, maple syrup, and beta-carotene. A review of the recipe suggests that a formula made using the recipe would have several deficiencies including too few calories and a nutrient content that would be insufficient, or in some cases too high. In addition, the instructions for use are imprecise and susceptible to error.

I Have Seen Bottled Water Marked for Use in Preparing Infant Formula. What Does This Mean?

The manufacturers of infant formula provide directions for mixing their products with water and usually do not specify the source of water other than to indicate that the water should be safe to drink. In most situations, it is safe to mix formula using ordinary cold tap water that is brought to a boil and boiled for one minute or as directed on the label of the infant formula. Some water companies wish to make available bottled waters which are marketed for infants and for use in mixing with infant formula. When manufacturers label their water as intended for infants, the water must meet the same standards established for tap water by the Environmental Protection Agency. The label must also indicate that the bottled water is not sterile. As with tap water, consumers should boil bottled water one minute before mixing with infant formula. Water that is sterilized by the manufacturer and intended for use with infants must meet certain strict FDA standards.

Chapter 16

Good Nutrition for the High Chair Set

"Open the hangar and let the airplane fly in," mother coaxes her reluctant 6-month-old, spoon circling in mid-air. Baby opens her mouth and "airplane," with its spinach cargo, zooms toward the opening—only to collide with a mouth snapped shut faster than the speed of sound. The green goo dribbles down baby's chin onto her bib. But mother notes with some consolation that baby is tentatively licking some spinach off her lips.

The trials and tribulations of feeding infants are sometimes compounded by uncertainties about when to introduce certain foods and whether homemade varieties offer any benefit over those that are commercially prepared.

About 25 years ago, it was commonly recommended that babies be given "solid" food beginning at 6 weeks of age or sometimes younger. But a generation of experience has led pediatric experts to conclude that 6 weeks is too early for even cereal mixed with milk, the first traditional solid food. Today the common recommendation is that babies should receive only breast milk or infant formula until they are at least 4 to 6 months old.

Reasons for this are several. Contrary to previous theory, experts now advise that solid food does not make a baby anymore likely to sleep through the night than a diet of only formula or breast milk. Such a liquid diet can appease the hunger of an infant under 4 to 6 mont hs of age. The nervous system also needs to mature so the baby

FDA Consumer, September 1985, revised January 1992, last updated March 1997.

can recognize a spoon, coordinate swallowing, and signal if hungry or full. Feeding solids before the baby has these skills is really a kind of force-feeding. Introducing solids too early may contribute to over-feeding and result in food allergies, which can cause gastrointestinal and other problems.

To make baby food more nutritious when babies are ready for it, manufacturers, over the years, have made a number of changes in their products. For example, precooked cereals marketed for infants and usually first offered when the baby is 4 to 6 months old are forti-fied with iron and B vitamins. Although some forms of iron added to food are not as available to the body as iron naturally present, manu-facturers of precooked baby cereals add a form of iron that is absorbed as well as other non-heme (non-meat) iron naturally present in food. Babies need added iron at this age because the iron they had at birth from their mothers is just about used up. Therefore, babies are usu-ally given supplemental iron in the form of drops, or in formula or baby cereal. Most precooked baby cereals contain 45 percent of the U.S. Daily Recommended Allowance (U.S. RDA) of iron per serving.

When cereal is first fed to babies, to find out if they are allergic to any one type, the single-grain varieties of rice, oatmeal and barley should be given first. Mixed cereals and wheat cereals should be added when the baby is several months older. Cereal made from wheat is a more frequent cause of allergy than the other grains and is slightly rougher on the stomach.

Once they've mastered cereal slurping, babies can be offered a va-riety of other foods. But these foods must be strained to a very soft, semi-liquid consistency because infants, lacking teeth, cannot yet chew properly and because their swallowing reflex has not yet matures.

For years, commercially prepared baby foods were available on in jars. Then, foil-lined canisters containing dehydrated flakes for mix-ing with water were introduced. After being opened, baby food jars lasts about three days in the refrigerator. The flakes do not have to be refrigerated and remain good for about two weeks after opening.

Though it's a time-consuming task, some parents prepare foods at home for their babies in the hope that what they strain and puree (usually with the help of a blender or food processor) may be nutri-tionally superior to the commercially prepared foods. Often these parents are most concerned about the possible addition of salt, sugar, and other additives to commercial baby foods. A certain amount of sodium is necessary to an infant's health, but an excessive intake is not desirable. Before 1970, baby foods in jars often contained added sodium in the form of salt and monosodium glutamate (MSG). Then the National Academy of Sciences and the American Academy of Pediatrics pointed out that the amount of sodium in baby foods was often far in excess of body needs and that additives (other than vitamins and minerals) were not necessary to the proper nourishment of infants. In response to these points and to the growing concern that high sodium intake early in life might lead to high blood pressure later on, manufacturers of baby food began to limit the amount of added sodium. By 1978, they had entirely stopped adding MSG and salt to products meant for babies under 1 year.

Concerns about sugar and other additives, such as preservatives, have similarly motivated manufacturers to limit the amount of these substances added to their products. Today, commercially prepared baby foods rarely contain preservatives. Sterilization during the manufacturing process contributes to their long shelf life. In most lines of baby food, refined sugar is added only to custards and puddings.

A parent who wants to know what is in baby food need go no further than the label. FDA regulates the labeling of all baby foods with the exception of strained meats, which come under the jurisdiction of U.S. Department of Agriculture. FDA requires labeling on "infant" food (for babies under a year a old) to be more complete than that of the other foods so that parents may be well-informed about what they are feeding their youngster. While the labeling of other foods may list spices and additives simply as such, the labels on infant food must list each ingredient by name, including each spice, flavoring and coloring. In addition, the labeling must specify the plant or animal source of an ingredient. For example, rather than vegetable oil, the label must say "coconut oil" or "palm oil." As with other foods, ingredients are listed in descending order of predominance. Most manufacturers also include on the label the amounts (or percentages of U.S. RDAs) of calories, protein, carbohydrates, fat, sodium, vitamins, and minerals.

Along with solid foods, parents usually start to feed babies fruit juices at about 6 to 7 months of age. Initially, fruit juices for babies were marketed in cans. However, concern about lead from the cans getting into the juice after the can was opened and left partly filled caused manufacturers to switch to small glass bottles. (Unopened cans do not pose this problem.) The juices are fortified with vitamin C (as are many strained fruits), and most brands do not contain added refine sugar. Juice should not be served to the baby in a cup. It is especially important not to put a baby to bed with a bottle of fruit juice because if, as the baby dozes, its mouth remains in contact with the fruit juice, the acid and natural sugars have more of a chance to promote tooth decay.

A separate line of products is marketed for babies over a year old. These are commonly referred to as "toddler" foods. Chunkier than infant foods, these foods help in the transition to regular table food. Unlike infant foods, the sodium content of some toddler foods has not been significantly reduced. The National Academy of Sciences has set 325 to 975 milligrams of sodium as the safe and adequate daily dietary intake for children 1 to 3 years old. Yet some products marketed for this age group have 500 to 700 milligrams of sodium per serving, so that a child eating more than one serving a day might get an excessive amount of sodium. FDA has been encouraging manufacturers to reduce the amount of sodium in these products. The U.S. Department of Agriculture, which regulates the meat products that compose the majority of "toddler" food lines, is also working with manufacturers on this problem.

Because children under 4 years old not have a full set of teeth and therefore cannot chew as well as older children, extra care is needed when giving them toddler foods such as meat sticks and biscuits. The same precautions should be taken when feeding them "finger" foods, such as hot dogs, nuts, and hard candies.

In response to these concerns, the following was added to the labeling of toddler biscuits:

- "For Your Information: Biscuits, cookies, toast and crackers should be eaten in an upright position—never while lying down—to reduce the possibility of choking on crumbs."

The following has been added to the labeling of toddler meat sticks:

- "This product is intended for children with teeth. To reduce the possibility of choking, serve these sticks only to toddlers who have learned to chew solid foods properly. It is important the mealtime and snack time of small children be supervised. They should be fed in an upright position and never during vigorous activities."

Despite these few problems, commercially prepared baby and toddler foods offer an adequate and safe alternative that most parents prefer to home-prepared foods for babies. FDA continues to monitor these foods and shares parents' concern that what zooms into their babies' mouths be safe and nutritious as possible.

Introducing Baby to Solid Foods

Foods are usually (but not necessarily) introduced in the order shown in Table 16.1, with several weeks between different types of foods. Ages of introduction are approximate and may vary with individual babies. The baby's doctor is the best source for advice on when and how often any particular food is appropriate for that baby. Cereals should be mixed with formula or breast milk.

Table 16.1. Ages at which Solid Foods are Typically Introduced

Age	Food	Frequency
4-6 months	precooked baby cereal	twice a day
	baby juices	between meals
5-6 months	strained single fruits	twice a day
6-7 months	strained vegetables	once a day
7-8 months	strained meats	once a day
	plain yogurt	once a day
	baby juices	between meals
8-9 months	egg yolk, strained	once a day

—by Judith Willis

Judith Willis is editor of *FDA Consumer*.

Chapter 17

Childhood and Adolescent Nutrition: Milk Matters

Good health starts with good nutrition. Good nutrition can protect against disease later in life. The Food Guide Pyramid and the Dietary Guidelines for Americans are national recommendations to help people choose diets that promote health and reduce disease risks. A healthy diet should include food from the major food groups: grains (bread, cereal, rice, and pasta); vegetables; fruits; dairy products; meat (poultry, fish, dry beans, eggs and nuts). Fats and oils, located at the top of the food pyramid, should be used sparingly.

Recent studies show that few American children are meeting all of the recommendations outlined in the food pyramid. Teenage girls, on average, failed to meet any of them. One essential nutrient lacking in the diets of many children and teens is calcium, found primarily in dairy products and in dark, leafy green vegetables. Calcium plays a role in the proper functioning of the heart, muscles, and nerves and in maintaining blood flow. But most calcium is used in building bone mass in order to support physical activity throughout life and to reduce the risk of bone fracture, especially that due to osteoporosis, the weakening of bone that can occur late in adulthood.

Building Strong Bones

Though they appear hard, rigid, and lifeless, bones are actually growing and alive. Exercise and adequate calcium both influence bone

National Institute of Child Health and Human Development (NICHD), May 1998.

mass. Weight-bearing exercise, such as dancing, weightlifting, or running, determines bone mass, shape, and strength. Smoking, unhealthy eating patterns, and alcohol use detract from bone mass. Excessive salt intake may increase the amount of calcium lost in the urine, and therefore, increase the body's need for calcium.

Scientists agree that diets deficient in calcium during childhood and adolescence contribute to the development of osteoporosis, which is not visible until late in life. A positive calcium balance—taking in more than is lost throughout childhood, adolescence, and young adulthood—will allow bones to develop to their maximum density. But it is during the teen years that optimal calcium intake is most important. Bones grow and incorporate calcium most rapidly then. Soon after, by the age of 17, approximately 90% of the adult bone mass will be established. By the age of 21 or soon after, calcium is no longer added to bones and a few years later, a steady process of loss of calcium from bones begins. Genetically, people differ in how much calcium is in their bones when they reach maturity, but how much calcium they eat while they are growing has an important influence. The more calcium that is in the bones when loss begins, the longer it will take before the bones become fragile and fracture easily.

No Bones about It, Kids and Teens Can't Do Without It

Research sponsored by the National Institute of Child Health and Human Development (NICHD) has shown that a "window of

Table 17.1. Calcium: Who Gets Enough?

Age Group	% Getting the 1989 RDA
Under 5 (males and females)	45.4
Males (6-11)	53.3
Males (12-19)	35.1
Males (20-29)	45.0
Females (6-11)	43.1
Females (12-19)	14.4
Females (20-29)	17.8

Source: USDA Continuing Survey of Food Intakes by Individuals, 1994. This Survey was evaluated using 1989 Recommended Dietary Allowance (RDA); new calcium guidelines, Dietary Reference Intakes, were issued in August 1997 and generally, set a higher intake standard.

opportunity" exists to add to the bone bank during the teen years. NICHD researchers have found that supplementing the daily diets of girls, ages 12 to 16, with an extra 350 mg of calcium, produced a 14% increase in their bone density, in comparison to unsupplemented girls. If this 14% increase in their bone density could be maintained, its impact would be striking. For every 5% increase in bone density, the risk of later bone fracture declines by 40%. It is becoming increasingly evident that adequate calcium intake is critical during adolescent years.

Kids and Calcium: How Much Do They Need?

The new federal calcium guidelines, the Dietary Reference intakes, recommend that children ages 4-8 get 800 mg of calcium per day, or the equivalent of 2-3 glasses of low-fat milk. Adolescents and young adults, ages 9-18, whose bones are growing very fast, need more calcium. They should have 1300 mg, or about 4-5 glasses of low-fat milk per day.

Kids and Calcium: Who Gets Enough?

Unfortunately, most children and teens do not meet dietary calcium recommendations. National nutrition surveys say that more than one-half of all children under 5—and nearly seven-eighths of girls ages 12-19—do not meet the 1989 federal recommendations for calcium. In fact, teenage girls only average about 800 mg of calcium per day, well below the amount needed for normal growth and development.

Table 17.2. Recommended Levels of Calcium

Age Group	1997 Adequate Intake Values (mg)
Birth to 6 months	210
6-12 months	270
1-3 years	500
4-8 years	800
9-13 years	1,300
14-18 years	1,300
Pregnant or lactating teens	1,300

Recommendations based on the Dietary Reference intakes for Calcium, National Academy of Sciences, 1997.

This is especially critical since the new Dietary Reference Intakes set even higher calcium levels than the 1989 guidelines. Individuals with inadequate intake of dietary calcium may increase their risk for bone fractures and development of osteoporosis.

Where Is the Calcium?

The NICHD believes low-fat milk or low-fat milk products are the best sources of calcium because they contain large amounts of calcium, along with additional nutrients to help the body better absorb calcium. They are also already part of most American diets. Along with calcium, milk provides other essential nutrients, including vitamin D, potassium, and magnesium, all essential for optimal bone health and

Table 17.3. Sources of Calcium

Types of Milk (8oz.)	Approximate Calcium (mg)
Fat-free/non-fat	300
Lowfat, 2%	300
Whole	300
Chocolate milk, lowfat, 2%	300

...fat-free, lowfat, whole or chocolate...all have about 300 mg of calcium!

Other Sources of Calcium

Serving Size	Food Item	Calcium (mg)
8 fluid oz.	Yogurt, plain, lowfat	415
1 oz.	Cheese, cheddar	204
1 cup	Broccoli, cooked, fresh	136
½ cup	Ice cream, soft serve	118
1 slice	Bread, white or whole wheat	20
1	Orange, medium	52
½ cup	Macaroni and cheese*	180
1 slice	Pizza, cheese*	220
8 fluid oz.	Calcium fortified orange juice	300

Calcium content varies, depending on ingredients
Sources: American Dietetic Association, USDA Handbook 8, and National Dairy Council.

human development. Green leafy vegetables are healthy sources of calcium too, but it takes at least 5 servings of collards a day to get the same amount of calcium that is in 3-4 glasses of milk.

Table 17.4. Types of Milk

8 oz. Milk	Calories	Fat (g)	Saturated Fat (g)	Calcium (mg)
Skim/non-fat	80	0	0	300
½% fat	90	1	1	300
1% fat	100	2.5	1.5	300
2% fat	120	5	3	300
Whole	150	8	5	300

Lactose Intolerance

Some parents may think that their child or teen is lactose intolerant. Lactose intolerance is the inability to properly digest lactose, a sugar found in milk and other dairy foods. Lactose intolerance results in symptoms of bloating, gas, stomach cramping, and diarrhea after eating dairy products. However, most children can tolerate lactose. African-American, Mexican-American, and American Indian children and Asian Pacific Islanders are more likely than Caucasian children to be lactose intolerant. Recent studies show, however, that even children diagnosed with lactose intolerance can drink one to two cups of milk each day without suffering abdominal discomfort.

For children and teens with lactose intolerance, milk is often better tolerated when consumed with a meal. Some dairy foods, such as hard cheeses, or yogurt, contain less lactose than milk and cause fewer symptoms. In addition, lactose-reduced and lactose-free milk products are now readily available in most supermarkets. For those who cannot tolerate any milk, dietary calcium can come from non-dairy sources such as green vegetables like broccoli and spinach. Alternatively, calcium-fortified foods, such as orange juice, or calcium tablets, which provide 200-500 mg per tablet, can serve as the source of necessary calcium.

Solving the Calcium Crunch

Children and teens can get enough calcium in their daily diets by drinking 3-4 glasses of milk throughout the day, in breakfast cereal, with lunch, dinner, or as a snack. Making milk the standard and routine drink with meals throughout childhood and adolescence, and even through the adult years, is the best way to assure adequate calcium intake. For children over the age of two, low-fat or non-fat milk is recommended because it will add calcium to the diet without the fat. There are now a variety of milk products available, ranging from whole milk to non-fat or skim milk—but an 8 oz. glass of any variety still contains about 300 mg of calcium. Teens and young adults concerned about calorie intake and weight gain should know that 12 oz. of fat-free milk contains less calories than a 12 oz. soft drink, and provides 1/3 of daily calcium needs as well as many other important nutrients.

The NICHD recognizes inadequate calcium consumption among children and adolescents to be a growing problem and a serious threat to their later healthy growth and development. NICHD researchers are working to develop methods to prevent osteoporosis both through physical activity and through dietary means in childhood. Although adequate calcium benefits bones of all ages, children and teens need more calcium today to protect against bone fractures tomorrow.

Chapter 18

Healthy Eating Is a Family Affair

What your family eats has a large impact, not only on their blood cholesterol levels, but on their general health as well. All children and teenagers need to eat a nutritious diet. They need to eat a variety of foods that provide enough calories and nutrients—carbohydrates, protein, fat, vitamins, and minerals. This helps them grow and develop properly. It is also important as they become more physically active. A nutritious and "heart-healthy" diet is also low in saturated fat, total fat, and dietary cholesterol. As you know, this type of diet is important to lower blood cholesterol and maintain it at acceptable levels.

Help Your Child Eat Right and Exercise

Telling children and teenagers to eat right and exercise is good; showing them is better. Here are some tips to help your children develop healthful habits.

- **Be a model**. Set a good example. Adults, particularly parents, are a major influence on children's behavior. Children are also influenced by television, radio, magazines, newspapers, ads, friends, brothers and sisters, and others who may not conform to your ways. So, eat a heart-healthy diet and your children will be more likely to do the same. Exercising with your child also sets a good example.

Excerpted from *Cholesterol in Children: Healthy Eating Is a Family Affair*, National Heart, Lung, and Blood Institute, NIH Pub. No. 92-3099, November 1992.

- **Know the dietary guidelines to lower blood cholesterol.** Knowing how diet, blood cholesterol, and heart disease are related will help you guide your family to lower their blood cholesterol levels. Knowing the basics on choosing foods low in saturated fat, total fat, and cholesterol is important to your success.

- **Know the food groups.** Know the tips food groups and the low-saturated fat, low-cholesterol choices within each group. This will help you buy and provide such foods and snacks at home.

- **Stock the kitchen.** Stock the kitchen with low-saturated fat, low-cholesterol foods from each of the food groups. Prepare these foods in large quantities to be frozen for quick use later. Foods such as casseroles, soups, and breads can be frozen in individual servings for a quick meal. The whole family will then have low-saturated fat, low-cholesterol meals on hand. Teach children how to choose healthy snacks.

- **Teach basic food preparation skills.** Teach children how to clean vegetables, make salads, and safely use the stove, oven, microwave, and toaster. Children who have basic cooking skills appreciate food more and are more inclined to try new foods.

- **Let children help.** Let children help with or even do the grocery shopping. The supermarket is an ideal place to teach children about foods. Teach them how to read food labels. Involve children in meal planning and preparation. Encourage them to prepare snacks, bag lunches, and breakfast. This will help them become responsible and fulfill a need for independence.

- **Plan family meals.** Eating meals together as a family can really help foster heart-healthy eating habits in children. The more you create a "family setting" where everyone shares the same nutritious meals, the more children will accept healthful eating as a way of life. Try to maintain regular family meals every day—breakfast, lunch or dinner, or all three. This way, the whole family can learn about healthful eating and build good eating habits.

- **Encourage physical activity.** Make time for physical activity. Encourage children to get some exercise throughout the day and especially on the weekends. Take trips that involve activities like hiking, swimming, and skiing. Join in the fun. Ride bikes, run, skate, or walk to places close by. Give your child a splash or dance party. Use your backyard or park for basketball, baseball, football, badminton, or volleyball.

Know the Dietary Guidelines for Lowering Blood Cholesterol Levels

In order to help your family eat in a way that is lower in saturated fat and cholesterol, you need to know some dietary guidelines. They are consistent with the "Dietary Guidelines for Americans" and include choosing a variety of foods that provide the following nutrients:

- Less than 10 percent of calories from saturated fat,
- An average of no more than 30 percent of calories from fat,
- Less than 300 milligrams of dietary cholesterol a day,
- Enough calories to support growth, and to reach or maintain a healthy weight.

The whole family (except infants under 2 years who need more calories from fat) should follow these guidelines.

Heart-Healthy Meals and Snacks

Heart-Healthy Meals Can Be Fun and Taste Good

Children as they get older, especially girls, may often skip breakfast. It is important to begin the day with a good breakfast. Breakfast is an easy meal to introduce good-tasting heart-healthy foods.

- Serve toast (whole-grain types), English muffins, bagels, and hot or cold cereal with skim milk. These are quick and easy to prepare.

- Serve unsweetened or barely sweetened cereals as often as you can. Adding fruit to unsweetened cereal makes it special, and at the same time, increases nutrients and fiber without adding fat.

- For special events or weekend treats, try pancakes, muffins, or French toast made with egg whites or egg substitutes and skim milk. Add some sweet syrup or fruit sauce, neither of which contains fat, to make it more appealing to children.

- For a more hearty breakfast, add some low-fat meat such as sliced poultry or lean ham to a bagel or an English muffin.

Lunch

Choosing lunch at school gives children the chance to make the right food choices for themselves. Packing a lunch offers them the chance to plan their own heart-healthy meals. Whether your child buys a school lunch or takes a packed lunch, discuss some tips for eating right. Try some of these:

- Sliced turkey, lean roast beef, chicken, or tuna fish are good choices for lower-fat sandwiches. Even add a bit of sliced processed low-fat cheese.

- Peanut butter and jelly is also okay, especially on whole grain bread. For more nutritional punch, create peanut butter and mashed bananas with raisins or carrots.

- Whole-wheat, rye, pumpernickel, or bran breads add more fiber to a sandwich and taste good too.

- Try some of last night's pasta salad or cold baked chicken with herbs for a switch from sandwiches for lunch.

- Pack some snacks such as apples, bananas, grapes, raisins, nuts, or seeds. Also, put in prepackaged juices or other types of unsweetened beverages.

Some lunches provided at school may be high in saturated fat and cholesterol. Check the menu in advance. If low-fat choices are not available on a certain day, you and your child can pack a lunch. However, if your child's school never offers heart-healthy choices, try to arrange that it does so. Work with your PTA or school system to promote a school lunch program which offers heart-healthy choices.

Dinner

Dinner may pose a problem for busy parents who have little time to shop and cook. Many rely on high-fat convenience foods like creamy, canned soups and boxed macaroni and cheese dinners. Replace these with foods lower in saturated fat and cholesterol that are quick and easy to prepare:

- Chicken breasts, fish fillets, and lean hamburgers take little time to prepare. Broil, bake, or microwave, rather than fry.

- Vegetables can be steamed or microwaved in minutes.

- Vegetable stew can be made with rice or pasta and shavings of lean meat instead of a lot of chunks. Meat contributes protein, vitamins, and minerals like iron. Children should not avoid eating meat. It is a good idea to "stretch" meat by using it in a combination dish, like stew.

- Many ethnic dishes can also be low in fat and quick and easy to prepare. Try Chinese stir fries of rice, peppers, mushrooms, and water chestnuts with thin strips of beef or chicken. Pizza can be made with low-fat cheese and vegetable toppings rather than sausage or pepperoni.

- Some TV dinners and other convenience meals can be low in saturated fat and cholesterol. Look for dinners that provide foods from different food groups including vegetables, fruits, and breads. Choose less often those that contain battered, fried, or deep fried items. Read the labels and compare. Choose the one lowest in total fat and saturated fat.

Snacking Is Okay

Snacking is not a bad word. What your child eats matters more than when it is eaten. Children are growing quickly and need calories. Young children's appetites and stomachs may be small, so they may tend to eat smaller amounts at one time. They may not be able to eat enough calories at a meal to meet their energy needs. So, snacks may need to be part of their eating pattern.

Preteens and teenagers also may need extra nutrition and calories to get them through their growth spurts or athletic programs. Snacks can help meet their energy needs without being high in saturated fat and cholesterol. Instead, they can be rich in carbohydrates and fiber.

Plan for snacks. We all tend to eat what's handy. So, stock your kitchen with nutritious, low-saturated fat, low-cholesterol snack foods from all of the food groups.

Let the snack foods you serve at home be the "good eating guide" when your child is away from home. Some of these snacks are now also found in vending machines. Your child just needs to choose them.

Low-Saturated Fat, Low-Cholesterol Snacks

- Snack mix of cereal, dried fruit, and small amounts of nuts and seeds
- Cold cereal, dry or with low-fat milk
- Peanut butter and jelly sandwich
- Fruit juice and vegetable juice
- Peanuts in a shell or other dry roasted nuts
- Toast with jam or jelly
- Fruit leather

- Low-fat cheese pizza on English muffin
- Celery stalk filled with peanut butter
- Vegetable soup and low-fat crackers
- Candy (nonchocolate fat-free types)
- Skim milk with graham crackers
- Raisins and other dried fruit
- Frozen grapes or bananas
- Flavored low-fat yogurt
- Low-fat cookies

Like anything else, snacking can be overdone. If snacking leads to eating too much, it can lead to weight gain. Or, if snacks come mainly from the "Sweets and Snacks" group, your child may not get enough of the nutrients provided by other foods.

Convenience Foods and Fast Foods Can Be Heart Healthy

Stopping now and then at a fast-food restaurant with friends or family does no harm. However, these days children may be eating fast and convenience foods three or more times a week. By serving heart-healthy meals and snacks at home, you can plan for fast-food meals once in a while. Also, some fast and convenience foods are now lower in saturated fat and cholesterol than they used to be.

Here are some ways to avoid eating too much saturated fat and cholesterol while enjoying convenience. Try some of these tips:

- Order a small plain hamburger. It is lower in fat than fried or battered fish and chicken or anything with cheese.

- Try lean roast beef and grilled or broiled chicken sandwiches or pita pockets filled with small pieces of meat and vegetables.

- Select the small serving; order the regular hamburger instead of the jumbo.

- Order a plain baked potato instead of French fries.

- Create a salad at the salad bar. Limit toppings of cheese, fried noodles, bacon bits, and salads made with mayonnaise. Also, limit salad dressings that add saturated fat and cholesterol.

- Try ethnic cuisine—many such as Chinese and mid-Eastern are becoming fast food.

- Choose pizza with vegetable toppings such as mushrooms, onions, or peppers. Avoid extra cheese, pepperoni, or sausage.

- Create convenience foods at home by freezing low-fat casseroles, soups, and leftovers in single serving sizes.

You Can Lead Your Child to Food, But You Can't Make Him Eat

The most carefully planned heart-healthy meal is no good if your child does not eat it. Younger children may just be picky eaters going through a stage. Older children may have "reasons" for being picky. Children can be encouraged to eat foods lower in saturated fat and cholesterol but should not be made to eat them. You need to be creative and give them choices:

- Let your child help fix the meal. Helping makes eating more fun.
- Make the meal attractive. For younger children, make a face on top of casserole or cut foods with a cookie cutter to make fun shapes.
- If your child doesn't like a certain lower fat food, serve it with something your child does like. Disguise an unliked food in other foods. For example, add the food to casseroles or soups, or bake it into muffins or quick breads.
- Above all, be a good role model yourself—let your eating patterns be the example for others.

Choosing to eat in a heart-healthy way is a family affair. It becomes even more important if someone in the family has high blood cholesterol. If your child has high blood cholesterol, talk to them about it. They may not understand why they need to eat this way and may be afraid of sudden changes. Encourage children to eat for the health of their heart, yet don't make too big a deal about it. If your child is growing well, he or she is probably getting enough to eat. So don't worry about it. If your child gets stuck on one food or refuses to make any changes, discuss the problem with your doctor or a dietitian.

HELP!

If you want more help in planning low-saturated fat, low-cholesterol eating patterns, visit a registered dietitian or other qualified nutritionist. They can help you design an eating pattern suited to your own child's needs and likes. Dietitians may be found at local hospitals, and state and district chapters of the American Dietetic Association (ADA). The ADA keeps a list of registered dietitians. By calling the Division of Practice (312-899-0040), you can request names of dietitians in your area. Others can be found in public health departments, health maintenance organizations, cooperative extension services, and colleges. You can also call the ADA's consumer nutrition hotline at 800-366-1655.

Dietitians can help you by giving further advice on shopping and preparing foods, eating away from home, and changing your child's eating habits to help maintain the new eating pattern. Their skill will help you and your child set short-term targets for change. This will help your child reach the blood cholesterol goal without greatly changing your family's eating patterns and lifestyle.

The National Cholesterol Education Program has produced booklets for children of different age groups: ages 7 to 10, 11 to 14, and 15 to 18. These booklets are designed to help children understand blood cholesterol levels and the need to eat in a way that is low in saturated fat, total fat, and cholesterol. To order these booklets and others for adults with high blood cholesterol, contact:

National Cholesterol Education Program
NHLBI Information Center
P.O. Box 30105
Bethesda, Maryland 20824-0105

Chapter 19

How Does Living Alone Affect Dietary Quality?

In the United States, the number of single-person households is increasing. According to the U.S. Bureau of the Census, 25 percent of American households consisted of one person in 1990, up from 17 percent in 1970. An understanding of the eating habits and the nutritional needs of these people as well as an awareness of their related demographic, socioeconomic, and diet- and health-related characteristics assists policy makers in determining governmental policies and programs related to nutrition, food assistance, and health issues. This understanding also helps nutritionists in educating Americans to recognize the link between diet and health and to choose a more healthful diet and helps researchers in determining dietary survey and methodology needs for future research.

USDA has conducted the Nationwide Food Consumption Survey (NFCS) since 1955. The survey collects information on individual and household characteristics as well as food and nutrient intakes from households in the 48 contiguous States. The most recent NFCS was conducted in 1987-88. The survey was designed as a self-weighted sample of the American population, but the response was much lower than expected (less than 35 percent). This raised concern about the representativeness of the sample. A weighting scheme was developed to adjust for nonresponse; however, because the possibility of nonresponse bias may still exist, we caution against generalization of the results from our sample of 6,080 adults to the American population.

United States Department of Agriculture (USDA), Research Report Number 51, October 1994.

This report uses information from NFCS 1987-88 to compare the dietary quality of individuals in single-person households to that of those in multiperson households. Dietary quality was measured in terms of total energy intake, nutrient intake, nutrient density (amount of nutrient per 1,000 kilocalories), and the contribution of each food group to the total diet. Additionally, to obtain more insight into the possible reasons for differences in the diets between the two household types, we compared dietary quality of these types in terms of weekly food expenditure and selected demographic, socioecomonic, and diet- and health-related characteristics.

Overall, population averages of food and nutrient intakes tend to hide the fact that some sex-age groups within the population consume significantly more or less of a nutrient or food group than others. Accordingly, we divided adult women and men in single-person and in multiperson households into subgroups defined by age: 19-34 years, 35-54 years, 55-64 years, 65-74 years, and 75 years and older. We then compared the dietary quality of adults who live alone to that of adults who live in multiperson households within each subgroup.

The diets of adults living alone were significantly lower in food energy, protein, total fat, saturated fatty acids, calcium, phosphorus, and sodium. However, the diets of women living alone were significantly more nutrient dense in carbohydrate, vitamins A, C, E, and B_6, carotenes, riboflavin, niacin, folate, magnesium, iron, and fiber than diets of women living in multiperson households. Diets of men living alone were more nutrient dense in niacin, vitamin B_6, and folate than diets of men in multiperson households.

Few significant differences between the dietary quality of adults living alone and those living in multiperson households were identified for the selected socioeconomic, demographic, and health-related characteristics. Notable exceptions were dietary supplement use, reported health status, and years of formal education. Both men and women who lived alone were more likely to take vitamin and mineral supplements regularly. The youngest single women and the oldest single men were more likely to report "excellent" or "good" health status; but overall, single women were less likely to rate their health status as excellent or good than women living in multiperson households. Both of these differences may indicate a special interest in nutrition or a concern about the adequacy of dietary intake or general health by singles.

Younger men and women living alone were more likely to have more years of education, but this does not appear to have influenced their dietary quality.

Nutrient Intakes

Overall, the diets of adults living alone were significantly lower in food energy, protein, total fat, saturated fatty acids, calcium, phosphorus, and sodium than the diets of adults living in multiperson households. In addition to these differences, single women had significantly lower intakes of thiamin, niacin, and zinc and significantly higher intakes of vitamin A. Which nutrients show significant differences depends on age as well as sex. Tables in this chapter indicate which nutrients show significant differences in intake by persons who live alone in each age group compared to their counterparts in multiperson households.

In each age group, the nutrient intakes by the single women were generally lower than those of their counterparts in multiperson households (Table 19.1, Table 19.3). For example, in addition to the differences seen in the group overall, young single women 19-34 years of age had significantly lower intakes of riboflavin, vitamin B_6, and iron.

Similarly, nutrient intakes by single men in each age group were generally lower than their counterparts in multiperson households (Table 19.2, Table 19.4). Single men 35-54 years of age had significantly lower nutrient intakes of calcium and sodium as well as of vitamin C, vitamin E, and thiamin and significantly higher intakes of cholesterol than did their counterparts in multiperson households. Single men 65-74 years of age had significantly lower intakes of carotenes, vitamin E, and dietary fiber and significantly higher intakes of cholesterol than did men in this age group living in multiperson households. The oldest single men (75 years of age and older) had significantly lower intakes of protein, calcium, phosphorus, and zinc than did their counterparts in multiperson households.

Food Group Contributions

Fruits and vegetables made up more of the diets of single women than of the diets of women in multiperson households—23 percent and 19 percent, respectively. This helps to explain higher nutrient intakes of vitamin A, carotenes, and vitamin C by single women. These results suggest that women may prefer fruits and vegetables. The reason for thinking this is that women who live alone generally need to consider only their own preferences, while women in multiperson households have to consider the tastes of men and children. Thus single women can eat more of the foods they prefer.

Results were different for men. Grain and cereal products made less of a contribution to the diets of men living alone than to the diets of men living in multiperson households. However, intakes of nutrients associated with this group, with the exception of dietary fiber, were not significantly lower for single men. Additionally, intakes of milk and milk products were lower for single men of all ages and significantly

Table 19.1. Nutrient Intakes: Women living alone as compared to women living with others.

[L: significantly lower; H: significantly higher. From weighted mean 3-day intakes; significant at p<.05. Blank cells indicate no statistically significant relation]

Nutrient	Age (years)					
	All ages	19-34	35-54	55-64	65-74	75+
Food energy........	L	L	-	-	-	-
Carbohydrate	-	-	-	-	-	-
Protein................	L	L	-	L	-	L
Fat......................	L	L	-	L	-	-
Saturated fat	L	L	L	-	-	-
Vitamin A............	H	-	-	H	-	-
Carotenes	-	-	-	-	-	-
Vitamin C	-	-	-	-	-	-
Vitamin E............	-	-	-	-	-	-
Thiamin	L	L	-	-	-	-
Riboflavin	-	L	-	-	-	-
Niacin.................	L	L	-	-	-	-
Vitamin B_6	-	L	-	-	-	-
Vitamin B_{12}.........	-	-	-	-	-	-
Folate.................	-	-	-	-	-	-
Phosphorus.........	L	L	-	-	-	-
Calcium..............	L	L	-	-	-	-
Magnesium	-	-	-	-	-	-
Iron....................	-	L	-	-	-	-
Zinc	L	L	-	L	-	-
Cholesterol.........	-	-	-	-	-	-
Fiber..................	-	-	-	-	-	-
Sodium...............	L	L	-	-	-	L

lower for the oldest single men. Milk intake may increase and decrease with increases and decreases in intake of cereals, and this relationship between milk and cereals may help to explain the lower intakes of calcium, phosphorus, and protein in single men.

Table 19.2. Nutrient Intakes: Men living alone as compared to men living with others.

[L: significantly lower; H: significantly higher. From weighted mean 3-day intakes; significant at $p<.05$. Blank cells indicate no statistically significant relation]

Nutrient	All ages	Age (years) 19-34	35-54	55-64	65-74	75+
Food energy	L	-	-	-	-	-
Carbohydrate	-	-	-	-	-	-
Protein	L	-	-	-	-	L
Fat	L	-	-	-	-	-
Saturated fat	L	L	-	-	-	-
Vitamin A	-	-	-	-	-	-
Carotenes	-	-	-	-	L	-
Vitamin C	-	-	L	-	-	-
Vitamin E	-	-	L	-	L	-
Thiamin	-	-	L	-	-	-
Riboflavin	-	-	-	-	-	-
Niacin	-	-	-	-	-	-
Vitamin B_6	-	-	-	-	-	-
Vitamin B_{12}	-	L	-	-	-	-
Folate	-	-	-	-	-	-
Phosphorus	L	-	-	-	-	L
Calcium	L	-	L	-	-	L
Magnesium	-	-	-	-	-	-
Iron	-	-	-	-	-	-
Zinc	-	-	H	-		L
Cholesterol	-	-	-	-	-	-
Fiber	-	-	-	-	L	-
Sodium	L	-	L	L	-	-

Table 19.3. Mean nutrient intakes by women, by household type.

Nutrient	Single-person household, by age						Multiperson household, by age					
	All ages	19-34	35-54	55-64	65-74	75+	All ages	19-34	35-54	55-64	65-74	75+
Food energy (kcal)	1,311.01	1,288.13	1,370.49	1,337.51	1,322.22	1,267.82	1,474.54	1,537.17	1,431.74	1,452.01	1,424.95	1,412.92
Carbohydrate (g)	157.93	151.91	156.10	169.08	161.34	155.76	172.01	180.78	165.66	164.58	167.57	169.88
Protein (g)	54.56	50.79	59.89	57.06	56.63	51.29	61.24	61.61	60.24	63.99	61.24	58.04
Fat (g)	51.69	51.60	53.56	50.00	52.42	50.82	60.61	63.23	58.83	60.15	57.70	57.35
Saturated fat (g)	18.25	18.50	18.08	16.66	18.63	18.66	21.70	23.06	20.94	20.86	19.67	21.42
Vitamin A (μg RE)	1,065.76	777.87	1,301.56	1,216.42	1,224.05	953.78	883.44	830.09	852.67	991.85	993.24	1,104.26
Carotenes (μg RE)	484.98	313.46	613.35	535.05	611.70	421.03	399.07	361.57	388.21	435.96	504.02	523.89
Vitamin C (mg)	89.57	71.89	101.10	113.61	100.93	75.34	81.87	76.78	81.03	89.61	94.15	89.81
Vitamin E (mg α-TE)	6.68	5.83	7.01	7.06	7.20	6.57	6.70	6.73	6.44	7.06	7.20	5.80
Thiamin (mg)	1.03	0.91	0.97	1.02	1.13	1.11	1.13	1.12	1.09	1.18	1.13	1.11
Riboflavin (mg)	1.39	1.27	1.35	1.38	1.49	1.46	1.43	1.46	1.37	1.49	1.46	1.47
Niacin (mg)	15.29	13.50	16.70	16.20	15.92	14.95	16.23	16.02	16.16	17.33	16.53	15.48
Vitamin B_6 (mg)	1.27	1.01	1.27	1.32	1.48	1.31	1.27	1.23	1.24	1.34	1.42	1.35
Vitamin B_{12} (μg)	5.21	5.25	7.54	6.29	4.31	3.76	4.48	4.35	4.48	5.24	3.89	4.67
Folate (μg)	204.46	170.83	194.49	209.67	236.44	212.33	193.10	188.33	186.86	207.14	218.32	197.34
Phosphorus (mg)	864.92	834.06	894.82	881.61	906.49	829.21	945.12	973.52	916.65	959.04	930.62	894.71
Calcium (mg)	550.31	547.24	504.55	523.84	588.38	566.93	598.75	638.83	562.05	584.19	584.00	585.09
Magnesium (mg)	202.15	173.53	224.82	216.81	224.45	189.49	202.15	191.31	203.67	221.23	221.23	199.75
Iron (mg)	10.04	9.10	9.97	10.22	10.53	10.42	10.57	10.35	10.34	11.42	11.07	11.03
Zinc (mg)	7.75	6.52	8.34	7.70	7.84	8.34	8.55	8.56	8.34	9.03	8.77	8.60
Cholesterol (mg)	225.37	216.62	236.03	230.01	230.57	219.25	241.77	246.40	239.54	244.73	231.79	227.85
Fiber (g)	11.32	9.31	12.02	12.07	12.87	11.00	10.78	9.98	10.78	11.80	12.88	11.25
Sodium (mg)	2,076.43	2,086.36	2,227.82	2,167.81	2,049.73	1,937.73	2,423.95	2,516.78	2,346.51	2,422.87	2,333.56	2,352.53

Weighted mean 3-day data from 1987-88 NFCS

Table 19.4. Mean nutrient intakes by men, by household type.

Nutrient	Single-person household, by age						Multiperson household, by age					
	All ages	19-34	35-54	55-64	65-74	75+	All ages	19-34	35-54	55-64	65-74	75+
Food energy (kcal)	1,934.53	2,170.96	1,861.41	1,680.88	1,775.51	1,701.71	2,090.74	2,218.96	2,070.71	1,946.37	1,885.98	1,912.75
Carbohydrate (g)	219.55	257.00	195.25	178.89	213.31	209.35	233.95	251.68	228.73	211.82	211.06	223.90
Protein (g)	78.61	86.60	76.56	77.99	74.58	58.56	85.58	88.47	85.61	82.72	78.21	82.02
Fat (g)	77.41	84.56	77.64	72.29	67.25	65.09	87.60	92.22	87.37	83.52	78.61	77.40
Saturated fat (g)	27.08	28.97	27.06	26.69	24.21	23.34	31.17	33.72	30.83	28.89	26.46	26.91
Vitamin A (μg RE)	1,110.06	974.91	868.53	1,402.63	1,116.13	2,389.24	1,053.39	976.33	1,028.64	1,084.34	1,433.30	1,178.13
Carotenes (μg RE)	375.27	387.83	303.70	530.82	333.57	512.05	443.35	370.32	455.41	503.31	629.77	461.65
Vitamin C (mg)	99.51	114.44	69.01	100.64	119.34	132.21	96.92	93.35	96.50	103.54	101.06	105.76
Vitamin E (mg α-TE)	8.60	10.10	7.40	9.10	7.95	7.50	9.18	9.25	8.82	9.18	10.62	8.60
Thiamin (mg)	1.45	1.60	1.25	1.56	1.48	1.43	1.55	1.57	1.53	1.58	1.51	1.63
Riboflavin (mg)	1.83	1.94	1.58	2.06	1.94	1.98	1.92	2.01	1.84	1.84	1.93	2.05
Niacin (mg)	22.65	24.94	21.69	21.19	20.56	21.10	22.45	22.78	22.67	21.73	21.89	20.83
Vitamin B_6 (mg)	1.77	1.91	1.58	1.87	1.88	1.76	1.75	1.77	1.71	1.87	1.84	1.78
Vitamin B_{12} (μg)	6.76	5.01	6.28	6.49	6.19	17.49	6.42	7.01	6.09	5.53	6.61	5.91
Folate (μg)	260.04	275.32	216.34	289.99	299.48	287.84	250.41	248.88	249.35	249.35	263.59	259.46
Phosphorus (mg)	1,176.01	1,334.07	1,079.24	1,173.67	1,116.93	974.53	1,298.81	1,383.55	1,251.98	1,223.44	1,175.45	1,286.68
Calcium (mg)	678.56	783.64	579.83	761.25	680.37	539.96	802.32	899.33	739.68	733.50	726.47	786.74
Magnesium (mg)	265.55	287.55	252.91	256.69	248.00	256.49	269.69	270.20	265.27	274.62	273.20	280.74
Iron (mg)	13.74	14.22	13.00	14.87	13.00	14.62	14.29	14.46	14.18	13.90	14.66	13.97
Zinc (mg)	11.45	12.21	10.94	11.46	12.25	9.09	12.23	12.32	12.51	11.69	11.62	11.88
Cholesterol (mg)	320.45	317.71	307.97	405.24	348.54	254.10	348.28	353.52	357.69	331.57	316.12	334.00
Fiber (g)	14.32	15.55	13.83	12.55	12.52	15.32	14.73	14.68	14.16	14.91	16.09	16.53
Sodium (mg)	2,998.56	3,236.55	2,904.78	2,736.08	2,908.35	2,757.06	3,691.92	3,821.85	3,676.77	3,665.56	3,448.52	3,225.27

Weighted mean 3-day data from 1987-88 NFCS

Nutrient Densities

Both single women and single men had diets significantly more nutrient dense in niacin, vitamin B_6, and folate than did their counterparts in multiperson households. Single women had diets significantly more nutrient dense in a number of other nutrients—carbohydrate, vitamin A, carotenes, vitamin C, vitamin E, riboflavin, magnesium, iron, and dietary fiber—and less nutrient dense in total fat and saturated fatty acids (Table 19.5). In particular, single women 55-64 years of age had significantly higher nutrient densities of vitamin C and lower nutrient densities of total fat and saturated fatty acids, and single women 65-74 years of age had significantly higher nutrient densities of vitamin A, carotenes, riboflavin, vitamin B_6, folate, and magnesium (Table 19.5, Table 19.7). The oldest single women—75 years of age and older—had significantly higher nutrient densities of vitamin E and folate.

In addition to having diets significantly more dense in niacin, vitamin B_6, and folate, single men's diets were less nutrient dense in sodium. Single men 55-64 years of age had significantly higher nutrient densities for a number of nutrients—thiamin, riboflavin, folate, calcium, iron, and cholesterol—than did their counterparts in multiperson households (Table 19.6, Table 19.8). Men aged 75 and over living alone had significantly lower nutrient densities for calcium and phosphorus than men of the same age in multiperson households. These men were also less likely to consume milk and milk products than their counterparts in multiperson households.

The nutrient densities of vitamin A, carotenes, vitamin C, vitamin E, riboflavin, vitamin B_6, vitamin B_{12}, folate, magnesium, and dietary fiber were at least 10 percent higher for single women than for women in multiperson households. In fact, for virtually all nutrients, densities for single women of all ages were higher than for women in multiperson households; the exceptions were total fat, saturated fatty acids, and sodium.

For single men the nutrient densities of carbohydrate, vitamin B_6, and folate were at least 10 percent higher for men in single-person households than for men in multiperson households. The difference in carbohydrate density may be related to lower fat and higher carbohydrate intake. For both single women and single men there is a tendency to have diets less dense in total fat, saturated fatty acids, and sodium, and more dense in carbohydrate, vitamins A and C, and fiber. As with nutrient intakes, this dietary behavior suggests that adults living alone have a greater awareness of current dietary recommendations and make a greater effort to follow such advice than adults living in multiperson households.

Table 19.5. Nutrient Densities: Women living alone as compared to women living with others.

[L: significantly lower; H: significantly higher. From weighted mean 3-day intakes; significant at p<.05. Blank cells indicate no statistically significant relation]

Nutrient	All ages	19-34	35-54	55-64	65-74	75+
Carbohydrate......	H	-	-	H	-	-
Protein	-	-	-	-	-	-
Fat	L	-	-	L	-	-
Saturated fat	L	-	-	L	-	-
Vitamin A	H	-	-	-	H	-
Carotenes	H	-	-	-	H	-
Vitamin C	H	-	-	H	-	-
Vitamin E	H	-	-	-	-	H
Thiamin...............	-	-	-	-	-	-
Riboflavin............	H	-	-	-	H	-
Niacin..................	H	-	-	-	-	-
Vitamin B_6...........	H	-	-	-	H	-
Vitamin B_{12}	-	-	-	-	-	-
Folate..................	H	-	-	-	H	H
Phosphorus	-	-	-	-	-	-
Calcium...............	-	-	-	-	-	-
Magnesium.........	H	-	-	-	H	-
Iron	H	-	-	-	-	-
Zinc.....................	-	L	-	-	-	-
Cholesterol	-	-	-	-	-	-
Fiber	H	-	H	-	-	-
Sodium	-	-	-	-	-	-

161

Table 19.6. Nutrient Densities: Men living alone as compared with men living with others.

[L: significantly lower; H: significantly higher. From weighted mean 3-day intakes; significant at $p<.05$. Blank cells indicate no statistically significant relation]

Nutrient	Age (years)					
	All ages	19-34	35-54	55-64	65-74	75+
Carbohydrate	-	-	-	-	-	-
Protein	-	-	-	-	-	-
Fat	-	-	-	-	-	-
Saturated fat	-	-	L	-	-	-
Vitamin A	-	-	-	-	-	-
Carotenes	-	-	-	-	L	-
Vitamin C	-	-	L	-	-	-
Vitamin E	-	-	-	-	-	-
Thiamin	-	-	-	H	-	-
Riboflavin	-	-	-	H	-	-
Niacin	H	H	-	-	-	-
Vitamin B_6	H	-	-	-	-	-
Vitamin B_{12}	-	L	-	-	-	-
Folate	H	-	-	H	-	-
Phosphorus	-	-	-	-	-	L
Calcium	-	-	-	H	-	L
Magnesium	-	-	-	-	-	-
Iron	-	-	-	H	-	-
Zinc	-	-	-	-	-	-
Cholesterol	-	-	-	H	-	-
Fiber	-	-	-	-	L	-
Sodium	L	-	-	-	-	-

Table 19.7. Mean nutrient densities of women, by household type.

Nutrient	Single-person household, by age						Multiperson household, by age					
	All ages	19-34	35-54	55-64	65-74	75+	All ages	19-34	35-54	55-64	65-74	75+
Carbohydrate (g)	120.94	117.70	113.74	127.82	122.29	123.91	116.56	117.59	115.75	112.72	117.91	121.45
Protein (g)	42.58	40.64	44.74	43.75	43.74	41.28	42.43	40.77	43.09	45.44	43.74	41.68
Fat (g)	38.87	39.67	38.98	36.28	39.15	39.22	40.69	40.81	40.66	41.14	40.12	39.74
Saturated fat (g)	13.67	14.21	13.10	11.93	13.93	14.30	14.52	14.86	14.43	14.22	13.66	14.59
Vitamin A (µg RE)	831.04	560.52	1,101.79	843.12	996.13	748.98	614.75	561.67	609.10	694.58	703.68	755.31
Carotenes (µg RE)	374.12	232.71	460.12	406.80	487.20	332.47	286.67	256.56	284.30	323.40	355.87	346.19
Vitamin C (mg)	69.24	52.52	76.61	91.00	78.25	60.13	57.57	51.21	59.47	63.58	68.01	64.41
Vitamin E (mg α-TE)	5.01	4.43	5.28	5.27	5.24	5.02	4.56	4.43	4.49	4.85	5.24	4.10
Thiamin (mg)	0.80	0.72	0.72	0.77	0.86	0.88	0.77	0.74	0.78	0.83	0.86	0.81
Riboflavin (mg)	1.08	0.97	1.07	1.01	1.17	1.15	0.98	0.96	0.97	1.04	1.04	1.05
Niacin (mg)	12.09	11.04	12.67	12.59	12.35	12.16	11.20	10.72	11.77	12.36	11.93	11.16
Vitamin B_6 (mg)	0.99	0.80	0.96	0.99	1.16	1.05	0.88	0.82	0.89	0.94	1.01	0.97
Vitamin B_{12} (µg)	4.05	3.55	6.91	4.24	3.58	2.87	3.07	2.87	3.17	3.55	2.78	3.41
Folate (µg)	159.11	128.41	152.92	156.29	187.48	169.09	134.43	124.96	135.39	144.76	157.67	140.05
Phosphorus (mg)	665.91	652.63	670.22	662.79	692.14	655.00	648.44	640.28	647.95	672.32	658.29	640.98
Calcium (mg)	417.45	417.10	382.44	384.47	444.56	436.92	409.53	421.29	393.49	405.82	409.44	414.24
Magnesium (mg)	158.08	134.77	170.88	165.07	176.50	151.47	141.47	127.79	148.15	156.02	157.99	142.61
Iron (mg)	7.82	7.34	7.41	7.76	8.12	8.32	7.32	6.90	7.39	7.92	7.95	7.84
Zinc (mg)	5.96	5.12	6.14	6.07	6.13	6.41	5.92	5.69	5.95	6.34	6.22	6.08
Cholesterol (mg)	176.85	172.59	183.81	170.58	179.79	176.96	164.89	160.21	168.87	170.55	163.94	163.17
Fiber (g)	8.74	7.26	8.90	9.19	9.94	8.73	7.46	6.58	7.72	8.30	9.20	7.93
Sodium (mg)	1,604.01	1,668.40	1,654.92	1,643.68	1,558.51	1,527.66	1,668.16	1,660.40	1,672.06	1,685.12	1,652.39	1,693.82

Weighted mean 3-day data from 1987-88 NFCS

163

Table 19.8. Mean nutrient densities of men, by household type.

Nutrient	Single-person household, by age						Multiperson household, by age					
	All ages	19-34	35-54	55-64	65-74	75+	All ages	19-34	35-54	55-64	65-74	75+
Carbohydrate (g)	133.32	117.86	104.10	112.30	120.21	123.21	111.96	114.20	109.53	109.40	111.53	119.43
Protein (g)	41.47	40.93	42.23	45.30	42.32	35.32	41.81	40.46	42.32	43.50	43.01	42.69
Fat (g)	39.67	38.96	41.18	41.02	39.15	39.22	41.67	41.28	42.21	42.36	41.39	39.48
Saturated fat (g)	13.85	13.35	14.25	15.02	13.42	13.82	14.77	15.03	14.89	14.61	13.85	13.74
Vitamin A (µg RE)	583.37	442.23	485.52	877.18	631.65	1,227.40	531.89	448.99	535.87	588.42	756.04	618.64
Carotenes (µg RE)	208.63	183.87	244.08	326.09	195.43	324.97	228.92	171.70	244.08	283.39	334.83	256.32
Vitamin C (mg)	52.80	55.10	37.15	61.71	70.76	73.06	48.61	44.61	48.12	56.01	54.40	56.71
Vitamin E (mg α-TE)	4.52	4.60	4.32	5.13	4.69	4.23	4.45	4.25	4.29	4.79	5.61	4.38
Thiamin (mg)	0.76	0.74	0.69	0.95	0.83	0.87	0.76	0.73	0.74	0.83	0.81	0.85
Riboflavin (mg)	0.96	0.87	0.88	1.29	1.08	1.12	0.93	0.92	0.90	0.96	1.04	1.07
Niacin (mg)	12.05	11.83	12.16	12.75	11.60	12.45	11.06	10.55	11.23	11.60	11.99	10.86
Vitamin B$_6$ (mg)	0.95	0.88	0.89	1.19	1.05	1.06	0.85	0.81	0.84	0.91	0.99	0.92
Vitamin B$_{12}$ (µg)	3.40	2.28	3.29	3.69	3.64	8.16	3.19	3.30	3.10	2.86	3.59	2.96
Folate (µg)	139.03	123.99	125.87	182.32	171.42	167.64	124.19	114.69	124.52	134.96	143.63	138.01
Phosphorus (mg)	608.97	611.58	586.42	696.31	625.15	575.37	627.09	630.46	611.28	638.57	637.08	674.52
Calcium (mg)	349.62	346.74	322.71	464.90	366.99	326.69	383.20	403.68	358.32	377.76	384.29	415.75
Magnesium (mg)	140.10	133.72	137.96	159.65	141.06	154.73	131.70	122.51	131.03	145.16	148.78	148.42
Iron (mg)	7.32	6.65	7.20	8.92	7.26	9.14	7.01	6.68	6.99	7.35	7.94	7.39
Zinc (mg)	6.05	5.72	6.12	6.66	6.80	5.53	5.95	5.59	6.16	6.12	6.40	6.17
Cholesterol (mg)	175.17	155.33	171.87	257.09	208.49	140.98	169.44	159.93	177.78	173.49	170.00	173.78
Fiber (g)	7.40	7.18	7.12	7.70	7.19	9.52	7.16	6.62	6.96	7.79	8.67	8.82
Sodium (mg)	1,553.16	1,506.84	1,534.69	1,609.29	1,637.80	1,653.09	1,795.10	1,747.93	1,798.26	1,924.75	1,841.70	1,749.34

Weighted mean 3-day data from 1987-88 NFCS

Measures of Dietary Quality

Dietary quality depends on the intake of numerous nutrients and dietary components that provide variety and promote health and well-being. Assessing dietary quality in terms of the three measures—nutrient intake, nutrient density, and food group contribution to the total diet—not only considers the intake of many nutrients and foods but also the reliance by individuals on certain food groups. This gives a more complete picture of the dietary behavior of adults than assessing only nutrient intakes.

The results show that lower nutrient intakes do not necessarily mean lower nutrient densities, nor do they necessarily indicate a diet of poorer quality than one with higher intakes. A more nutrient dense diet may make it easier to obtain important nutrients. For example, single women had higher nutrient density for vitamin A, and this helped them to achieve a higher total intake of vitamin A, even though they consumed fewer kilocalories. However, adequate absolute amounts of nutrients need to be consumed to avoid nutrient deficiencies and to obtain adequate kilocalories for normal activity. Single women also had a higher nutrient density for iron, but their total iron intake was lower.

Examination of these results suggests a positive relationship between nutrient density and absolute nutrient intake of a given nutrient when consumption of foods rich in that nutrient play a major part of the diet. Although specific nutrient intakes or densities are higher in one household type than the other, adults from both single-person and multiperson households have some common problems in meeting dietary guidance objectives. Women had low intakes of calcium, iron, zinc, and dietary fiber. Men had high intakes of cholesterol. Total fat and saturated fatty acid intakes were higher than dietary recommendations for both women and men. All would benefit from nutritional intervention programs.

Food Expenditures

Single-person households share common characteristics that can affect dietary behavior. For example, single-person households tend to spend more money per capita on food.

In this study, single-person households had a lower total food bill than multiperson households. Single persons spent an average of 13.4 percent of their household income on food, while multiperson households spent 16.1 percent of household income on food (Table 19.9).

However, as might be expected, per-person food expenditures by singles were 25 percent higher than in multiperson households. Food expenditure per person tends to decline as household size increases because larger households can take advantage of economies of scale, such as buying in bulk.

Table 19.9. Food expenditures, by household type

	Single-person	Multiperson
Food Cost:	--------------per week------------	
At home...............................	$28.33	$68.10
Away from home	$13.34	$33.08
Total.......................................	$41.69	$101.27
Per person.............................	$41.69	$34.11
Income:	--------------per year------------	
Household	$16,123.00	$32,681.00
Per person.............................	$16,123.00	$11,574.00
Percentage of annual income		
spent on food.........................	13.4%	16.1%

Socioeconomic, Demographic, and Diet and Health-Related Characteristics

Few significant differences were found in the socioeconomic, demographic, and health-related characteristics studied. People living alone used vitamin and mineral supplements more frequently than those in multiperson households. Two-fifths of the women and one-third of the men in single-person households reported using supplements frequently, while one-third of the women and one-fourth of the men in multiperson households did.

The youngest female and the oldest male singles were more likely to report an "excellent" or "good" health status. Overall, however, single women were less likely to rate their health status as excellent or good than were women living in multiperson households. These differences may indicate that single women have a special interest in nutrition or a concern about the adequacy of dietary intake or general health.

There was no overall significant difference in the reported health status between men living alone and men in multiperson households.

Men and women 19-34 years of age who live alone had more years of education than did their counterparts in multiperson households. The level of education did not appear to relate to improved dietary intakes for either group. In fact, young single women with more years of education had lower intakes for many nutrients than did other single women or women living in multiperson households (Table 19.3).

Overall, it appears that in this study, supplement use and reported health status are the socioeconomic, demographic, and health-related characteristics which may have the strongest relation to the dietary quality of adults living in these two types of households.

—by Shirley A. Gerrior, Joanne F. Guthrie, Jonathan J. Fox, Steven M. Lutz, Thomas P. Keane, and P. Peter Basiotis, Agricultural Research Service, U.S. Department of Agriculture.

Additional Readings

Blaylock, J.R., D.M. Smallwood, and N. Blisard. 1991. Per capita food spending. *Food Rev.* July-September, pp. 28-32.

Davis, M.A., S.P. Murphy, J.M. Neuhaus, and D. Lein. 1990. Living arrangements and dietary quality of older U.S. adults. *J. Amer. Dietet. Assoc.* 90:1667-1672.

Murphy, S.P., M.A. Davis, J.M. Neuhaus, and D. Lein. 1990. Factors influencing the dietary adequacy and energy intake of older Americans. *J. Nutr. Educ.* 22:284291.

Senauer, B.H., E. Asp, and J. Kinsey. 1991. Food trends and the changing consumer. St. Paul, Minnesota: *Eagan Press*, pp. 385.

Sexauer, B.H., and J.S. Mann. 1979. Food spending in single-person households. *Natl. Food Rev.* 1:32-33.

Chapter 20

Special Advice for Older Adults

As you age, health conditions may limit what you can eat. This can make eating a balanced diet more difficult. You may need to pay more attention to getting adequate nutrients and fluids and to achieving and maintaining a healthy weight. You may also need to consider possible interactions between foods and medications.

Meeting Your Nutrient Needs

Until recently, research on nutritional requirements has focused on younger people. No one really knows enough about how nutritional needs change as people age. Researchers believe you need the same variety of foods as younger people, but different quantities of some nutrients. Furthermore, individual health and level of activity differ widely among the older population. The best strategy is to figure out a balanced approach to eating that fits your general health and preferences.

Use the guide in Figure 20.1 to help you remember what foods and how much to eat each day. Each of the food groups in the three lower levels of the Pyramid supplies specific vitamins and minerals, so it's important to include them all to get the nutrients you need for good health. Try to have at least the lowest number of suggested servings from each of these food groups every day. The lowest number of servings, with modest amounts of fat and sweets, provides about 1,600 calories— right for many older women. Older men need somewhat more (see

Excerpted from *Food Facts for Older Americans,* U.S. Department of Agriculture, Human Nutrition Information Service, Home and Garden Bulletin No. 251, April 1993.

Table 20.2). But remember, individual needs vary, depending on your body size, health, and how active you are. If you need more food, eat more from each of these food groups, and go easy on foods from the fats, oils, and sweets group.

What Counts as 1 Serving?

Breads, Cereals, Rice, and Pasta
1 slice of bread
½ cup of cooked rice or pasta
½ cup of cooked cereal
1 ounce of ready-to-eat cereal

Fruits
1 piece of fruit or melon wedge
¾ cup of juice
½ cup of canned fruit
¼ cup of dried fruit

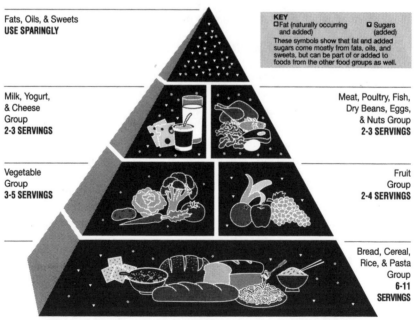

Source: U.S. Department of Agriculture/U.S. Department of Health and Human Services

Figure 20.1. A Guide to Daily Food Choices.

Vegetables
½ cup of chopped raw or cooked vegetables
1 cup of leafy raw vegetables

Milk, Yogurt, and Cheese
1 cup of milk or yogurt
1½ to 2 ounces of cheese

Meat, Poultry, Fish, Dry Beans, Eggs, and Nuts
2½ to 3 ounces of cooked lean meat, poultry, or fish
Count ½ cup of cooked beans or 1 egg or 2 tablespoons of peanut butter as 1 ounce of lean meat (about one-third of a serving)

Fats, Oils, and Sweets
Limit calories from these especially if you need to lose weight.

The amount you eat might be more than one serving. For example,
a dinner portion of spaghetti would count as two or three servings of
pasta.

Table 20.2. Suggested numbers of servings for older adults

Food Group	Suggested Number of Servings*
Bread group	6-9
Vegetable group	3-4
Fruit group	2-3
Milk group	2
Meat group	2

**Lower numbers of servings are suggested for older women. The higher
numbers are suggested for older men.*

A Closer Look at Fat and Added Sugars

The small tip of the Pyramid (see Figure 20.1) shows fats, oils, and
sweets. These are foods such as salad dressings, cream, butter, margarine, sugars, soft drinks, candies, and sweet desserts. Alcoholic
beverages are also part of this group. These foods provide calories but
few vitamins and minerals. Most people should go easy on foods from
this group.

Some fat or sugar symbols are shown in the other food groups. That's to remind you that some foods in these groups can also be high in fat and added sugars, such as cheese or ice cream from the milk group, or french fries from the vegetable group. When choosing foods for a healthful diet, consider the fat and added sugars in your choices from all the food groups, not just fats, oils, and sweets from the Pyramid tip.

Did You Know

Learning to estimate serving sizes can be helpful in following the guide to food choices. Here are some typical portion sizes:

- a ¼-inch-thick slice of cooked lean meat or poultry measuring about 3 x 4 inches weighs about two ounces.

- a 3-ounce, cooked, lean hamburger patty starts out as 4 ounces or ¼ pound of raw meat. The cooked patty will measure about 3 inches across and about ½ inch thick, about the size of the palm of a woman's hand, or the size of a large mayonnaise jar lid.

- a 1-inch cube of hard cheese, like cheddar or Swiss, weighs about ½ ounce.

- a cooked chicken breast half, without skin, weighs about 3 ounces.

Of Special Interest for Older Adults—Calcium and Vitamin D

All nutrients are important for good health at any age, but some that have been mentioned in the news lately have special importance for older adults. For example, inadequate calcium has been linked to osteoporosis, a condition in which hones become weak and brittle. The exact cause of osteoporosis is not known. Several nutrients in addition to calcium are involved.

However, many scientists believe that women particularly need to get adequate amounts of calcium throughout life. Milk, yogurt, cheese, and other dairy products are the best sources of calcium. Some dark-green leafy vegetables, canned fish eaten with the hones (canned sardines and salmon), and tofu also provide calcium.

To absorb calcium, your body needs vitamin D. Vitamin D is added to most fluid milk; it can also be made by your skin when exposed to sunlight. Dietary supplements of vitamin D are usually not necessary.

Your doctor or dietitian should advise you on your need for additional vitamin D. If they recommend supplements, they should tell you how much you should take. Generally, vitamin D supplements should not exceed the U.S. Recommended Daily Allowance (U.S. RDA) of 400 International Units (IU) per day, because continued use of high doses is harmful. (U.S. RDAs are nutrient standards developed for food product labels by the U.S. Government.)

In addition to getting adequate calcium and vitamin D, it's important to note that moderate exercise that places weight on your bones, such as walking, helps maintain and may even increase bone density and strength in older adults.

Who's at Risk for Osteoporosis?

Anyone can get osteoporosis, but women are at greatest risk, especially white women who are thin, fair-skinned, and small in build. Aging itself, extreme immobility, and genetics, as well as smoking and drinking alcoholic beverages, are believed to contribute to risk for osteoporosis. Loss of calcium from the bones increases in women after menopause, when levels of the hormone estrogen decrease. Estrogen replacement therapy can be prescribed by a doctor to help decrease bone loss after menopause. Because estrogens may have negative side effects in some women, the decision to take estrogen should be made by each woman with the help of her doctor.

How to Get Enough Calcium If You Don't Drink Milk

Milk is the most obvious and popular source of both calcium and vitamin D, but some people don't drink it and need to consider other ways to get calcium. Some people have trouble digesting lactose, the sugar occurring naturally in milk. If you have trouble digesting milk:

- Drink milk that has had lactase added or add it yourself. Lactase is an enzyme that breaks down milk sugar. It can be purchased at many drug stores.

- Drink only a small amount of milk at a time.

- Eat yogurt or cheese. Lactose has been partially broken down in these foods.

- Try cooked foods made with milk such as soups, puddings, or custards.

173

If you don't like milk, eat more of other foods with calcium, such as:

- foods made with milk or cheese.

- tofu, a soy product that is sometimes made with calcium sulfate (check the label); ½ cup (4 ounces) of tofu made with calcium sulfate has about the same amount of calcium, protein, and fat as 1 cup of whole milk.

- dark-green leafy vegetables, such as kale, collards, and broccoli.

- tortillas made with cornmeal that is fortified with calcium; label may state that the cornmeal is processed with lime, or may list the cornmeal as "masa harina."

- canned or dried fish with edible bones, such as salmon and sardines.

Should You Take a Vitamin Supplement?

Thirty-seven percent of American adults take a daily multivitamin pill. Some even take extra vitamins and minerals as well, especially vitamin C. Yet most of these supplements are unnecessary for people of any age. A well-balanced diet should provide all of your nutritional needs. High doses of some vitamins, such as A and D, can be harmful. Large amounts of some supplements can upset the natural balance of nutrients normally maintained by the body. Large doses, called megavitamins, containing 10 to 100 times the RDA for a vitamin or mineral, can act like drugs, with potentially serious results.

While researchers continue to learn more about how nutrient requirements change during aging, eating a balanced diet containing foods from each food group is the best approach to getting the nutrients you need. Supplements may be beneficial for people who cannot eat a balanced diet or who do not eat enough food, or people who take medicines that interact with nutrients. Before you decide to take a nutritional supplement, discuss it with your doctor or dietitian. If you have specific health problems, or likes and dislikes that greatly limit your food choices, consult a registered dietitian (R.D.) for help in planning the best diet for you.

Drink Enough Fluids

The sense of thirst declines with age, so older people may not drink enough water and other fluids. Sometimes people intentionally drink less to avoid going to the bathroom often. But if you aren't getting enough fluids you can become dehydrated, especially during hot weather.

Drinking plenty of fluids is important to help your body flush out wastes—it's worth a few more trips to the bathroom. Most adults should drink at least eight glasses of water a day. This water can come from any beverage—juice, coffee, tea, milk, or soft drinks—as well as from soup. However, the caffeine in coffee and other drinks may increase your urge to urinate. The sugar in regular soft drinks is an added source of calories you may not need. Plain water, unsweetened fruit juices, and lowfat milk are better choices. Or, for a refreshing carbonated drink, mix fruit juice with club soda or seltzer water. To make plain water more appealing, try it chilled with a twist of lemon or lime.

What about Constipation?

Constipation bothers many older adults. The frequency of bowel movements among healthy people varies from three a day to three a week. Know what is normal for you and avoid relying on laxatives. Drinking enough fluids; eating plenty of fruits, vegetables, and whole-grain products for fiber; and exercising regularly can help with this condition.

Prevention of Constipation Is the Best Approach

- Eat foods with dietary fiber, such as whole-wheat breads and cereals, fruits, and vegetables every day.

- Drink plenty of liquids.

- Exercise regularly.

- Go to the bathroom when you feel the need. Don't delay.

Facts about Fiber

Dietary fiber (sometimes called "roughage") is the part of plant foods that humans can't digest. The fiber passes through the intestines, forming bulk for the stool. There are two major types of fiber—insoluble and soluble. Each has different health benefits, so both are needed in the diet. Insoluble fiber is most often found in whole-grain products, such as whole-wheat bread and cereals, fruits and vegetables with their peels, and dry beans and peas. Insoluble fiber helps prevent constipation. Diets high in insoluble fiber and low in fat may also reduce your risk of colon cancer.

Soluble fiber is found in fruits, vegetables, dry beans and peas, and some cereal products such as oatmeal, oat bran, and rice bran. Some research indicates that diets that are low in fat and saturated fat and rich in soluble fiber may help reduce blood cholesterol levels.

How Much Fiber Should You Eat?

It isn't clear yet exactly how much fiber you should eat each day. Some health experts have suggested that an increase to a range of 20 to 30 grams is a good idea. That's about twice what the average adult eats now. Because plant foods differ in the types and amounts of fiber they contain, it's a good idea to eat different kinds of foods rich in fiber. You can get about 20 grams of fiber if you eat three servings of whole-grain foods, two to three servings of fruit, and three to four servings of vegetables daily. You don't need to take fiber supplements or sprinkle bran on all your foods.

Are You Getting Enough Fiber in Your Diet?

How often do you eat:

1. Three or more servings of breads and cereals made with whole grains?
2. Starchy vegetables such as potatoes, corn, peas, or dishes made with dry beans or peas?
3. Several servings of other vegetables?
4. Whole fruit with skins and/or seeds (berries, apples, pears, etc.)?

The best answer is ALMOST DAILY. Whole-grain products, fruits, and vegetables provide fiber. Eating a variety of these foods daily will provide you with adequate fiber, both soluble and insoluble types.

Five Quick Tips to Increase Fiber in Your Diet

1. Try a whole-grain breakfast cereal, hot or cold. It doesn't have to be 100-percent bran—look for a cereal with at least 2 grams of dietary fiber per serving.
2. Choose baked goods made with whole grains, such as corn muffins; cracked wheat bread; graham crackers; oatmeal

bread or muffins; and whole-wheat, pumpernickel or rye breads, rolls, and bagels.

3. Eat fresh fruit or stewed fruit—an orange, half a grapefruit, prunes, or apricots—instead of drinking fruit juice.

4. Eat fruits and vegetables with their peels—apples, pears, peaches, potatoes, or summer squash.

5. Add cooked or canned dry beans, split peas, and lentils to your favorite soups, stews, and salads.

If you're not used to eating foods with fiber, increase fiber gradually to avoid gas or cramping. Be sure to drink enough water or other fluids when you eat more high-fiber foods.

Avoiding Problems When Medications and Foods Don't Mix

Many older adults take several medications, both prescription and over-the-counter types. It's important to find out from your doctor or pharmacist if these medicines are affected by food or beverages. Some medicines must be taken with meals, while others work better on an empty stomach. Some medicines may have serious or unpleasant side effects or may not work as well if taken in combination with certain foods or alcoholic beverages. Writing out a schedule for your meals and medicines can help you take your medicines properly and get adequate nutrition—both are important to your health.

Ask your doctor or pharmacist if there are special instructions about diet and if there are foods you should avoid when taking your medicine. You may need special advice about diet and:

- diuretics and other high blood pressure medicines,
- some antibiotics,
- some pain relievers,
- some antidepressants,
- anticoagulants (drugs for blood thinning),
- antacids.

Do You Take Medicines Properly?

When you get a new prescription medicine, be sure you understand when to take it, how much to take, how long to take it, and what to do if you miss a dose.

Tell your doctor about any other medicines you may be taking, including those prescribed by other doctors, over-the-counter medicines, and any vitamins or other supplements.

Ask whether there are foods or over-the-counter medicines you should not take with your new prescription.

Contact your doctor or pharmacist right away if you experience any side effects. If you are taking several medicines for long periods, ask your doctor every once in a while if you should still be taking all of them. Don't stop taking any prescribed medicines without consulting your doctor.

Make sure you understand the name of the drug and directions printed on the container. Ask your pharmacist to use large type if necessary. If child-proof containers are hard to handle, ask for easy-to-open containers.

Discard old prescription medicines and expired over-the-counter drugs. Never take drugs that were prescribed for a friend or relative, even though your symptoms may be the same.

Planning a Menu Using the Food Guide

The sample menu in Figure 20.3 shows how you might use the Food Guide Pyramid (shown in Figure 20.1). The 1,600-calorie menu includes the lower numbers of servings from the food groups, and the 2,400-calorie menu includes the higher numbers of servings shown in Table 20.2. Jelly, margarine, sherbet, and lemonade are extras, from the Fats, Oils, and Sweets group. Listed below are nutrient values for the two menus:

	1,600 Calorie Menu	2,400 Calorie Menu
Total fat, grams	46	75
% of calories	26	28
Saturated fat, grams	18	24
% of calories	10	9
Cholesterol, mg	185	235
Sodium, mg	2,190	3,010
Dietary fiber, grams	18	30

Menu

1,600 calories		2,400 calories
BREAKFAST		
1/2 medium	Grapefruit	1/2 medium
2 slices	Whole-wheat toast	2 slices
1 tsp.	Margarine, soft	2 tsp.
None	Jelly	1 tbsp.
1 cup	Milk, skim	1 cup
LUNCH		
6 fl. oz.	Vegetable juice, no salt added	6 fl. oz.
	Luncheon salad:	
1 oz.	Turkey	2 oz.
1 oz.	Ham	1 oz.
1-1/2 oz.	Swiss cheese	1-1/2 oz.
1-1/2 cups	Mixed greens	1-1/2 cups
1 tbsp.	French dressing, low calorie	1-1/2 tbsp.
2 small	Corn muffins	3 small
1 medium	Peach, fresh	2 medium
DINNER		
3 oz.	Sirloin steak, broiled (lean only)	3 oz.
1/2 cup	Yellow corn, fresh or frozen	1 cup
1/2 cup	Stewed tomatoes, no salt added	1/2 cup
1 small	Whole-grain roll	2 small
1 tsp.	Margarine, soft	1 tsp.
1/2 cup	Lime sherbet	1/2 cup
As desired	Coffee, tea, or water	As desired
SNACKS		
None	Peanut butter sandwich	1 sandwich
	2 slices of whole-wheat bread	
	2 tbsp. of peanut butter	
	2 tsp. of jelly	
3 squares	Graham crackers	None
8 fl. oz.	Lemonade	8 fl. oz.

Figure 20.3. Sample Menu for 1,600 calories and 2,400 calories

Ask Yourself

- Do I eat foods from all the food groups each day?

- Am I getting enough calcium-rich foods?

- Do I need to take a vitamin supplement, or can I add foods to my diet that will provide me with the nutrients I need?

- Have I discussed the vitamins I take with my doctor or dietitian?

- How much fluid do I drink each day?

- Are these fluids high in calories?

- Do I know how all of the medications I am taking interact with foods or drinks?

Questions Older People Ask

New information about nutrition seems to come out each day. Often, the information does not address the concerns of older adults. This section answers some common questions older people ask about nutrition.

Are There Any Foods or Vitamins That Can Help Prevent Memory Loss?

As of now, there is no reliable evidence that any foods or vitamins can help prevent memory loss such as occurs in Alzheimer's disease. Choline and lecithin have been tried to treat Alzheimer's, but neither was successful. People with Alzheimer's are at a greater risk for developing nutritional deficiencies, which can cause additional problems. Other kinds of severe memory loss and confusion are caused by excessive alcohol intake or by a deficiency of vitamin B_{12} or folate. A B_{12} deficiency can sometimes be reversed by injections of this vitamin. It's important for anyone showing signs of memory loss and confusion to have a complete checkup, including a nutritional evaluation. Ask your health care provider.

Is There Such a Thing as "Good Cholesterol"?

You may have heard the terms "good cholesterol" and "bad cholesterol." These terms refer to substances called lipoproteins, which are "transport vehicles" that carry cholesterol in the blood. There are several kinds of lipoproteins. High-density lipoprotein (HDL) is often called the "good" kind because it removes cholesterol from the bloodstream, carrying it to the liver. The "bad" kind of cholesterol is transported by low-density lipoprotein (LDL). This is the cholesterol that gets deposited inside the arteries, where it may build up over time and eventually block the flow of blood. High levels of LDL increase your risk of heart disease, while high HDL levels lower your risk.

Diet can affect levels of LDL and HDL in the blood, but there are no foods that contain these substances. A cholesterol screening usually tells you the total amount of cholesterol circulating in your blood, but not how much of it comes from HDL and LDL. If your total cholesterol level is over 200 mg/dl and you have other risk factors for heart disease, your doctor may request another blood test to find out what your HDL and LDL levels are. This test must be done after you fast for 12 hours. Talk with your doctor about how the various components of blood cholesterol affect your risk.

I Have Trouble with My Teeth and Gums and Have Difficulty Eating Raw Vegetables. How Can I Get Enough Fiber?

Cooked vegetables and fruits also supply fiber in your diet, as do cooked cereals and baked goods that contain whole grains. These will be much easier to chew. See your dentist or ask for a referral to one who specializes in dental problems of older adults. Much can be done to help your teeth and gums to make eating a variety of foods more enjoyable.

Things Just Don't Taste Good to Me, So I Have No Interest in Eating. What Can I Do to Perk Up My Appetite?

People often find that their senses of taste and smell get duller as they age. As a result, they may overload their food with salt or even lose interest in food. Be creative with herbs, spices, and lemon juice. They all add flavor that can perk up your taste again. Experiment with different spices to see what appeals to you. You may even want to try growing fresh herbs, either in your garden or in a pot on a sunny windowsill. Trying new recipes and choosing colorful foods in a variety of textures may also add interest to your meals.

I Hate Eating Alone and as a Result, I Often Skip Meals. How Can I Make Eating Interesting?

Eating alone can be boring and sometimes even depressing. Many people don't want to spend time preparing meals just for themselves. Make an effort to make meals enjoyable. Try some of these ideas:

- Plan meals, set the table, light candles, play music, or eat when a television show you like is on. You deserve the same effort and care in preparing your own meals as the guests you might serve for a dinner party.

- Invite friends over for meals. You could each bring a part of the meal or trade portions of "planned leftovers."

- Eat out once a week or so. Many restaurants have lower prices and smaller portions at lunchtime. Some may offer reduced prices for older adults. Plan a daytime outing with a friend—go to lunch and visit a museum or attend an afternoon concert or theater performance.

- Visit a senior center at lunchtime; participate in meals offered through your local agency on aging.

- Form a gourmet club with others who eat alone.

I've Never Liked Eating Breakfast. Do I Need to Eat Breakfast to Have a Healthy Diet?

It's not necessary to eat a big meal first thing in the morning. The important goal is to eat a balanced diet that includes foods from all the food groups each day. Set an eating pattern that works for you. For example, perhaps you like a mid-morning snack instead of a formal breakfast. Just be sure to make it a healthy snack, such as fruit and a muffin or toast. Often, people who skip meals eat too many snacks filled with empty calories.

What Can I Eat to Help My Arthritis?

Unfortunately, there is no food that relieves the pain of arthritis, but scientists are doing a lot of research in this area. You may see advertisements for food products or supplements that promise relief, but in truth they won't help you. A balanced diet will contribute to your overall good health, and avoiding too much weight will put less strain on your joints. There are also many simple tools such as jar openers that you can use to help you with everyday tasks. Contact your local chapter of the Arthritis Foundation, listed in the telephone book, for more information.

Can I Always Believe What I Read in the Newspaper?

New research about diet and health often gets in the newspaper or appears on the evening news, but no matter how promising or discouraging this news may be, making changes in your diet based on a single report is not wise. Government agencies and health organizations, such as the U.S. Departments of Agriculture and of Health and Human Services (USDA and DHHS), the National Academy of Sciences, and the American Heart Association, base their recommendations on dozens of studies carried out over many years. These groups continuously review new research findings and make recommendations only when there is widespread agreement among experts.

How Do I Know When a Claim That a Food Product or Supplement Cures Diseases Is True?

These claims can be dangerous because they often prevent users from getting the medical help they need. They also create false hopes and waste money. In general, if it sounds too good to be true, it is. Suspect a product if it:

- makes outrageous claims, like curing a disease or reversing the aging process. No product or food has yet been proven to do either.
- promises immediate or fast results.
- does not list ingredients.
- cites only one study or a preliminary study as proof of results.
- does not give information about possible side effects.
- claims to be a secret formula.
- is available only from one source.

I Don't Eat Many Dairy Products. How Can I Get Enough Calcium?

People who have trouble digesting milk can usually drink it in small amounts or can drink milk to which the enzyme lactase has been added. Buttermilk, yogurt, or cheese are good alternatives and are easier to digest. Other people simply don't like milk or dairy products. Calcium can be found in other foods. It's found naturally in leafy green vegetables like kale and broccoli. It's also added to some products such as fruit juice. It's best to get as much calcium as you can from the food you eat. If you feel you are not getting enough from foods, discuss whether you should take a calcium supplement (and what kind) with your doctor or dietitian.

I Take Diuretics. How Can I Get Enough Potassium?

First of all it's important to know if the diuretic you take is one that depletes potassium or one that has little effect on it. Generally, the more potent diuretics produce significant potassium losses. You should discuss the specific drug you are taking with the doctor who prescribed it for you. Most people's diets do not provide enough potassium to make up for what is lost due to the diuretic. However, proper choice of foods can effectively replace potassium losses.

Most foods provide some potassium. Fruits, vegetables, milk, and yogurt are among the best sources. Some meats, poultry, and fish are good sources too. Here are some common foods that are good sources of potassium:

- bran cereals
- cooked dried fruit such as apricots, peaches, prunes
- bananas
- potatoes, baked or boiled
- sweet potatoes, pumpkin, winter squash
- stewed tomatoes
- lima beans
- cooked dry beans, peas, lentils
- milk and yogurt (all types)

Did You Know?

One baked potato (even without the skin) has 610 mg of potassium; one banana (well-known as a good source of potassium) has 450 mg.

Chapter 21

Malnutrition in the Elderly: A National Crisis

18 Facts about Malnutrition in the Elderly

1. Malnutrition occurs too frequently in the elderly (65 years of age and over)—fueling the health care crisis even though it is preventable.

   - One in four elderly in the community are malnourished.
   - 35–55% of elderly patients in acute care hospitals are malnourished.
   - Two in five elderly in long term care facilities are malnourished.

2. 85% of older Americans have chronic diseases that could be helped by nutritional intervention according to the U.S. Senate Committee on Education and Labor.

3. Malnutrition compromises the immune system and contributes to the development of infection, poor wound healing, serious complications, sepsis, multi-system organ failure, disability, longer hospital stays, death, and catastrophic health care costs.

4. Malnutrition significantly increases hospital stay and direct medical costs.

Excerpted from *Malnutrition in the Elderly: A National Problem*, Region X, U.S. Administration on Aging, Seattle Washington, 1996.

5. Socio-economic factors, such as poverty and social isolation, increase risk of malnutrition in the elderly. Statistics of the elderly show:

   - 33% live alone

   - 20% skip at least one meal a day

   - 42% women and 17% men have annual incomes of less than $6000/year, making it difficult to budget for food.

6. Polypharmacy increases risk of drug-induced malnutrition due to alteration of appetite, absorption and metabolism of nutrients. It also increases risk of drug-drug interactions and drug-nutrient interactions. Statistics show that the elderly, 65 years and older:

   - Use multiple prescription drugs

   - Consume 25% of all prescription medication

   - Use 40 to 90% of over-the-counter drugs (non-prescription)

7. The signs of malnutrition and inactivity mimic the effects of aging, leading to delayed recognition of poor nutrition in the elderly.

8. Physical inactivity is associated with many of the leading causes of death and disability in the U.S. Maintaining musculoskeletal mass in the elderly is critical to preventing disability, falls, and hip fractures.

9. Medical and nursing schools place little emphasis on nutrition. In a 1988 survey, only 27% of medical schools required a nutrition course. Consequently, there is widespread lack of education among health care professionals and the public regarding:

   - Risk factors, major and minor indicators of poor nutritional health

   - How to do nutritional screening

   - How to initiate intervention strategies

   - The critical role nutrition plays in health promotion and disease prevention

10. Obesity masks malnutrition and is associated with increased risk for diabetes mellitus, hypertension, cardiovascular disease, stroke, sleep apnea, gout, and osteoarthritis. 25% or more elderly are overweight.

11. Billions of dollars can be saved by a five-year delay in onset of age-related diseases or hip fractures.

12. America is graying. By the year 2010, one in seven Americans will be 65 or older and by 2030, this will increase to one in five.

13. Few health insurance policies offer reimbursement for routine nutrition screening and early intervention.

14. Fragmentation and lack of interdisciplinary collaboration in health care practice exists. The expertise of dietitians, pharmacists, and physical therapists is poorly utilized.

15. Health care professionals are unaware of programs funded under the Older American's Act and the important role these programs play in providing continuum of health care.

16. "Healthy People 2000' calls for at least 75% of primary care providers to provide nutrition assessment and counseling.

17. Mental, oral, physical, and nutritional health are all intricately dependent upon each other. Oral problems affecting kinds and amounts of food eaten can affect physical, mental, and nutritional health, or vice versa. Many dementias have been caused by metabolic disorders, drug toxicity, dehydration, B_{12} deficiency, and malnutrition.

18. Malnutrition is a major factor in readmission to hospitals.

What Is Malnutrition?

In order to further discuss the causes, risks, consequences of, and solutions to malnutrition, we offer you definitions of malnutrition and nutrition.

As defined in Webster's New World Dictionary:

- Malnutrition is... "faulty or inadequate nutrition; poor nourishment resulting from insufficient food, improper diet, etc."

- Nutrition is... "A nourishing or being nourished; especially the series of processes by which an organism takes in and assimilates food for promoting and replacing worn or injured tissues."

As defined in Mosby's Medical Dictionary:

- Malnutrition is... "any disorder of nutrition. It may result from an unbalanced, insufficient, or excessive diet or from the impaired absorption, assimilation or use of foods."

- Nutrition is... "the sum of the processes involved in the taking in of nutrients and in their assimilation and use for proper body functioning and maintenance of health. The successive stages include ingestion, digestion, absorption, assimilation, and excretion."

Types of malnutrition (poor nutritional status) in varying combinations and degrees include:

- Deficiencies of nutrients
- Imbalances of nutrients
- Excesses of nutrients

What Causes Malnutrition/Poor Nutritional Status?

Malnutrition is caused by anything that interferes with the body's supply of adequate nutrient(s) at the cellular level:

- Ingestion
- Digestion
- Absorption
- Metabolism
- Assimilation (utilization—getting nutrients to the tissues)
- Excretion

Deficiencies, imbalances, and excesses of nutrient(s) in varying combinations and degrees are included. Stress, illness, and medication can alter the needs of the body.

Risk factors for malnutrition are multifactorial and multifaceted. They include:

- Physiological factors (including age-related factors)
- Socioeconomic factors
- Psychological factors

Inherent in these factors are risk factors and major and minor indicators.

Risk Factors

- Inappropriate food intake
- Poverty
- Social isolation
- Dependency/disability

- Acute/chronic diseases or conditions
- Chronic medication use
- Advanced age (80+)

Major Indicators

- Weight loss of 10 lbs. +
- Underweight/overweight
- Serum albumin below 3.5 g/dl
- Change in functional status
- Inappropriate food intake
- Mid-arm muscle circumference <10th percentile
- Triceps skinfold <10th percentile or >95th percentile
- Obesity
- Nutrition-related disorders
  - —Osteoporosis
  - —Osteomalacia
  - —Folate deficiency
- B_{12} deficiency

Minor Indicators

- Alcoholism
- Cognitive impairment
- Chronic renal insufficiency
- Multiple concurrent medications
- Malabsorption syndromes
- Anorexia, nausea, dysphagia
- Change in bowel habit
- Fatigue, apathy, memory loss
- Poor oral/dental status
- Dehydration
- Poorly healing wounds
- Loss of subcutaneous fat or muscle mass
- Fluid retention
- Reduced iron, ascorbic acid, zinc

Medical Practices Which Contribute to Malnutrition

- Inadequate surveillance of nutritional status, both in and out of the hospital or institution

- Prolonged use of glucose and saline intravenous fluids as the only source of nutrition

- Failure to evaluate and record weight loss or gain
- Failure to observe patient food intake
- Failure to identify oral problems or mental health problems that can affect nutritional status and physical health of the elderly
- Withholding meals for diagnostic tests
- Surgery on undernourished patients without nutritional intervention
- Failure to recognize increased metabolic needs of illness, stress, injury
- Failure to give nutritional support after surgery
- Prolonged bedrest and inactivity

How Do Physiological Factors and Age-Related Changes Affect Nutritional Status?

Aging is a process, not a disease. Everyone ages but at different rates and in different ways. The cumulative effects of malnutrition and lack of exercise are often mistakenly contributed to "old age."

Changes in body composition occur with aging. The body makes fewer metabolically active cells (protein and bone). This means that there is a reduction in total body protein (muscle, organs, skeletal tissue, protein compartments, immune functions, antigens, and red and white blood cells). Adequate nutrition, exercise, and muscle toning have been proven to slow this process or vice versa.

Changes in Body Composition Occur with Aging

- The body makes fewer metabolically active cells
  - Protein
  - Bone

- Reduction in total body protein, bone mass, and bone density
  - Muscle
  - Organs
  - Immune cells
  - Blood cells
  - Bones

- Body fat increases as muscle mass decreases. (Obesity can mask loss of muscle mass.)

- Strength decreases as muscle mass decreases.
- Decrease in total body water (related to a decrease in lean body mass). (Approximately 72% of muscle and organ cell tissue is made up of water.)

Caloric needs decline as people lose lean body mass, but other nutrient requirements stay the same.

- Protein
- Fiber
- Water
- Vitamins & minerals
- Trace elements
- Carbohydrates
- Fat

Problems affecting intake of needed nutrients:

- Physiological
  - Chronic illness
  - Oral/dental problems
  - Medication use
  - Sensory changes
  - Physical disabilities
  - A Socioeconomical
  - Poverty
  - Social isolation
  - Dependency
- Psychological
  - Depression
  - Mental/Cognitive problems
- Lack of nutritional knowledge

How Does Malnutrition Affect the Body?

The human body consists of billions of specialized cells that make up the various organs, body systems, and structure. They require adequate food, air, water, and exercise to live and function properly. When these basic needs are not provided:

- Cells die
- Immune system becomes depressed

- Illness/disease/disability ensue
- Catastrophic costs are generated

The Body Cannibalizes Itself in an Effort to Survive

Figure 21.1 illustrates the cascading effects of protein-calorie malnutrition in which the body cannibalizes itself, breaks down its own lean body mass in an effort to survive. Proteins are broken down for energy. Nutrition screening will identify individuals at risk of poor nutritional status and pinpoint needed intervention. Early intervention will prevent the illness, disease, disability, and catastrophic costs generated by protein-calorie malnutrition.

Consequences of Inactivity & Malnutrition: Inactivity Breeds Disability

With inactivity and malnutrition, muscles atrophy, bones lose their density and become porous. When muscle mass atrophies, it leads to:

- Functional disability: increased falls and injuries
- Compromised immune system
- Compromised respiratory function

Normal aging is associated with:

- A progressive decrease in body protein
- A progressive decrease in lean body mass at the cellular and tissue levels
- A progressive reduction in bone mass

Prevention of age-related disabilities is possible through:

- Nutrition screening/ intervention
- Nutrition programs
- Exercise and muscle toning program

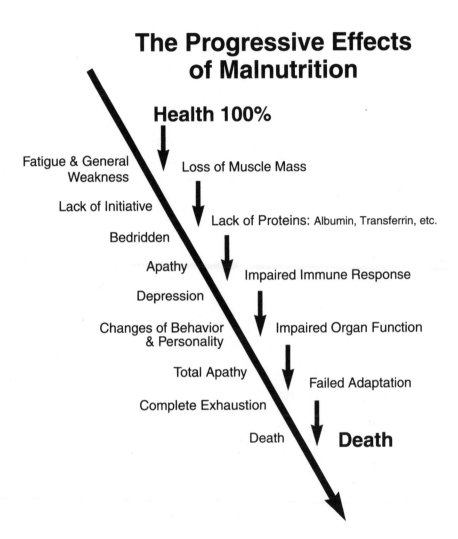

Figure 21.1. The cascading effects of protein-caloric malnutrition.

Part Three

Nutrition for People with Specific Medical Concerns

Chapter 22

Coping with Food Allergies

Do you start itching whenever you eat peanuts? Does seafood cause your stomach to churn? Symptoms like these cause millions of Americans to suspect they have a food allergy.

But true food allergies affect a relatively small percentage of people: Experts estimate that only 2 percent of adults, and from 2 to 8 percent of children, are truly allergic to certain foods. Food allergy is different from food intolerance, and the term is sometimes used in a vague, all-encompassing way, muddying the waters for people who want to understand what a real food allergy is.

"Many people who have a complaint, an illness, or some discomfort attribute it to something they have eaten. Because in this country we eat almost all the time, people tend to draw false associations between food and illness," says Dean Metcalfe, M.D., head of the Mast Cell and Physiology Section at the National Institute of Allergy and Infectious Diseases.

Allergy and Intolerance—Different Problems

The difference between an allergy and an intolerance is how the body handles the offending food. In a true food allergy, the body's immune system recognizes a reaction-provoking substance, or allergen, in the food—usually a protein—as foreign and produces antibodies to halt the "invasion." As the battle rages, symptoms appear

"Food Allergies: Rare But Risky," *FDA Consumer*, May 1994; updated June 1997.

197

throughout the body. The most common sites are the mouth (swelling of the lips), digestive tract (stomach cramps, vomiting, diarrhea), skin (hives, rashes or eczema), and the airways (wheezing or breathing problems). People with allergies must avoid the offending foods altogether.

Cow's milk, eggs, wheat, and soy are the most common sources of food allergies in children. Allergists believe that infant allergies are the result of immunologic immaturity and, to some extent, intestinal immaturity. Children sometimes outgrow the allergies they had as infants, but an early peanut allergy may be lifelong. Adults are usually most affected by tree nuts, fish, shellfish, and peanuts.

Food intolerance is a much more common problem than allergy. Here, the problem is not with the body's immune system, but, rather, with its metabolism. The body cannot adequately digest a portion of the offending food, usually because of some chemical deficiency. For example, persons who have difficulty digesting milk (lactose intolerance) often are deficient in the intestinal enzyme lactase, which is needed to digest milk sugar (lactose). The deficiency can cause cramps and diarrhea if milk is consumed. Estimates are that about 80 percent of African-Americans have lactose intolerance, as do many people of Mediterranean or Hispanic origin. It is quite different from the true allergic reaction some have to the proteins in milk. Unlike allergies, intolerances generally intensify with age.

Dangerous Dishes

For people with true food allergies, the simple pleasure of eating can turn into an uncomfortable—and sometimes even dangerous—situation. For some, food allergies cause only hives or an upset stomach; for others, one bite of the wrong food can lead to serious illness or even death.

Food intolerance may produce symptoms similar to food allergies, such as abdominal cramping. But while people with true food allergies must avoid offending foods altogether, people with food intolerance can often eat some of the offending food without suffering symptoms. The amount that may be eaten before symptoms appear is usually very small and varies with each individual.

When Food Additives Are a Problem

Over the years, people have reported to FDA adverse reactions to certain food additives, including aspartame (a sweetener), monosodium glutamate (a flavor enhancer), sulfur-based preservatives, and tartrazine, also known as FD&C Yellow No. 5 (a food color). The federal Food, Drug, and Cosmetic Act requires that FDA ensure the safety of all substances added to foods, but individual health conditions sometimes cause problems with certain additives.

Aspartame

After reviewing scientific studies, FDA determined in 1981 that aspartame was safe for use in foods. In 1987, the General Accounting Office investigated the process surrounding FDA's approval of aspartame and confirmed the agency had acted properly. However, FDA has continued to review complaints alleging adverse reactions to products containing aspartame. To date, FDA has not determined any consistent pattern of symptoms that can be attributed to the use of aspartame, nor is the agency aware of any recent studies that clearly show safety problems.

Carefully controlled clinical studies show that aspartame is not an allergen. However, certain people with the genetic disease phenylketonuria (PKU), those with advanced liver disease, and pregnant women with hyperphenylalanine (high levels of phenylalanine in blood) have a problem with aspartame because they do not effectively metabolize the amino acid phenylalanine, one of aspartame's components. High levels of this amino acid in body fluids can cause brain damage. Therefore, FDA has ruled that all products containing aspartame must include a warning to phenylketonurics that the sweetener contains phenylalanine.

Monosodium glutamate

Monosodium glutamate (MSG) has been used for many years in home and restaurant foods, and in processed foods. People sensitive to MSG may have mild and transitory reactions when they eat foods that contain large amounts of MSG (such as would be found in heavily flavor-enhanced foods). Because MSG is commonly used in Chinese cuisine, these reactions were initially referred to as "Chinese restaurant syndrome."

FDA believes that MSG is a safe food ingredient for the general population. It is regarded by the agency as among food ingredients that are "generally recognized as safe." FDA has studied adverse reaction reports and other data concerning MSG's safety. The agency also has an ongoing contract with the Federation of American Societies for Experimental Biology to re-examine the scientific data on possible adverse reactions to glutamate in general. MSG must be declared on the label of any food to which it is added.

Sulfites

Of all the food additives for which FDA has received adverse reaction reports, the ones that most closely resemble true allergens are sulfur-based preservatives. Sulfites are used primarily as antioxidants to prevent or reduce discoloration of light-colored fruits and vegetables, such as dried apples and potatoes, and to inhibit the growth of microorganisms in fermented foods such as wine.

Though most people don't have a problem with sulfites, they are a hazard of unpredictable severity to people, particularly asthmatics, who are sensitive to these substances. FDA uses the term "allergic-type responses" to describe the range of symptoms suffered by these individuals after eating sulfite-treated foods. Responses range from mild to life-threatening.

FDA's sulfite specialists say scientists, at this time, are not sure how the body reacts to sulfites. To help sulfite-sensitive people avoid problems, FDA requires the presence of sulfites in processed foods to be declared on the label, and prohibits the use of sulfites on fresh produce intended to be sold or served raw to consumers.

FD&C Yellow No. 5

Color additives must go through the same safety approval process as food additives. But one color, FD&C Yellow No. 5 (listed as tartrazine on medicine labels), may prompt itching or hives in a small number of people.

Since 1980 (for drugs taken orally) and 1981 (for foods), FDA has required all products containing Yellow No. 5 to list it on the labels so sensitive consumers could avoid it. (As of May 8, 1993, food labels must list all certified colors as part of the requirements of the Nutrition Labeling and Education Act of 1990.)

True Allergies

Heredity may cause a predisposition to have allergies of any type, and repeated exposure to allergens starts sensitizing those who are susceptible. Some experts believe that, rarely, a specific allergy can be passed on from parent to child. Several studies have indicated that exclusive breast-feeding, especially with maternal avoidance of major food allergens, may deter some food allergies in infants and young children. (Smoking during pregnancy can also result in the increased possibility that the baby will have allergies.) Most patients who have true food allergies have other types of allergies, such as dust or pollen, and children with both food allergies and asthma are at increased risk for more severe reactions.

Life-Threatening Reactions

The greatest danger in food allergy comes from anaphylaxis, a violent allergic reaction involving a number of parts of the body simultaneously. Like less serious allergic reactions, anaphylaxis usually occurs after a person is exposed to an allergen to which he or she was sensitized by previous exposure (that is, it does not usually occur the first time a person eats a particular food). Although any food can trigger anaphylaxis (also known as anaphylactic shock), peanuts, tree nuts, shellfish, milk, eggs, and fish are the most common culprits. As little as one-fifth to one-five-thousandth of a teaspoon of the offending food has caused death.

Anaphylaxis can produce severe symptoms in as little as 5 to 15 minutes, although life-threatening reactions may progress over hours. Signs of such a reaction include: difficulty breathing, feeling of impending doom, swelling of the mouth and throat, a drop in blood pressure, and loss of consciousness. The sooner that anaphylaxis is treated, the greater the person's chance of surviving. The person should be taken to a hospital emergency room, even if symptoms seem to subside on their own.

There is no specific test to predict the likelihood of anaphylaxis, although allergy testing may help determine what a person may be allergic to and provide some guidance as to the severity of the allergy. Experts advise people who are susceptible to anaphylaxis to carry medication, such as injectable epinephrine, with them at all times, and to check the medicine's expiration date regularly. Doctors can instruct patients with allergies on how to self-administer epinephrine. Such prompt treatment can be crucial to survival.

Injectable epinephrine is a synthetic version of a naturally occurring hormone also known as adrenaline. For treatment of an anaphylactic reaction, it is injected directly into a thigh muscle or vein. It works directly on the cardiovascular and respiratory systems, causing rapid constriction of blood vessels, reversing throat swelling, relaxing lung muscles to improve breathing, and stimulating the heartbeat.

Epinephrine designed for emergency home use comes in two forms: a traditional needle and syringe kit known as Ana-Kit, or an automatic injector system known as Epi-Pen. Epi-Pen's automatic injector design, originally developed for use by military personnel to deliver antidotes for nerve gas, is described by some as "a fat pen." The patient removes the safety cap and pushes the automatic injector tip against the outer thigh until the unit activates. The patient holds the "pen" in place for several seconds, then throws it away.

While Epi-Pen delivers one premeasured dosage, the Ana-Kit provides two doses. Which system a patient uses is a decision to be made by the doctor and patient, taking into account the doctor's assessment of the patient's individual needs.

Advice from Study

Hugh A. Sampson, M.D., and colleagues at Johns Hopkins University School of Medicine in Baltimore, MD., published a study of anaphylactic reactions in children in the August 6, 1992, issue of the *New England Journal of Medicine*. The study involved 13 children who had severe allergic reactions to food: Six died, and seven nearly died. Among the study's conclusions:

- Asthma, a disease with allergic underpinnings, was common to all children in the study.

- Epinephrine should be prescribed and kept available for those with severe food allergies.

- Children who have an allergic reaction should be observed for three to four hours after a reaction in a medical center capable of dealing with anaphylaxis.

Anne Munoz-Furlong, who founded The Food Allergy Network for people with food allergies in 1991 after struggling to deal with her own child's allergies, comments: "My youngest daughter was diagnosed with milk and egg allergies when she was 9 months old, nine years ago. We tried to lead a life around her restricted diet. For example, we had Jell-O mold for her first birthday because I didn't know it was possible to create a cake without milk or eggs. I knew there must be other families struggling with the same issue."

Finding the Forbidden

Because there is no "cure" for food allergies other than strict avoidance of an offending food, one of the biggest problems those with food allergies face is verifying whether a forbidden product is contained in a particular food. For example, in Sampson's study, all six deaths occurred because either the child or the parent was unaware the food contained a substance to which the child was allergic. Munoz-Furlong says the Nutrition Labeling and Education Act, which requires more complete food labeling, should greatly help people with food allergies to avoid dangerous foods.

"The new labeling changes will make it easier for the consumer to readily identify things they could be allergic to," says Linda Tollefson, D.V.M., chief of the epidemiology branch at FDA's Center for Food Safety and Applied Nutrition. "Before this law was passed, true allergens were required to be on the label, but the exceptions were standardized foods, which will now have to list all ingredients."

According to Elizabeth J. Campbell, director of the center's division of programs and enforcement policy, the principle underlying standardized foods originally was that people basically knew what was in various foods.

"Originally, food standards were adopted to ensure uniformity. If you saw a product labeled mayonnaise, food standardization meant it had to be mayonnaise. People used to know what was in mayonnaise; nowadays they have to be told that mayonnaise contains both eggs and oil," Campbell says. "Years ago, when the law was first written to provide for standards of identity for certain foods, it only required that optional ingredients be declared. The new law stipulates that all ingredients in standardized foods must be declared."

Campbell believes that once the labeling is in place, consumers will have the information they need to make correct food choices. "In most cases, ingredients have to be labeled simply because they are ingredients, not because they are unsafe," she stresses. "For those with food allergies, I think it is more of a patient education problem."

Food additives, such as sulfites and certain colors, can also cause problems for people sensitive to them.

"If you have a food allergy, you really have to alter your life," Tollefson says. "You have to really read labels, and really be careful about what you eat."

Steve Taylor, Ph.D., a professor and head of Department of Food Science and Technology at the University of Nebraska in Lincoln, says the biggest problem for people with food allergies is restaurant food. Historically, restaurants have been regulated by local heath departments and have not had to label foods.

"For many restaurants, labeling of food products they serve would cause horrendous problems...what about chalkboard menus? How would you include all the ingredients? Enforcement would be a nightmare," he admits.

But steps are being taken to better educate restaurant employees. The Food Allergy Network and The American Academy of Allergy and Immunology, along with the National Restaurant Association, recently produced a pamphlet on food allergies, which has been distributed to 30,000 members of the association. The brochure explains what restaurants can do to help customers who need to avoid certain foods, defines anaphylaxis, and advises employees on what to do if food allergy incidents occur.

John A. Anderson, M.D., director of the Allergy and Immunology Training Program at Henry Ford Hospital in Detroit, says changes in food habits may be responsible for the feeling some physicians have that food allergies may be on the rise.

"You could make a case for the fact that we are introducing peanuts, in the form of peanut butter, to people at a very young age, which would affect the prevalence rate for people who are sensitive to that allergen," he notes. "In Japan, where they use more soy, there is a higher prevalence of soy allergy. My feeling is that as soy, a cheap protein supplement, is put in a lot of commercial foods you will see an increase in the rate sensitivity worldwide."

Metcalfe says that if food allergies are rising, it is due to more common use of foods that tend to be allergenic. He cites milk as a source of protein supplement in many prepared foods, and points out that people are eating more exotic seafood and more fish.

"But it's important to remember that the majority of people with true food allergies are allergic to three or fewer foods," Metcalfe says.

Other than advising anyone with a known or suspected severe food allergy to carry and know how to self-administer epinephrine, there is no treatment for food allergy other than to eliminate the offending food. But Metcalfe is optimistic about the future.

"I don't think it is likely a drug will be found to prevent food allergies. But I do think within 10 years we will see allergy shots available for some of the more common food allergies, because we are learning to identify and purify food allergens. I think we will see some development of immunotherapy for food allergies," he says.

Food Allergies and Biotechnology

People with food allergies have expressed the concern that new varieties of food, developed through the new techniques of biotechnology (such as gene splicing), may introduce allergens not found in the food before it was altered.

FDA addressed this concern in its 1992 biotechnology policy statement and said it will regulate whole foods developed through biotechnology by applying the same rigorous safety standards as for all other foods. The agency is taking steps to ensure that foods developed though biotechnology do not pose any new risks for consumers.

Under the new policy guidelines, a protein copied by genetic engineering from a food commonly known to cause an allergic reaction is presumed to be allergenic unless clearly proven otherwise. Any food product of biotechnology that contains such proteins must list the allergen on the label.

Labeling would not be required if the manufacturer could demonstrate that the allergen was not transferred. For example, if a food company were to breed potatoes containing a genetically engineered soy protein (to which some people might be allergic), the labeling on the potatoes would have to disclose the presence of the soy protein. But labeling would not be required if scientific data clearly showed that the protein had been changed and no longer contained the soy allergen.

To ensure that FDA has state-of-the-art information for its food biotechnology policy, the agency will sponsor a scientific conference in the spring of 1994 to discuss what makes a substance a food allergen.

How to Cope

What should you do if you suspect you have a food allergy?

The Food Allergy Network's Anne Munoz-Furlong suggests keeping a food diary as a first step, writing down everything you eat or drink for a one- or two-week period. Note any symptoms and how long it took for such symptoms to develop.

But Furlong and other experts agree that those who suspect food allergies also need to be evaluated by a physician with intensive specialty training in allergy and immunology. Be sure to discuss what diagnostic and treatment plan is anticipated, and the costs.

Ask if the tests have been proven effective by accepted standards of scientific evaluation.

"Go to a board-certified physician who is an allergy expert," advises Paul C. Turkeltaub, M.D., associate director of the division of allergenic products and parasitology at FDA's Center for Biologics Evaluation and Research. "Be very wary of claims of food allergy to explain chronic, common complaints."

The diagnosis of food allergy requires a careful history, physical exam, appropriate exclusion diet, and diagnostic test to rule out other conditions. Tests can include direct allergy skin tests, blood tests, or "elimination and challenge" tests for suspected foods.

The most accurate kind of test is a controlled challenge test, often done in "blind" or "double-blind" fashion to eliminate psychological factors. In a blind challenge, the patient is given either a sample of the food, without being told what it is, or a placebo, an inert substance used as a control in the test. The observer (a doctor or assistant), however, knows what the substance is. Both patient and observer record any symptoms of allergic reaction. In a double-blind challenge, neither the patient nor the observer knows if the patient is given the food (allergen) or the placebo.

In recent years, unproven tests such as "food cytotoxic blood tests" and "sublingual provocation food testing" have been promoted as supposed "diagnostic" tools to detect food allergies. FDA believes that food cytotoxic blood tests are not supported by well-controlled studies and clinical trials.

In food cytotoxic testing, a test tube of blood is taken from the patient. The white cells (leukocytes) are mixed with plasma and sterile water and placed on microscope slides coated with dried extracts of a particular food. The reaction of the cells is then examined under a microscope; if they change shape, disintegrate, or collapse—or the person examining them says they do—the patient is supposedly allergic to that particular food. Test results may be interpreted by a "nutritional counselor" working on commission, who recommends vitamins and minerals (often available on site) that the patient needs to correct his or her "allergic condition." But FDA and other experts emphasize there is no evidence that such tests are valid in diagnosing food allergies.

Sublingual provocation food testing dates back to 1944. The test consists of placing three drops of an allergenic extract under a patient's tongue and waiting 10 minutes for any symptoms to appear. When the doctor is satisfied he has determined the cause of the symptoms, he administers a "neutralizing" dose, which is usually three drops of a diluted solution of the same allergenic extract. The symptoms are then expected to disappear in the same sequence in which they appeared. Advocates claim that if the neutralizing dose is given before a challenge test (for instance, eating a meal containing the offending food), the person will not have symptoms.

But after careful study of existing data, The American Academy of Allergy and Immunology says no controlled clinical studies demonstrate either diagnostic or therapeutic effects of sublingual provocation food testing. The academy concludes that use of the tests should be reserved for experiments in well-designed trials.

If you are diagnosed with a food allergy, scrutinize food labels to detect potential sources food allergens. When eating out, ask about ingredients if you are unsure about a particular food; ask to talk to the manager of the restaurant about ingredients in specific dishes.

Keep epinephrine with you and know how to administer it. If you do experience a reaction, seek medical attention immediately, even if the symptoms are mild or seem to subside. Mild symptoms may be followed 10 to 60 minutes later by the onset of severe problems.

More Information

For more information about food allergies, contact the following groups:

The Food Allergy Network
10400 Eaton Place, Suite 107
Fairfax, VA 22030
(703) 691-3179
(1-800) 929-4040

American Academy of Allergy, Asthma and Immunology
611 East Wells St.
Milwaukee, WI 53202
(414) 272-6071
Physician Referral Hotline
(1-800) 822-ASMA

The American Dietetic Association
216 W. Jackson Blvd.
Chicago, IL 60606-6995
(1-800) 877-1600

Chapter 23

Eating to Lower Your High Blood Cholesterol

Introduction

Anyone can have high blood cholesterol. But, because there are no warning signs, you may have been surprised to learn that you have high blood cholesterol. The good news is that you can take steps to lower it. The best way to lower your high blood cholesterol is to eat foods low in saturated fat, total fat, and cholesterol; be more physically active; and lose weight, if you are overweight.

What Is Blood Cholesterol—and Why Does It Matter?

High blood cholesterol is a serious problem: it is a "risk factor" for heart disease. That means that having high blood cholesterol increases your chance, or risk, of getting heart disease. The higher your blood cholesterol, the greater your risk of getting heart disease. And heart disease is the number one killer of both men and women in the United States.

Two specific kinds of blood cholesterol are called low density lipoproteins (LDL) and high density lipoproteins (HDL). LDL-cholesterol, sometimes called "bad" cholesterol, causes the cholesterol to build up in the walls of your arteries. Thus, the more LDL you have in your blood, the greater your heart disease risk. In contrast, HDL-cholesterol,

Excerpted from *Step by Step: Eating to Lower Your High Blood Cholesterol*, National Heart, Lung, and Blood Institute (NHLBI), NIH Pub. No. 94-2920, August 1994.

sometimes called "good" cholesterol, helps your body get rid of the cholesterol in your blood. Thus, if your levels of HDL are low, your risk of heart disease increases.

Every adult, ages 20 and older, should have his or her blood cholesterol checked at least once every 5 years. Here's a quick look at the numbers and what they mean.

Total Cholesterol. Your total cholesterol level falls into one of these categories (for anyone 20 years of age or older):

1. Desirable Blood Cholesterol: less than 200 mg/dL
2. Borderline-High Blood Cholesterol: 200-239 mg/dL
3. High Blood Cholesterol: 240 mg/dL and above

Cholesterol levels less than 200 mg/dL are considered desirable while levels of 240 mg/dL or above are high and require more specific attention. Levels from 200-239 mg/dL also require attention especially if your HDL-cholesterol is low or if you have two or more other risk factors for heart disease.

HDL-Cholesterol. Unlike total and LDL-cholesterol, the lower your HDL, the higher your risk for heart disease. An HDL level less than 35 mg/dL is considered low and increases your risk for heart disease. The higher your HDL, the better. An HDL level of 60 mg/dL or above is high.

LDL-Cholesterol. Your doctor will likely check your LDL-cholesterol level if your:

- HDL-cholesterol is low,
- total cholesterol is high, OR
- total cholesterol is borderline-high, and you have two or more other risk factors for heart disease.

Your LDL level gives a better picture of your risk for heart disease than your total cholesterol. Here are the categories for LDL levels (for anyone 20 years of age or older without heart disease):

1. Desirable: less than 130 mg/dL
2. Borderline-High Risk: 130-159 mg/dL
3. High Risk: 160 mg/dL and above

Lowering LDL is the main aim of treatment for a cholesterol problem. If your LDL level puts you at high-risk and you have fewer than two other risk factors for heart disease, then your treatment goal is an LDL level of less than 160 mg/dL. However, if you have two or more other risk factors for heart disease, your LDL goal should be less than 130 mg/dL. If you already have heart disease, your LDL should be even lower—100 mg/dL or less.

Risk Factors for Heart Disease

Factors You Can Do Something about

- Cigarette smoking
- High blood cholesterol (high total cholesterol and high LDL-cholesterol)
- Low HDL-cholesterol
- High blood pressure
- Diabetes
- Obesity/overweight
- Physical inactivity

Factors You Cannot Control

- Age: 45 years or older for men; 55 years or older for women
- Family history of early heart disease—heart attack or sudden death: Father or brother stricken before age of 55; mother or sister stricken before the age of 65.

What You Need to Do to Lower Blood Cholesterol

Now that you know about blood cholesterol, get set to lower it. All healthy Americans, regardless of their blood cholesterol level, should eat in a heart-healthy way. This is true beginning with toddlers (about age 2) on up to their parents, grandparents, and even great-grandparents The whole family should also be physically active. And if you have a high blood cholesterol level—whether due to what you eat, heredity, or both—it is even more important to eat healthfully and to be physically active. Adopting these behaviors also can help control high blood pressure as well as diabetes.

Choose Foods Low in Saturated Fat

All foods that contain fat are made up of a mixture of saturated and unsaturated fats. Saturated fat raises your blood cholesterol level more than anything else that you eat. It is found in greatest amounts in foods from animals, such as fatty cuts of meat, poultry with the skin, whole-milk dairy products, lard, and in some vegetable oils like coconut, palm kernel, and palm oils. The best way to reduce your blood cholesterol level is to choose foods low in saturated fat. One way to do this is by choosing foods such as fruit, vegetables, and whole grain foods naturally low in fat and high in starch and fiber.

Choose Foods Low in Total Fat

Since many foods high in total fat are also high in saturated fat, eating foods low in total fat will help you eat less saturated fat. When you do eat fat, you should substitute unsaturated fat for saturated fat. Unsaturated fat is usually liquid at room temperature and can be either monounsaturated or polyunsaturated. Examples of foods high in monounsaturated fat are olive and canola oils, those high in polyunsaturated fat include safflower, sunflower, corn, and soybean oils. Any type of fat is a rich source of calories, so eating foods low in fat will also help you eat fewer calories. Eating fewer calories can help you lose weight—and, if you are overweight, losing weight is an important part of lowering your blood cholesterol.

Choose Foods High in Starch and Fiber

Foods high in starch and fiber are excellent substitutes for foods high in saturated fat. These foods—breads, cereals, pasta, grains, fruits, and vegetables—are low in saturated fat and cholesterol. They are also usually lower in calories than foods that are high in fat. Foods high in starch and fiber are also good sources of vitamins and minerals.

Diets low in saturated fat and cholesterol, and high in fruits, vegetables, and grain products—like oat and barley bran and dry peas and beans—may help to lower blood cholesterol.

Choose Foods Low in Cholesterol

Dietary cholesterol also can raise your blood cholesterol level, although usually not as much as saturated fat. So, it is important to choose foods low in dietary cholesterol. Dietary cholesterol is found only in foods that come from animals. Many of these foods also are high in saturated fat. Foods from plant sources do not have cholesterol but can contain saturated fat.

Move It...Be More Physically Active

Moving it—being physically active—helps your blood cholesterol levels: It can raise HDL and may lower LDL. Being more active also can help you lose weight, lower your blood pressure, improve the fitness of your heart and blood vessels, and reduce stress.

Lose Weight, If You Are Overweight

People who are overweight tend to have higher blood cholesterol levels than people of desirable weight. And overweight people with an "apple" shape—bigger (pot) belly—tend to have a higher risk for heart disease than those with a "pear" shape—bigger hips and thighs.

Whatever your body shape, when you cut the fat in your diet, you cut down on the richest source of calories. An eating pattern high in starch and fiber instead of fat is a good way to lose weight: many starchy foods have little fat and are lower in calories than high fat foods. If you are overweight, losing even a little weight can help to lower LDL-cholesterol and raise HDL-cholesterol. You don't need to reach your desirable weight to see a change in your blood cholesterol levels.

Heart-Healthy Eating: The Step I and Step II Diets

All Americans should follow the general rules to lower blood cholesterol. In fact, this is a way that the whole family can eat (except infants under 2 years who need more calories from fat), because these guidelines are similar to those recommended for the general population. And if the whole family eats in this way, it will help you make your blood cholesterol-lowering diet your everyday way of eating.

If you have high blood cholesterol, you will have to pay attention to what you eat by following either the Step I diet or Step II diet, as advised by your doctor.

Step I Diet

On the Step I diet, you should eat:

- 8-10 percent of the day's total calories from saturated fat.
- 30 percent or less of the day's total calories from fat.
- Less than 300 milligrams of dietary cholesterol a day.
- Just enough calories to achieve and maintain a healthy weight. (You may want to ask your doctor or registered dietitian what is a reasonable calorie level for you.)

Step II Diet

If you do not lower your blood cholesterol enough on the Step I diet or if you are at high risk for heart disease, your doctor will ask you to follow the Step II diet. If you already have heart disease, you should start on the Step II diet right away. The Step II diet helps you cut down on saturated fat and cholesterol even more than the Step I diet. This helps lower your blood cholesterol even more.

On the Step II diet, you should eat:

- Less than 7 percent of the day's total calories from saturated fat.
- 30 percent or less of the day's total calories from fat.
- Less than 200 milligrams of dietary cholesterol a day.
- Just enough calories to achieve and maintain a healthy weight. (You may want to ask your doctor or registered dietitian what is a reasonable calorie level for you.)

To get the full benefits of the Step II diet, you should have help from a registered dietitian or other qualified nutritionist. If your levels do not go down enough, you may need to take medicine along with your diet.

Amount of Fat

The recommendations for saturated fat and total fat are based on a percentage of the calories you eat; the actual amount you should eat daily will vary depending on how many calories you eat. See the Table 23.1 to get an idea of the number of grams of saturated fat and total fat you should be eating.

A Word about Sodium

If you have high blood pressure as well as high blood cholesterol (and many people do), your doctor may tell you to cut down on sodium or salt. As long as you are working on getting your blood cholesterol number down, this is a good time to work on your blood pressure, too. Try to limit your sodium intake to 2,400 milligrams a day.

What Kind of Success Can You Expect?

Generally your blood cholesterol level should begin to drop a few weeks after you start on a cholesterol-lowering diet. How much your level drops depends on the amounts of saturated fat and cholesterol you used to eat, how high your high blood cholesterol is, how much weight you lose if you are overweight, and how your body responds to the changes you make. Over time, you may reduce your blood cholesterol level by 10-50 mg/dL or even more.

Table 23.1. Counting Saturated Fat and Total Fat on the Step I and Step II Diets

If you eat this many calories....

	1,200	1,500	1,800	2,000	2,500

This is the recommended amount of fat for each day:

Saturated Fat (grams)*

	1,200	1,500	1,800	2,000	2,500
Step I	12	15	18	20	25
Step II	8	10	12	13	17

Total Fat (grams)**

	1,200	1,500	1,800	2,000	2,500
Step I and Step II	40	50	60	65	80

*Amounts are equal to 9 percent of total calories for Step I and 6 percent of total calories for Step II. Remember 1 gram of fat equals 9 calories.

**Amounts are equal to 30 percent of total calories (rounded down to the nearest 5); your intake should be this much or less.

NOTE: On average, women consume about 1,800 calories a day and men consume about 2,500 calories a day.

Table 23.2. Sample Menu for Step I and Step II Diets with Traditional American-Style Foods—2,500 calories

STEP I—*2,500 calories*	STEP II—*2,500 calories*
Breakfast	**Breakfast**
1 medium bagel	1 medium bagel
2 teaspoons low fat cream cheese	*2 teaspoons jelly*
1 1/2 cups shredded wheat cereal	1 1/2 cups shredded wheat cereal
1 small banana	1 small banana
1 cup 1 percent milk	*1 cup skim milk*
3/4 cup orange juice	3/4 cup orange juice
1 cup coffee	1 cup coffee
2 tablespoons 1 percent milk	*2 tablespoons skim milk*
Lunch	**Lunch**
1/2 cup minestrone soup, canned	1/2 cup minestrone soup, canned
1 lean roast beef sandwich	1 lean roast beef sandwich
2 slices whole wheat bread	2 slices whole wheat bread
3 ounces lean roast beef, unseasoned	*2 ounces lean roast beef,*
3/4 ounce American cheese, low fat	*unseasonsed*
1 leaf lettuce	3/4 ounce American cheese, low fat
3 slices tomato	1 leaf lettuce
2 teaspoons mayonnaise, low fat	3 slices tomato
1 cup fresh mixed fruit salad	*2 teaspoons tub margarine*
1 cup lemonade	1 cup fresh mixed fruit salad
	1 cup lemonade
Snack	
1 fresh large apple	**Snack**
	1 fresh large apple
Dinner	
3 ounces salmon	**Dinner**
1 medium baked potato	*3 ounces flounder*
2 teaspoons tub margarine	*1 teaspoon vegetable oil*
1/2 cup green beans	1 medium baked potato
1/2 teaspoon tub margarine	2 teaspoons tub margarine
1/2 cup carrots	1/2 cup green beans
1/2 teaspoon tub margarine	1/2 teaspoon tub margarine
1 medium white dinner roll	1/2 cup carrots
1 teaspoon tub margarine	1/2 teaspoon tub margarine
1 cup ice milk	1 medium white dinner roll
1 cup iced tea, unsweetened	1 teaspoon tub margarine
	1 cup frozen yogurt
Snack	1 cup iced tea, unsweetened
3 cups popcorn	
1 tablespoon tub margarine	**Snack**
	3 cups popcorn
	1 tablespoon tub margarine

Note: No salt is used when making the food.

	Step I	Step II
Calories	2,471	2,453
Percent calories from fat	29	28
Percent Calories from saturated fat	8	7
Cholesterol (milligrams)	162	144
Sodium (milligrams)	2,400	2,426

Table 23.3. Sample Menu for Step I and Step II Diets with Traditional American-Style Foods—1,800 calories

STEP I—*1,800 calories*	STEP II—*1,800 calories*
Breakfast	**Breakfast**
1/2 medium bagel	1/2 medium bagel
1 teaspoon low fat cream cheese	*1 teaspoon jelly*
1 cup shredded wheat cereal	1 cup shredded wheat cereal
1 small banana	1 small banana
1 cup 1 percent milk	*1 cup skim milk*
3/4 cup orange juice	*1 cup orange juice*
1 cup coffee	1 cup coffee
2 tablespoons 1 percent milk	*2 tablespoons skim milk*
Lunch	**Lunch**
1/2 cup minestrone soup, canned	1/2 cup minestrone soup, canned
1 lean roast beef sandwich	1 lean roast beef sandwich
2 slices whole wheat bread	2 slices whole wheat bread
3 ounces lean roast beef, unseasoned	*2 ounces lean roast beef, unseasoned*
3/4 ounce American cheese, low fat	3/4 ounce American cheese, low fat
1 leaf lettuce	1 leaf lettuce
3 slices tomato	3 slices tomato
2 teaspoons mayonnaise, low fat	*2 teaspoons tub margarine*
1 medium apple	1 medium apple
1 cup water	1 cup water
Dinner	**Dinner**
3 ounces salmon	*3 ounces flounder*
1 medium baked potato	*1 teaspoon vegetable oil*
1 teaspoon tub margarine	1 medium baked potato
1/2 cup green beans	1 teaspoon tub margarine
1/2 teaspoon tub margarine	1/2 cup green beans
1/2 cup carrots	1/2 teaspoon tub margarine
1/2 teaspoon tub margarine	1/2 cup carrots
1 medium white dinner roll	1/2 teaspoon tub margarine
1 teaspoon tub margarine	1 medium white dinner roll
1/2 cup ice milk	1 teaspoon tub margarine
1 cup iced tea, unsweetened	*1/2 cup low fat frozen yogurt*
	1 cup iced tea, unsweetened
Snack	**Snack**
2 cups popcorn	*3 cups popcorn*
1 teaspoon tub margarine	*2 teaspoons tub margarine*

Note: No salt is used when making the food.

	Step I	Step II
Calories	1,821	1,870
Percent calories from fat	30	29
Percent calories from saturated fat	9	7
Cholesterol (milligrams)	150	130
Sodium (milligrams)	2,046	2,148

Chapter 24

Dietary Approaches to Stop Hypertension (DASH)

This eating plan is from the "Dietary Approaches to Stop Hypertension" (DASH) study. It is rich in fruits, vegetables, and lowfat dairy foods, and low in saturated and total fat. In a report in the April 17, 1997, issue of *The New England Journal of Medicine*, the DASH diet lowered blood pressure and, so, may help prevent and control high blood pressure.

The research centers in DASH were the Brigham and Women's Hospital, Boston, MA; Center for Health Research, Portland, OR; Duke University Medical Center, Durham, NC; Johns Hopkins University, Baltimore, MD; and Pennington Biomedical Research Center, Baton Rouge, LA. The National Heart, Lung, and Blood Institute was both a partner in the research and provided funding for the study.

The DASH eating plan shown in this chapter is based on 2, 000 calories a day. Depending on your caloric needs, your number of daily servings in a food group may vary from those listed.

Tips on Eating the DASH Way

- Start small. Make gradual changes in your eating habits.
- Center your meal around carbohydrates, such as pasta, rice, beans, or vegetables.

This research was funded by the National Heart, Lung, and Blood Institute (NHLBI), with additional support by the National Center for Research Resources and the Office of Research on Minority Health, all units of the National Institutes of Health. DASH is also online at http:// dash.bwh.harvard.edu.

- Treat meat as one part of the whole meal, instead of the focus.
- Use fruits or low fat, low-calorie foods such as sugar free gelatin for desserts and snacks.

Table 24.1. The DASH Diet

Food Group	Daily Servings	1 Serving Equals:	Examples and Notes	Significance of each Food Group to the DASH Diet Pattern
Grains & grain products	7-8	1 slice bread 1/2 C dry cereal 1/2 C cooked rice, pasta, or cereal	whole wheat breads, English muffin, pita bread, bagel, cereals, grits, oatmeal	major sources of energy and fiber
Vegetables	4-5	1 C raw leafy vegetable 1/2 C cooked vegetable 6 oz vegetable juice	tomatoes, potatoes, carrots, peas, squash, broccoli, turnip greens, collards, kale, spinach, artichokes, beans, sweet potatoes	rich sources of potassium, magnesium, and fiber
Fruits	4-5	6 oz fruit juice 1 medium fruit 1/4 C dried fruit 1/2 C fresh, frozen, or canned fruit	apricots, bananas, dates, grapes, oranges, orange juice, grapefruit, grapefruit juice, mangoes, melons, peaches, pineapples, prunes, raisins, strawberries, tangerines	important sources of potassium, magnesium, and fiber
Low fat or nonfat dairy foods	2-3	8 oz milk 1 cup yogurt 1.5 oz cheese	skim or 1 % milk, skim or low fat buttermilk, nonfat or low fat yogurt, part skim mozzarella cheese, nonfat cheese	major sources of calcium and protein
Meats, poultry, fish	2 or less	3 oz cooked meats, poultry, or fish	select only lean; trim away visible fats; broil, roast, or boil, instead of frying; remove skin from poultry	rich sources of protein and magnesium
Nuts	1/2	1.5 oz or 1/3 C or 2 Tbsp seeds ½ C cooked legumes	almonds, filberts, mixed nuts, peanuts, walnuts, sunflower seeds, kidney beans, lentils	rich sources of energy, magnesium, potassium, protein, and fiber

Table 24.2. The DASH Diet: Number of Servings

Total number of servings in 2,000 calories/day menu:

Food Group	Servings
Grains	8
Vegetables	4
Fruits	5
Dairy Foods	3
Meats, Poultry, & Fish	2
Nuts	1
Fats & Oils	2.5

Table 24.3. Sample Menu (based on 2,000 calories/day).

Food	Amount	Servings Provided
Breakfast		
orange juice	6 oz	1 fruit
1% low fat milk	8 oz (1C)	1 dairy
corn flakes (with 1 tsp sugar)	1 C	2 grains
banana	1 medium	1 fruit
whole wheat bread (with 1 Tbsp jelly)	1 slice	1 grain
soft margarine	1 tsp	1 fat
Lunch		
chicken salad	3/4 C	1 poultry
pita bread	1/2 slice, large	1 grain
raw vegetable medley:		
carrot & celery sticks	3-4 sticks each	
radishes	2	1 vegetable
loose-leaf lettuce	2 leaves	
part skim mozzarella cheese	1.5 slice (1.5 oz)	1 dairy
1 % low fat milk	8 oz	1 dairy
fruit cocktail in light syrup	1/2 C	1 fruit
Dinner		
herbed baked cod	3 oz	1 fish
scallion rice	1 C	2 grains
steamed broccoli	1/2 C	1 vegetable
stewed tomatoes	1/2 C	1 vegetable
spinach salad:		
raw spinach	1/2 C	
cherry tomatoes	2	1 vegetable
cucumber	2 slices	
light Italian salad dressing	1 Tbsp	1/2 fat
whole wheat dinner roll	1 small	1 grain
soft margarine	1 tsp	1 fat
melon balls	1/2 C	1 fruit
Snacks		
dried apricots	1 oz (1/4 C)	1 fruit
mini-pretzels	1 oz (3/4 C)	1 grain
mixed nuts	1.5 oz (1/3 C)	1 nuts
diet ginger ale	12 oz	0

REMEMBER! If you use the DASH diet to help prevent or control high blood pressure, make it part of a lifestyle that includes choosing foods lower in salt and sodium, keeping a healthy weight, being physically active, and, if you drink alcohol, doing so in moderation. To learn more about high blood pressure, call 1-800-575-WELL or visit the NHLBI website at http://www.nhlbi.nih.gov/nhlbi/nhlbi.htm.

Chapter 25

I Have Diabetes: What Should I Eat?

How Can I Control My Diabetes?

You can help control your blood sugar (also called blood glucose) and diabetes when you eat healthy, get enough exercise, and stay at a healthy weight.

A healthy weight also helps you control your blood fats and lower your blood pressure.

Many people with diabetes also need to take medicine to help control their blood sugar.

How Can I Eat Healthy?

Using the food pyramid helps you eat a variety of healthy foods. When you eat different foods, you get the vitamins and minerals you need.

Eat different foods from each group each day. See how to do this in Table 25.1.

Table 25.1. Examples of different foods from same group.

	Day 1	Day 2
Fruit:	apple	banana
	orange	mango
Vegetable:	broccoli	salad
		green beans

National Institute of Diabetes and Digestive and Kidney Diseases (NIDDK), NIH Pub. No. 98-4192, November 1997.

What Are Starches?

Starches are bread, grains, cereal, pasta, or starchy vegetables. Eat some starches at each meal. People might tell you not to eat many starches, but that is no longer correct advice. Eating starches is healthy for everyone, including people with diabetes.

The number of servings you should eat each day depends on:

- The calories you need.
- Your diabetes treatment plan.

Starches give your body energy, vitamins and minerals, and fiber. Whole grain starches are healthier because they have more vitamins, minerals, and fiber. Fiber helps you have regular bowel movements.

The Food Pyramid

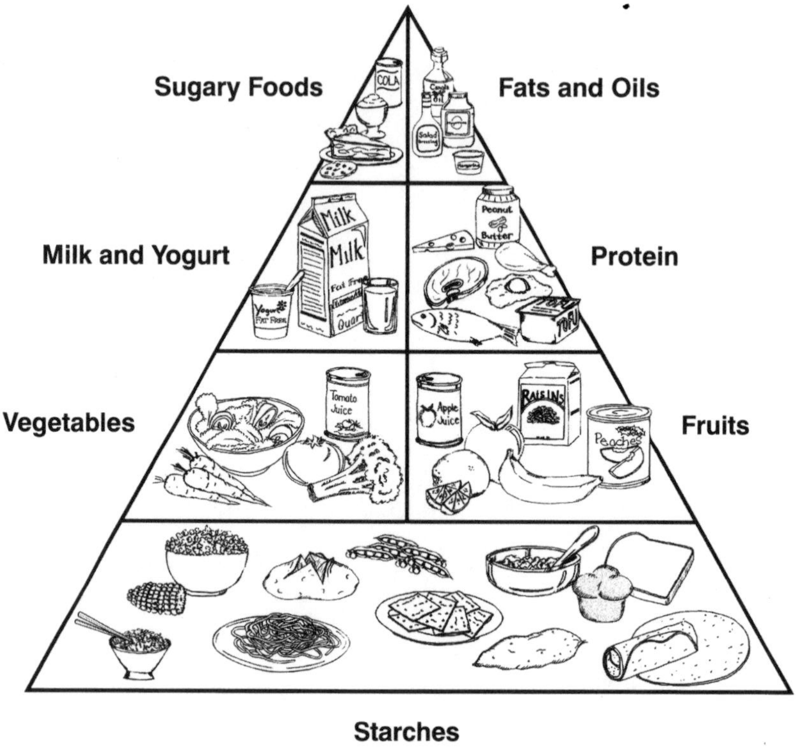

Figure 25.2. The Food Pyramid

How Much Is a Serving of Starch?

1 Serving

- 1 slice of bread or
- 1 small potato or
- ½ cup cooked cereal or
- ¾ cup dry flakes of cereal or
- 1 small tortilla

2 Servings

- 2 slices of bread or
- 1 small potato plus 1 small ear of corn

3 Servings

- 1 small roll plus ½ cup of peas plus 1 small potato or
- 1 cup of rice

You might need to eat one, two, or three starch servings at a meal. If you need to eat more than one serving at a meal, choose several different starches or have two or three servings of one starch.

What Are Healthier Ways to Buy, Cook, and Eat Starches?

- Buy whole grain breads and cereals.
- Eat fewer fried and high-fat starches such as regular tortilla chips and potato chips, french fries, pastries, biscuits, or muffins.
- Use low-fat or fat-free yogurt or fat-free sour cream instead of regular sour cream on a baked potato.
- Use mustard instead of mayonnaise on a sandwich.
- Use the low-fat or fat-free substitutes such as low-fat mayonnaise or light margarine on bread, rolls, or toast.
- Use vegetable oil spray instead of oil, shortening, butter, or margarine.
- Cook or eat cereal with fat-free (skim) or low-fat (1%) milk.
- Use no-sugar jelly, low-fat or fat-free cottage cheese, nonfat yogurt, or salsa.

What Are Vegetables?

Vegetables are healthy for everyone, including people with diabetes. Eat raw and cooked vegetables every day. Vegetables give you vitamins, minerals, and fiber, with very few calories.

The number of servings you should eat each day depends on:

- The calories you need.
- How you take care of your diabetes.

How Much Is a Serving of Vegetables?

1 Serving

- ½ cup carrots or
- ½ cup cooked green beans

2 Servings

- ½ cup carrots plus 1 cup salad or
- ½ cup vegetable juice plus ½ cup cooked green beans

3 Servings

- ½ cup cooked greens plus ½ cup cooked green beans and 1 small tomato or
- ½ cup broccoli plus 1 cup tomato sauce

You might need to eat one, two, or three vegetable servings at a meal. If you need to eat more than one serving at a meal, choose a few different types of vegetables or have two or three servings of one vegetable.

What Are Healthier Ways to Buy, Cook, and Eat Vegetables?

Eat raw and cooked vegetables with little or no fat. You can cook and eat vegetables without any fat.

- Try low-fat or fat-free salad dressing on raw vegetables or salads.
- Steam vegetables using a small amount of water or low-fat broth.
- Mix in some chopped onion or garlic.
- Use a little vinegar or some lemon or lime juice.
- Add a small piece of lean ham or smoked turkey.

- Sprinkle with herbs and spices. These flavorings add almost no fat or calories.

If you do use a small amount of fat, use canola oil, olive oil, or tub margarine instead of fat from meat, butter, or shortening.

What Are Fruits?

Fruit is healthy for everyone, including people with diabetes. Fruit gives you energy, vitamins and minerals, and fiber.

The number of servings you should eat each day depends on:

- The calories you need.
- How you take care of your diabetes.

How Much Is a Serving of Fruit?

1 Serving

- 1 small apple or
- ½ cup juice or
- ½ grapefruit

2 Servings

- 1 banana or
- ½ cup orange juice plus 1¼ cup whole strawberries

You might need to eat one or two fruit servings at a meal. If you need to eat more than one serving at a meal, choose different types of fruits or have two servings of one fruit.

How Should I Eat Fruit?

Eat fruits raw, as juice with no sugar added, canned in their own juice, or dried.

- Buy smaller pieces of fruit.
- Eat pieces of fruit rather than drinking fruit juice. Pieces of fruit are more filling.
- Buy fruit juice that is 100-percent juice with no added sugar.
- Drink fruit juice in small amounts.
- Save high-sugar and high-fat fruit desserts such as peach cobbler or cherry pie for special occasions.

What Are Milk and Yogurt Foods?

Fat-free and low-fat milk and yogurt are healthy for everyone, including people with diabetes. Milk and yogurt give you energy, protein, calcium, vitamin A, and other vitamins and minerals.

Drink fat-free (skim or nonfat) or low-fat (1%) milk each day. Eat low-fat or fat-free yogurt. They have less total fat, saturated fat, and cholesterol.

The number of servings you should eat each day depends on:

- The calories you need.
- How you take care of your diabetes.

Note: If you are pregnant or breastfeeding, eat four to five servings of milk and yogurt each day.

How Much Is a Serving of Milk and Yogurt?

1 Serving

- 1 cup fat-free plain yogurt or
- 1 cup skim milk

What Are Protein Foods?

Protein foods are meat, poultry, eggs, cheese, fish, and tofu. Eat small amounts of some of these foods each day.

Protein foods help your body build tissue and muscles. They also give your body vitamins and minerals.

The number of servings you should eat each day depends on:

- The calories you need.
- How you take care of your diabetes.

How Much Is a Serving of Protein Food?

1 Serving

- 2 to 3 ounces of cooked fish or
- 2 to 3 ounces of cooked chicken or
- 2 ounces of cheese or
- 4 ounces (½ cup) of tofu

The serving size you eat now may be too big.

One serving should weigh between 2 and 3 ounces after cooking, about the size of a deck of cards.

What Are Healthier Ways To Buy, Cook, and Eat Protein Foods?

- Buy cuts of beef, pork, ham, and lamb that have only a little fat on them. Trim off extra fat.
- Eat chicken or turkey without the skin.
- Cook protein foods in low-fat ways:
  - Broil
  - Grill
  - Stir-fry
  - Roast
  - Steam
  - Stew
- To add more flavor, use vinegars, lemon juice, soy or teriyaki sauce, salsa, ketchup, barbecue sauce, and herbs and spices.
- Cook eggs with a small amount of fat.
- Eat small amounts of nuts, peanut butter, fried chicken, fish, or shellfish. They are high in fat.

What Are Fats and Oils?

You find the fats and oils section at the tip of the food pyramid. This tells you to eat small amounts of fats and oils because they have lots of calories. Some fats and oils also contain saturated fats and cholesterol that are not good for you.

You also get fat from other foods such as meats and some dairy foods.

High-fat food is tempting. But eating small amounts of high-fat food will help you lose weight, keep your blood sugar and blood fats under control, and lower your blood pressure.

How Much Is a Serving of Fat or Oil?

1 Serving

- 1 strip of bacon or
- 1 teaspoon oil

2 Servings

- 1 tablespoon regular salad dressing or
- 2 tablespoons light salad dressing plus1 tablespoon light mayonnaise

Your meals may include one or two servings of fat.

What Are Sugary Foods?

You find the sugary foods and sweets section at the tip of the food pyramid. This tells you to eat small amounts of sugary foods.

Sugary foods have calories and do not have much nutrition. Sugary foods have lots of calories. Some sugary foods are also high in fat—like cakes, pies, and cookies. They also may contain saturated fats and cholesterol.

Sugary foods and sweets are tempting. But eating small amounts of sugary foods will help you lose weight, keep your blood sugar under control, control your blood fats, and lower your blood pressure.

How Much Is a Serving of Sugary Foods and Sweets?

1 Serving

- 3" diameter cookie or
- 1 plain cake doughnut or
- 4 chocolate kisses or
- 1 tablespoon maple syrup

Once in a while you can eat a serving of a sugary food. Talk to your diabetes teacher about how to fit sugary foods into your meal plan.

How Can I Satisfy My Sweet Tooth?

Eat a serving of sugar-free popsicles, diet soda, fat-free ice cream or yogurt, or sugar-free hot cocoa mix once in a while.

Remember, fat-free and low sugar foods still have some calories. Eat them as part of your meal plan.

Points to Remember

To follow a healthy eating plan:

- Choose foods from all six food groups each day

- Eat a wide variety of foods from each group to get all your vitamins and minerals.
- Eat enough starches, vegetables, fruits, and low-fat milk and yogurt.
- Eat smaller amounts of lower fat protein foods.
- Eat fewer fats, oils, and sugary foods.

How To Find More Help

Diabetes Teachers (nurses, dietitians, pharmacists, and other health professionals)

- To find a diabetes teacher near you, call the American Association of Diabetes Educators toll-free at 1-800 TEAMUP4 (1-800-832-6874).

Recognized Diabetes Education Programs (teaching programs approved by the American Diabetes Association)

- To find a program near you, call 1-800-DIABETES (1-800-342-2383) or look at its Internet home page <http://www.diabetes.org> and click on "Diabetes Info."

Dietitians

- To find a dietitian near you, call The American Dietetic Association's National Center for Nutrition and Dietetics at 1-800-366-1655 or look at its Internet home page <http://www. eatright. org> and click on "Find a Dietitian."

Two other booklets can help you learn more about food and diabetes:

- *I Have Diabetes: How Much Should I Eat?*
- *I Have Diabetes: When Should I Eat?*

For your convenience these two booklets are included in this volume. For free copies of these booklets:

- Call the National Diabetes Information Clearinghouse (NDIC) at (301) 654-3327.
- Write to NDIC, 1 Information Way, Bethesda, MD 20892-3560.

- E-mail NDIC at <ndic@info.niddk.nih.gov>

- Look at these booklets online at <http://www.niddk.nih.gov> under "Health Information."

Chapter 26

Celiac Disease and the Gluten-Free Diet

What Is Celiac Disease?

Celiac disease is a digestive disease that damages the small intestine and interferes with absorption of nutrients from food. People who have celiac disease cannot tolerate a protein called gluten, which is found in wheat, rye, barley, and possibly oats. When people with celiac disease eat foods containing gluten, their immune system responds by damaging the small intestine. Specifically, tiny fingerlike protrusions, called villi, on the lining of the small intestine are lost. Nutrients from food are absorbed into the bloodstream through these villi. Without villi, a person becomes malnourished—regardless of the quantity of food eaten.

Because the body's own immune system causes the damage, celiac disease is considered an autoimmune disorder. However, it is also classified as a disease of malabsorption because nutrients are not absorbed. Celiac disease is also known as celiac sprue, nontropical sprue, and gluten-sensitive enteropathy.

Celiac disease is a genetic disease, meaning that it runs in families. Sometimes the disease is triggered—or becomes active for the first time—after surgery, pregnancy, childbirth, viral infection, or severe emotional stress.

National Institute of Diabetes and Digestive and Kidney Diseases (NIDDK), NIH Publication No. 98-4225, April 1998.

What Are the Symptoms?

Celiac disease affects people differently. Some people develop symptoms as children, others as adults. One factor thought to play a role in when and how celiac appears is whether and how long a person was breastfed—the longer one was breastfed, the later symptoms of celiac disease appear, and the more atypical the symptoms. Other factors include the age at which one began eating foods containing gluten and how much gluten is eaten.

Symptoms may or may not occur in the digestive system. For example, one person might have diarrhea and abdominal pain, while another person has irritability or depression. In fact, irritability is one of the most common symptoms in children.

Symptoms of celiac disease may include one or more of the following:

- Recurring abdominal bloating and pain.
- Chronic diarrhea.
- Weight loss.
- Pale, foul-smelling stool.
- Unexplained anemia (low count of red blood cells).
- Gas.
- Bone pain.
- Behavior changes.
- Muscle cramps.
- Fatigue.
- Delayed growth.
- Failure to thrive in infants.
- Pain in the joints.
- Seizures.
- Tingling numbness in the legs (from nerve damage)
- Pale sores inside the mouth, called aphthus ulcers.
- Painful skin rash, called dermatitis herpetiformis.
- Tooth discoloration or loss of enamel.
- Missed menstrual periods (often because of excessive weight loss).

Anemia, delayed growth, and weight loss are signs of malnutrition—not getting enough nutrients. Malnutrition is a serious problem for anyone, but particularly for children because they need adequate nutrition to develop properly.

Some people with celiac disease may not have symptoms. The undamaged part of their small intestine is able to absorb enough nutrients to prevent symptoms. However, people without symptoms are still at risk for complications of celiac disease. (Complications are described below.)

How Is Celiac Disease Diagnosed?

Diagnosing celiac disease can be difficult because some of its symptoms are similar to those of other diseases, including irritable bowel syndrome, Crohn's disease, ulcerative colitis, diverticulosis, intestinal infections, chronic fatigue syndrome, and depression.

Recently, researchers discovered that people with celiac disease have higher than normal levels of certain antibodies in their blood. Antibodies are produced by the immune system in response to substances that the body perceives to be threatening. To diagnose celiac disease, physicians test blood to measure levels of antibodies to gluten. These antibodies are antigliadin, anti-endomysium, and antireticulin.

If the tests and symptoms suggest celiac disease, the physician may remove a tiny piece of tissue from the small intestine to check for damage to the villi. This is done in a procedure called a biopsy: the physician eases a long, thin tube called an endoscope through the mouth and stomach into the small intestine, and then takes a sample of tissue using instruments passed through the endoscope. Biopsy of the small intestine is the best way to diagnose celiac disease.

Screening

Screening for celiac disease involves testing asymptomatic people for the antibodies to gluten. Americans are not routinely screened for celiac disease. However, because celiac disease is hereditary, family members—particularly first-degree relatives—of people who have been diagnosed may need to be tested for the disease. About 10 percent of an affected person's first-degree relatives (parents, siblings, or children) will also have the disease. The longer a person goes undiagnosed and untreated, the greater the chance of developing malnutrition and other complications.

What Is the Treatment?

The only treatment for celiac disease is to follow a gluten-free diet—that is, to avoid all foods that contain gluten. For most people, following this diet will stop symptoms, heal existing intestinal damage, and prevent further damage. Improvements begin within days of starting the diet, and the small intestine is usually completely healed—meaning the villi are intact and working—in 3 to 6 months. (It may take up to 2 years for older adults.)

The gluten-free diet is a lifetime requirement. Eating any gluten, no matter how small an amount, can damage the intestine. This is true for anyone with the disease, including people who do not have noticeable symptoms. Depending on a person's age at diagnosis, some problems, such as delayed growth and tooth discoloration, may not improve.

A small percentage of people with celiac disease do not improve on the gluten-free diet. These people often have severely damaged intestines that cannot heal even after they eliminate gluten from their diets. Because their intestines are not absorbing enough nutrients, they may need to receive intravenous nutrition supplements. Drug treatments are being evaluated for unresponsive celiac disease. These patients may need to be evaluated for complications of the disease.

If a person responds to the gluten-free diet, the physician will know for certain that the diagnosis of celiac disease is correct.

The Gluten-Free Diet

A gluten-free diet means avoiding all foods that contain wheat (including spelt, triticale, and kamut), rye, barley, and possibly oats—in other words, most grain, pasta, cereal, and many processed foods. Despite these restrictions, people with celiac disease can eat a well-balanced diet with a variety of foods, including bread and pasta. For example, instead of wheat flour, people can use potato, rice, soy, or bean flour. Or, they can buy gluten-free bread, pasta, and other products from special food companies.

Whether people with celiac disease should avoid oats is controversial because some people have been able to eat oats without having a reaction. Scientists are doing studies to find out whether people with celiac disease can tolerate oats. Until the studies are complete, people with celiac disease should follow their physician or dietitian's advice about eating oats.

Plain meat, fish, rice, fruits, and vegetables do not contain gluten, so people with celiac disease can eat as much of these foods as they like. Examples of foods that are safe to eat and those that are not are provided in Table 26.1.

The gluten-free diet is complicated. It requires a completely new approach to eating that affects a person's entire life. People with celiac disease have to be extremely careful about what they buy for lunch at school or work, eat at cocktail parties, or grab from the refrigerator for a midnight snack. Eating out can be a challenge as the person with celiac disease learns to scrutinize the menu for foods with gluten and question the waiter or chef about possible hidden sources of gluten. However, with practice, screening for gluten becomes second nature and people learn to recognize which foods are safe and which are off limits.

A dietitian, a health care professional who specializes in food and nutrition, can help people learn about their new diet. Also, support groups are particularly helpful for newly diagnosed people and their families as they learn to adjust to a new way of life.

What Are the Complications of Celiac Disease?

Damage to the small intestine and the resulting problems with nutrient absorption put a person with celiac disease at risk for several diseases and health problems.

- Lymphoma and adenocarcinoma are types of cancer that can develop in the intestine.

- Osteoporosis is a condition in which the bones become weak, brittle, and prone to breaking. Poor calcium absorption is a contributing factor to osteoporosis.

- Miscarriage and congenital malformation of the baby, such as neural tube defects, are risks for untreated pregnant women with celiac disease because of malabsorption of nutrients.

- Short stature results when childhood celiac disease prevents nutrient absorption during the years when nutrition is critical to a child's normal growth and development. Children who are diagnosed and treated before their growth stops may have a catch-up period.

- Seizures, or convulsions, result from inadequate absorption of folic acid. Lack of folic acid causes calcium deposits, called calcifications, to form in the brain, which in turn cause seizures.

How Common Is Celiac Disease?

Celiac disease is the most common genetic disease in Europe. In Italy about 1 in 250 people and in Ireland about 1 in 300 people have celiac disease. It is rarely diagnosed in African, Chinese, and Japanese people.

Table 26.1. The Gluten Free Diet: Some Examples (Continued on next page.)

Following are examples of foods that are allowed and those that should be avoided when eating gluten-free. Please note that this is not a complete list. People are encouraged to discuss gluten-free food choices with a physician or dietitian who specializes in celiac disease. Also, it is important to read all food ingredient lists carefully to make sure that the food does not contain gluten.

Food Group	Allowed	Not Allowed
Beverages	Coffee, tea, carbonated drinks, wine made in U.S., rum, some root beer	Ovaltine, malted milk, ale, beer, gin, whiskey, flavored coffee, herbal tea with malted barley
Milk	Fresh, dry, evaporated, or condensed milk; cream; sour cream; whipping cream; yogurt	Malted milk, some commercial chocolate milk, some nondairy creamers
Meat, Fish, Poultry	Fresh meats, fish, other seafood, and poultry; fish in canned oil, brine, or water; some hot dogs and lunch meats	Prepared meat containing wheat, rye, oats, or barley; tuna canned in vegetable broth
Cheese	All aged cheese, such as cheddar, Swiss, edam, parmesan; cottage cheese; cream cheese; pasteurized processed cheese; cheese spreads	Any cheese product containing oat gum, some veined cheeses (bleu, stilton, roquefort, gorgonzola)
Potato or Other Starch	White and sweet potatoes, yams, hominy, rice, wild rice, gluten-free noodles, some oriental rice and bean thread noodles	Regular noodles, spaghetti, macaroni, most packaged rice mixes, seminola, spinach noodles, frozen potato products with wheat flour added
Cereals	Hot cereals made from cornmeal, Cream of Rice, hominy, rice; Puffed Rice, Kellogg's Corn Pops, cereals made without malt	All cereals containing wheat, rye, oats, or barley; bran; graham; wheat germ; durum; kaska; bulgar; buckwheat; millet; triticale; amaranth; spelt; teff; quinoa; kamut
Breads	Specially prepared breads using only allowed flours	All breads containing wheat, rye, oat, or barley flours and grains listed above
Flours and Thickening Agents	Arrowroot starch, corn bran, corn flour, corn germ, cornmeal, corn starch, potato flour, potato starch flour, rice bran, rice flour, rice polish, rice starch, soy flour, tapioca starch, bean and lentil flours, nut flours	Amaranth, wheat germ, bran, wheat starch; all flours containing wheat, rye, oats, or barley; buckwheat; spelt; quinoa; teff; kamut; millet

Table 26.1. The Gluten Free Diet: Some Examples (Continued from previous page.)

Source: Food and Nutrition Services, The University of Iowa Hospitals and Clinics. (1996) Gluten Restricted, Gliadin Free Diet. Iowa City, Iowa: The University of Iowa Hospitals and Clinics.

Food Group	Allowed	Not Allowed
Vegetables	All plain, fresh, frozen, or canned vegetables; dried peas and beans; lentils; some commercially prepared vegetables	Creamed vegetables, vegetables canned in sauce, some canned baked beans, commercially prepared vegetables and salads
Fruits	All fresh, frozen, canned, or dried fruits; all fruit juices; some canned pie fillings	Thickened or prepared fruits; some pie fillings; raisins and dried dates that have been dusted with flour
Fats	Butter, margarine, vegetable oil, nuts, peanut butter, hydrogenated vegetable oils, some salad dressings, mayonnaise, nonstick cooking sprays	Some commercial salad dressings, wheat germ oil, nondairy cream substitutes, most commercial gravies and sauces
Soups	Homemade broth and soups made with allowed ingredients, some commercially canned soups, specialty dry soup mixes	Most canned soups and soup mixes, bouillon and bouillon cubes with hydrolyzed vegetable protein
Desserts	Cakes, quick breads, pastries, and puddings made with allowed ingredients; cornstarch, tapioca, and rice puddings; some pudding mixes; custard; ice cream with few, simple ingredients; sorbet; meringues; mousse; sherbets; frozen yogurt	Commercial cakes, cookies; pies made with wheat, rye, oats, or barley; millet, amaranth, buckwheat, spelt, teff, quinoa, kamut; prepared mixes; puddings; ice cream cones; Jell-O instant pudding; cream fillings; products made with brown rice syrup
Sweets	Jelly, jam, honey, brown and white sugar, molasses, most syrups, some candy, chocolate, pure cocoa, coconut, marshmallows	Commercial candies dusted with wheat flour; butterscotch chips; flavored syrups; sweets containing malt/malt flavorings; some brown rice syrup; some corn syrup
Miscellaneous	Salt, pepper, herbs, herb extracts, food coloring, cloves, allspice, ginger, nutmeg, cinnnamon, chili powder, tomato puree and paste, olives, active dry yeast, bicarbonate of soda, baking powder, cream of tartar, dry mustard, some condiments, apple cider, rice or wine vinegar	Curry powder, dry seasonings mixes, gravy extracts, meat sauces, catsup, mustard, horseradish, chip dips, most soy sauce, some distilled white vinegar, instant dry baking yeast, some cinnamon, condiments made with wheat-derived distilled vinegars, communion wafers/bread, some alcohol-based flavoring extracts

An estimated 1 in 4,700 Americans have been diagnosed with celiac disease. Some researchers question how celiac disease could be so uncommon in the United States since it is hereditary and many Americans descend from European ethnic groups in whom the disease is common. A recent study in which random blood samples from the Red Cross were tested for celiac disease suggests that as many as 1 in every 250 Americans may have it. Celiac disease could be underdiagnosed in the United States for a number of reasons:

- Celiac symptoms can be attributed to other problems.
- Many doctors are not knowledgeable about the disease.
- Only a handful of U.S. laboratories are experienced and skilled in testing for celiac disease.

More research is needed to find out the true prevalence of celiac disease among Americans.

Diseases Linked to Celiac Disease

People with celiac disease tend to have other autoimmune diseases as well, including:

- Dermatitis herpetiformis.
- Thyroid disease.
- Systemic lupus erythematosus.
- Insulin-dependent diabetes.
- Liver disease.
- Collagen vascular disease.
- Rheumatoid arthritis.
- Sjogren's syndrome.

The connection between celiac and these diseases may be genetic.

Dermatitis Herpetiformis

Dermatitis herpetiformis (DH) is a severe itchy, blistering skin disease caused by gluten intolerance. DH is related to celiac disease since both are autoimmune disorders caused by gluten intolerance, but they are separate diseases. The rash usually occurs on the elbows, knees, and buttocks.

Although people with DH do not usually have digestive symptoms, they often have the same intestinal damage as people with celiac disease.

DH is diagnosed by a skin biopsy, which involves removing a tiny piece of skin near the rash and testing it for the IgA antibody. DH is treated with a gluten-free diet and medication to control the rash, such as dapsone or sulfapyridine. Drug treatment may last several years.

Additional Resources

American Celiac Society
58 Musano Court
West Orange, NJ 07052
(201) 325-8837

Celiac Disease Foundation
3251 Ventura Boulevard, #1
Studio City, CA 91604-1838
(818) 990-2354
Website: http://www.celiac.org/cdf
E-mail: cdf@primenet.com

Celiac Sprue Association/USA Inc.
P.O. Box 31700
Omaha, NE 68131-0700
(402) 558-0600
Website: http://www.csaceliacs.org/

Gluten Intolerance Group of North America
P.O. Box 23053
Seattle, WA 98102-0353
(206) 325-6980

National Center for Nutrition and Dietetics
American Dietetic Association
216 West Jackson Boulevard, Suite 800
Chicago, IL 60606-6995
(800) 366-1655

Gluten-Free Living *(a bimonthly newsletter)*
P.O. Box 105
Hastings-on-Hudson, NY 10706

Chapter 27

Ketogenic Diets for Seizure Control

Two dateline NBS segments and a TV movie starring Meryl Streep that aired earlier this year have put a special diet to control epileptic seizures in the public eye. The anti-seizure eating regimen, known as the ketogenic diet, has also been garnering more attention in the scientific community.

The potential benefits are enormous. According to study results, one third of people put on the regimen have a significant reduction in seizure incidence, sometimes to the point of becoming seizure-free. In the best-case scenarios, seizures are brought under control within 2 to 3 years, and patients can gradually be tapered off the diet without a recurrence of attacks—and without medications. A second third shows some benefit, while another third experiences no benefit or has side effects requiring that the regimen be discontinued.

Presently, the diet is used almost exclusively in children, who make up almost a third of the 2.5 million Americans with epilepsy. But research is underway to see if it can help adults, with some promising preliminary results.

This chapter includes text from "A Diet for Epilepsy Provides New Hope," © June 1997, reprinted with permission, *Tufts University Health & Nutrition Letter*, 50 Broadway, 15th Floor, New York, NY 10004; and "Frequently Asked Questions (FAQs) about the Ketogenic Diet," Stanford University School of Medicine, at www.stanford.edu/group/ketodiet, reprinted with permission.

243

Not an Easy, Do-It-Yourself Plan

Just about all the calories in the ketogenic diet come from fats such as butter or heavy whipping cream (which many patients find more palatable than less saturated cooking oils or margarine). Carbohydrates and protein are severely limited. That's because the aim of the diet is to get the body to use fat for energy rather than the usual blood sugar (a form of carbohydrate that can be synthesized from the carbohydrates or the proteins in food).

When fat is broken down for energy, some of it gets metabolized into substances called ketones (hence the name of the plan), which then enter the brain. Once there, the ketones act as a kind of sedative, preventing the sudden disturbances in the normal electrical functioning of the brain that lead to seizures.

But even the slightest "cheating," like eating just one cookie, can induce a seizure. In addition, only 70 to 80 percent of normal calorie consumption is allowed (poor growth among children is a serious concern), and fluids are strictly limited. And there can be side effects, ranging from drowsiness and vomiting to large increases in blood cholesterol and recurrent infections.

Because it's so hard to follow, the diet should be considered only for those who have more than 2 seizures a week despite treatment with at least 2 different anticonvulsant medications, according to the Johns Hopkins Pediatric Epilepsy Center.

For more information about epilepsy and the ketogenic diet, check the Web page of the Epilepsy Foundation of America at www.efa.org, or call 1-800-332-1000.

Common Questions from Parents Regarding the Ketogenic Diet

What type of seizures is the ketogenic diet effective for?

It appears to be effective for multiple types of seizures. However, we have found it to be most effective for myoclonic seizures and "minor motor" seizures. The diet also seems to be helpful for other type of seizures, such as tonic-clonic seizures and complex partial seizures.

Is my child a good candidate for the ketogenic diet?

We recommend that you consult your physician or neurologist about the appropriateness of the ketogenic diet for your child's seizure disorder. You should also contact other keto providers and families who have been on the diet. Usually the ketogenic diet is used as a secondary method of treatment, that is, when conventional anti-seizure medications do not seem to adequately control seizures. Also, if the adverse effects of the anti-seizure medications are too great, the diet can also be considered (so that medications can be reduced).

How do I locate an institution that is currently treating children successfully with the ketogenic diet?

Ask your child's neurologist for a referral to a, preferably close to home, site that will evaluate your child for appropriateness to start the ketogenic diet. Please note that as there are a limited number of institutions that have an active keto team, your child may have to wait a month or more to be admitted. You can find a partial list of centers/programs that are offering the ketogenic diet on the internet at www.stanford.edu/group/ketodiet/ketocenters.html.

How long will my child have to be in the hospital?

Uncomplicated hospital admissions scheduled to initiate the ketogenic diet are typically 4-5 days in duration (Monday-Friday).

How long does my child stay on the diet?

If the diet proves to be a worthwhile form of therapy, usually the diet is followed for 2 years and weaned in the third year, similar to what might be tried with an antiepileptic drug (AED).

How soon will we know if the diet is working?

The diet's effectiveness is seen in varying amounts of time among individuals. It can be immediate, while the diet is being initiated in the hospital, or it may take several months. Remember, seizures are different for all children; some have several daily and others only once every 6 months.

How can my child go on a ketogenic diet if he is allergic or intolerant to dairy products?

The ketogenic diet can be planned for children who cannot tolerate milk or milk products; this is true for either oral or gastrostomy fed keto kids. Heavy whip cream does not need to be a component of the diet, it can be replaced with other food sources of carbohydrate, fat, and protein and produce the same degree of ketosis. For children fed by a gastrostomy, nasogastric or jejunal feeding tube, RCF (Ross Carbohydrate Free) is recommended. The protein in dairy products, which is the allergen, is replaced by a soy protein in RCF, thus there is no allergic potential, as long as the child is not allergic [to the soy protein].

How will we be able to manage birthdays and holidays?

Most of us are used to celebrating special occasions with friends, family, fun and—yes—food. These days can still be special, but they do not need to be food centered for the ketogenic kids. For instance, at Halloween, trick or treat candy can be traded in for nickels to buy a new toy or rent a video. Birthday candles can be stuck into Play Dough and placed on a gift or the table. The rest of the family need not suffer through the holidays, however, being sensitive to a keto kid's unique diet therapy is warranted.

How will my child feel on this diet?

Children do seem to respond differently to the different stages of the ketogenic diet. A lot of this depends on what the child's baseline awake state is. Most often, during the fasting your child may feel sleepy, lethargic, and cranky. Then as the diet begins, lethargy may continue as well as nausea and vomiting. This may be due to excessive ketosis or the side effects of the change in metabolism from using glucose as a primary energy source to using fats instead. It may be also related to a change in drug levels. In time, children should return to their normal, or close to normal activity level; some keto kids even get more energetic with time. One common, side effect of a high-fat diet for everyone is a slower gastric emptying time; thus even though the portions may look smaller, the food will stay in the stomach longer and give a longer feeling of satiety.

What if my child "cheats" on the diet?

Cheating or mistakes happen for various reasons; it can be purposeful by the child or an incorrect amount of food weighed out and realized retrospectively. Trying to minimize this is important, but being prepared for what might likely occur at least once is equally important. Depending on how big the extra amount of food is/was depends on the treatment. Oftentimes, it is safe just to recognize the mistake and pick up with the regular ketogenic meal plan at the next meal.

Will anti-seizure medications be discontinued after my child goes on the diet?

Well, that depends on the individual circumstances. In most patients anti-seizure medications are reduced. If they are on polytherapy, we usually try to eliminate some of the medications, perhaps maintaining just one medication. If they start the diet while on just one medication, we may try to reduce the dosage. If the patient is on a barbiturate, we do routinely decrease the dose when they go on the diet, since the diet seems to raise the barbiturate levels.

If the diet seems to be working, how long will my child be on the diet?

If your child remains seizure-free for 2 years, most neurologists would recommend switching back to a normal diet. This "wean" off the ketogenic diet is analogous to weaning anti-seizure medication after a seizure-free interval. The success rates of the ability of children to remain seizure-free off the diet after a successful treatment (with the diet) are not well studied.

Can the ketogenic diet be used in adults?

In general, the diet does not seem to be as effective in adults. Most studies have been restricted to children and a few adolescents. In these studies, people have pointed out that the diet does not seem to work as well in older children, and seems to work best in children aged 1-10 years. The reason is not clear, but some have felt that older adolescents and adults may not make or use ketones quite so well. There are currently no published adult studies.

Can the ketogenic diet be used for conditions other than epilepsy?

So far, the only condition that the diet seems to be effective for is epilepsy. It also seems to be useful for treating seizures in a rare metabolic condition that begins in infancy (such as glucose transport protein defects). In this condition inadequate amounts of glucose (sugar) get transported to the brain. There is very little information on the use of the diet in other conditions, such as multiple sclerosis, diabetes, obesity, etc.

Chapter 28

Dietary Management for Phenylketonuria (PKU)

Introduction

Phenylketonuria, called PKU for short, is an inherited condition which prevents the affected individual from normally metabolizing—or using—phenylalanine (phe), one of the essential amino acids found in all protein foods. Unless the condition is detected and treatment is initiated soon after birth, this hereditary biochemical abnormality prevents normal brain development and usually results in severe mental retardation. Other manifestations such as skin rash, seizures, excessive restlessness, irritable behavior and a musty body odor may also be present.

Fortunately, detection of the condition shortly after birth through the use of a routine blood screening procedure has become standard practice in every state and Canadian province since 1991. Placing the baby on a phenylalanine-restricted diet within the first weeks of life, and maintaining good diet control thereafter, is effective in preventing the damaging effects of PKU. Treatment requires elimination of foods naturally high in protein. Special care must be taken to maintain enough-but not too much—phe in the child's diet. Such a balance is obtained only through careful nutritional, biochemical and medical supervision, and considerable effort by the parents.

Beginning at an early age, most children with PKU learn to discriminate between foods that are allowed on their diet from those that

Excerpted from *Education of Students with Phenylketonuria (PKU)*, National Institute of Child Health and Human Development, NIH Pub. No. 92-3318, November 1991.

249

are not. However, maintaining the diet may become more difficult when a child with PKU enrolls in school. "Swapping" lunch items may be a temptation; or students may try a diet soft drink which uses the artificial sweetener, NutraSweet (a product containing phe).

Screening, Diagnosis and Incidence

After its discovery in 1934 by Dr. A. Folling in Norway, and until the early 1960s, PKU was detected with a urine "wet diaper" test. This method has many disadvantages, and since 1964 has been replaced by a blood test which can be administered with great accuracy as early as the first few days of life. Infants initially screened before 24 hours of age should be rescreened by three weeks of age (American Academy of Pediatrics, 1982). When the baby has higher than normal levels of phe in the blood, confirmatory tests must be performed, and if the diagnosis is established, diet treatment begins as soon as possible. Results from the Collaborative Study of Children Treated for Phenylketonuria clearly indicate a loss in IQ scores if the baby is not put on the diet within the first 20 days of life and kept in good dietary control.

Approximately five children with PKU are born in the United States each week. This means an estimated incidence of one baby with PKU born in about 15,000 live births.

Diet Management

Proper diet management is essential in the treatment of PKU. This involves severely limiting the child's intake of all foods containing protein. Protein contains the amino acid, phenylalanine (phe), which the child cannot effectively utilize. Milk and other dairy products, meat, fish, eggs, dried beans and peas, and nuts are concentrated sources of phe; fruits, vegetables, and cereals contain smaller amounts. The only foods that do not contain phe are sugar, oil, pure starch, and water; and products made with these ingredients such as hard candy and soft drinks. Special medical foods which provide protein and important nutrients are an essential part of the food intake pattern of individuals with PKU. Special low protein foods and baking ingredients are available from several companies.

Normally, the body uses a small part of the phe from dietary protein for growth and repair of body tissue, and changes part of the phe into other useful chemical compounds such as tyrosine. Tyrosine is another amino acid and is needed to make proteins, hormones and neurotransmitters which control brain functions. Tyrosine also helps to make pigments for skin and hair coloring. The enzyme necessary to convert excess phe into tyrosine does not work effectively in the person with PKU. The absence of tyrosine combined with the excess phe and abnormal compounds circulating in the body leads to brain damage. This is particularly true in the first few years of life when dietary compliance is critical to prevent damage and to insure normal growth and development.

Even after reaching school age, continued use of a restricted-phe diet is indicated. The Collaborative Study of Children Treated for Phenylketonuria found that children with PKU who were taken off the diet began to show a drop in I.Q. scores and poorer school performance.

The special PKU diet is designed to give each individual the exact amount of phe required for adequate growth and to prevent buildup of harmful amounts. This delicate balance, unique to each person, is achieved by careful measuring of all food and calculating the phe intake on a daily basis. Nutritionists and parents have developed cookbooks and food lists to assist in this exacting task. Frequent blood tests are necessary to monitor the blood phe levels and to determine dietary effectiveness.

In order to supply the other essential elements of protein needed for normal growth and development, a special protein source is necessary. These sources of protein, called medical foods, contain all the amino acids except that most or all of the phe has been removed. Some of the products have added fat and carbohydrates, while all have been fortified with vitamins and minerals. These medical foods are generally taken as a liquid beverage. The medical food plus carefully selected foods low in protein provide a balanced diet for the child.

Special diet management problems may occur at school. For example, young children with PKU cannot have a high protein snack. Special events, such as a birthday, may involve a cake containing forbidden high-phe food ingredients. Because the child with PKU should not eat these foods, he/she may be identified as "different." Parents commonly provide alternatives for their child. However, teachers and administrators must be aware of potential problems and help the child with PKU to participate maximally in all activities, including snacktime and parties by notifying parents to send substitutes.

If a school lunch program is provided, some foods can be safely eaten by the child with PKU. It is often helpful to send the week's menu home so that parents can indicate which items (and in what quantity) are allowed, and which must be avoided, and return the menu to the teacher. By the time children with PKU reach middle school, and often earlier, they themselves will be able to identify foods that are on their diet. However, they may still require help in determining the appropriate quantity. The ability of children with PKU to participate in the same lunchroom program as their classmates, if appropriate, will lessen the feelings of being different, and thus contribute to the student's healthy social and emotional growth.

Glossary

Amino Acids. Organic compounds which combine to form proteins. An "essential" amino acid must be supplied by food; a "non-essential" amino acid can be produced within the body.

Medical Foods. These are special formulas designed to provide the person with PKU with the needed protein, but with little or no phenylalanine. Some of these products and their manufacturers are:

- "Lofenalac" (Mead Johnson), "'Analog XP" (Ross Laboratories), and "PKU 1", (Mead Johnson) are commonly used with infants with PKU;
- "Maxamaid XP" (Ross Laboratories), Phenyl-Free" (Mead Johnson), "PKU 2", "PKU 3" (Mead Johnson), and "PKU Aid" (Anglo-Dietetics Ltd.) provide school-aged children with the needed protein source.
- "Maxamum XP" (Ross Laboratories) and "PKU 3" (Mead Johnson) are utilized for pregnant PKU women.

Enzyme. A chemical compound which changes one substance into another (i.e., a catalyst). The enzyme, phenylalanine hydroxylase, is the one that is defective in individuals with PKU—thus they are unable to convert the amino acid, phenylalanine, into other products.

"Equal." An artificial sweetener containing aspartame, which is 56% phenylalanine (phe) and thus must be totally avoided by persons with PKU.

Hyperphenylalaninemia. The term used to designate a number of conditions (one of which is classical PKU) in which the individual exhibits elevated levels of phenylalanine in the blood.

Maternal PKU. The problems associated with pregnancy where the mother-to-be has PKU.

"Nutra-Sweet." A sugar substitute found in many "diet" products such as soft drinks. It is made of aspartame which contains 56%

phenylalanine; and, therefore, like "Equal," should not be used by persons with PKU.

Phenylketonuria. An inherited error of metabolism in which the individual cannot metabolize (or use) the essential amino acid, phenylalanine.

PKU. A common abbreviation for phenylketonuria.

Phenylalanine. The essential amino acid in all protein which a person with PKU cannot convert into useful products.

Phe. A common abbreviation for phenylalanine.

Protein. Compounds made of amino acids that are essential for all living cells in the body.

Tyrosine. A non-essential amino acid present in all protein foods. In persons with PKU it becomes an essential amino acid because the enzyme necessary for its production from phenylalanine is defective.

For Additional Information

For additional information or assistance beyond that presented in this chapter, the following sources are suggested:

Clinics or Treatment of PKU and Maternal PKU

A directory of the 115 PKU clinics in the United States is available in the publication, Schuett, V.E. (1990) National Survey of Treatment Programs for PKU and Selected Other Inherited Metabolic Diseases (DHHS Pub. No. HRS-M-CH-89-5) which can be obtained from:

National Center for Education in Maternal and Child Health
2000 15th St. North, suite 701
Arlington, VA 22201
(703) 524-7802
Website:http://ericps.crc.uiuc.edu/npin/reswork/workorgs/ncemch.html

The following regional contributing centers of the Maternal PKUCollaborative Study can also provide information and assistance concerning PKU and maternal PKU:

Northeast Region: Connecticut, Delaware, New Hampshire, Maine, Maryland, Massachusetts, New Jersey, New York, Pennsylvania, Rhode Island,Vermont, Virginia, West Virginia, District of Columbia.

Children's Hospital Medical Center
300 Longwood Avenue
Boston, Massachusetts 02115
(617) 355-6000
Website: http://web1.tch.harvard.edu/

Midwest Region: *Illinois, Indiana, Iowa, Kansas, Kentucky, Michigan, Minnesota, Missouri, Nebraska, North Dakota, Ohio, Oklahoma, South Dakota, Wisconsin.*

University of Illinois at Chicago
Human Nutrition and Dietetics
1919 West Taylor Street
Chicago, Illinois 60612
(312) 996-8055
Website: http://www.uic.edu/ahp/hnd/

Southeast Region: *Alabama, Arkansas, Florida, Georgia, Louisiana, Mississippi, North Carolina, South Carolina, Tennessee, Texas, Puerto Rico.*

University of Texas Medical Branch
Department of Pediatrics
Galveston, Texas 77550
(409) 772-1011
Website: http://www.utmb.edu/

Western Region: *Alaska, Arizona, California, Colorado, Hawaii, Idaho, Montana, Nevada, New Mexico, Oregon, Utah, Washington, Wyoming.*

PKU Section
Children's Hospital of Los Angeles
4650 Sunset Boulevard
Los Angeles, California 90027
(213) 669-2152

*All Provinces of **Canada.***

The Hospital for Sick Children
555 University Avenue
Toronto, Ontario M5G IX8, Canada
(416) 598-6356 or (416) 781-1805

Chapter 29

Eating Hints for Cancer Patients

Eating Well during Cancer Treatment

A nutritious diet is always vital for your body to work at its best. Good nutrition is even more important for people with cancer. Why?

- Patients who eat well during their treatment are able to cope better with the side effects of treatment. Patients who eat well may be able to handle a higher dose of certain treatments.

- A healthy diet can help keep up your strength, prevent body tissues from breaking down, and rebuild tissues that cancer treatment may harm.

- When you are unable to eat enough food or the right kind of food, your body uses stored nutrients as a source of energy. As a result, your natural defenses are weaker and your body cannot fight infection as well. Yet, this defense system is especially important to you now, because cancer patients are often at risk of getting an infection.

Can Good Nutrition Treat Cancer?

Doctors know that patients who eat well during cancer treatment are better able to cope with side effects. However, there is no evidence that any kind of diet or food can either cure cancer or stop it from

Excerpted from *Eating Hints for Cancer Patients*, National Cancer Institute (NCI), NIH Pub. No. 97-2079, January 1997.

coming back. In fact, some diets may be harmful, especially those that don't include a variety of foods. There is also no evidence that dietary supplements, such as vitamin or mineral pills, can cure cancer or stop it from coming back.

The National Cancer Institute (NCI) strongly urges you to eat nutritious foods and follow the treatment program prescribed by a doctor who uses accepted and proven methods or treatments. People who depend upon unconventional treatments may lose valuable treatment time and reduce their chances of controlling cancer and getting well.

The NCI also recommends that you ask your doctor, nurse, or registered dietitian before taking any vitamins or mineral supplements. Too much of some vitamins or minerals can be just as dangerous as too little. Large doses of some vitamins may even stop your cancer treatment from working the way it should. To avoid problems, don't take these products on your own. Follow your doctor's directions for safe results.

Managing Eating Problems during Treatment

All the methods of treating cancer—surgery, radiation therapy, chemotherapy, and biological therapy (immunotherapy)—are very powerful. Although treatments target the cancer cells in your body, they sometimes can damage normal, healthy cells. This may produce unpleasant side effects that cause eating problems.

Side effects of cancer treatment vary from patient to patient. The part of the body being treated, length of treatment, and the dose of treatment also affect whether side effects will occur. Ask your doctor about how your treatment may affect you.

The good news is that only about one-third of cancer patients have side effects during treatment, and most side effects go away when treatment ends. Your doctor will try to plan a treatment that minimizes side effects.

Cancer treatment also may affect your eating in another way. When some people are upset, worried, or afraid, they may have eating problems. Losing your appetite and nausea are two normal responses to feeling nervous or fearful. Such problems should last only a short time.

While you are in the hospital, members of the food or nutrition service, including a registered dietitian, can help you plan your diet. They also can help you solve your physical or emotional eating problems. Feel free to talk to them if problems arise during your recovery as well. Ask them what has worked for their other patients.

Don't be afraid to give food a chance. Not everyone has problems with eating during cancer treatment. Even those who have eating problems have days when eating is a pleasure.

Coping with Side Effects

The following offers practical hints for coping with treatment side effects that may affect your eating. These suggestions have helped other patients manage eating problems that can be frustrating to handle. Try all the ideas to find what works best for you. Share your needs and concerns with your family and friends, particularly those who prepare meals for you. Let them know that you appreciate their support as you work to take control of eating problems.

Loss of Appetite

Loss of appetite or poor appetite is one of the most common problems that occurs with cancer and its treatment. Many things affect appetite, including nausea, vomiting and being upset or depressed about having cancer. A person who has these feelings, whether physical or emotional, may not be interested in eating.

The following suggestions may help make meal times more relaxed so that you feel more like eating.

- Stay calm, especially at mealtimes. Don't hurry your meals.

- Involve yourself in as many normal activities as possible. If you feel uneasy and do not want to take part, don't force yourself.

- Try changing the time, place, and surroundings of meals. A candlelight dinner can make mealtime more appealing. Set a colorful table. Listen to soft music while eating. Eat with others or watch your favorite TV program while you eat.

- Eat whenever you are hungry. You do not need to eat just three main meals a day. Several small meals throughout the day may be even better.

- Add variety to your menu.

- Eat food often during the day, even at bedtime. Have healthy snacks handy. Taking just a few bites of the right foods or sips of the right liquids every hour or so can help you get more protein and calories.

Sore Mouth or Throat

Mouth sores, tender gums, and a sore throat or esophagus often result from radiation therapy, anticancer drugs, and infection. If you have a sore mouth or gums, see your doctor to be sure the soreness is a treatment side effect and not an unrelated dental problem. The doctor may be able to give you medicine that will control mouth and throat pain. Your dentist also can give you tips for care of your mouth.

Certain foods will irritate an already tender mouth and make chewing and swallowing difficult. By carefully choosing the foods you eat and by taking good care of your mouth, you can usually make eating easier. Here are some suggestions that may help:

- Try soft foods that are easy to chew and swallow, such as milk shakes; bananas, applesauce, and other soft fruits; peach, pear, and apricot nectars; watermelon; cottage cheese; mashed potatoes, macaroni and cheese; custards, puddings, and gelatin; scrambled eggs; oatmeal or other cooked cereals; pureed or mashed vegetables such as peas and carrots; pureed meats; liquids.

- Avoid foods that can irritate your mouth: citrus fruit or juice such as oranges, grapefruits, tangerines; spicy or salty foods; rough, coarse, or dry foods such as raw vegetables, granola, toast, crackers.

- Cook foods until they are soft and tender.

- Cut foods into small pieces.

- Mix food with butter, thin gravies, and sauces to make it easier to swallow.

- Use a blender or food processor to puree your food.

- Use a straw to drink liquids.

- Try foods cold or at room temperature. Hot and warm foods can irritate a tender mouth and throat.

- If swallowing is hard, tilting your head back or moving it forward may help.

- If heartburn is a problem, try sitting up or standing for about an hour after eating.

- If your teeth and gums are sore, your dentist may be able to recommend a special product for cleaning your teeth.

- Rinse your mouth with water often to remove food and bacteria and to promote healing.

- Ask your doctor about anesthetic lozenges and sprays that can numb the mouth and throat long enough for you to eat meals.

Changed Sense of Taste or Smell

Your sense of taste or smell may change during your illness or treatment. A condition called mouth blindness or taste blindness may give foods a bitter or metallic taste, especially meat or other high-protein foods. Many foods will have less taste. Chemotherapy, radiation therapy, or the cancer itself may cause these problems. Dental problems also can change the way foods taste. For most people, changes in taste and smell go away when their treatment is finished.

There is no "foolproof" way to improve the flavor or smell of food because each person is affected differently by illness and treatments. However, the tips given below should help make your food taste better. (If you also have a sore mouth, sore gums, or a sore throat, talk to your doctor or registered dietitian. They can suggest ways to improve the taste of your food without hurting the sore areas.)

- Choose and prepare foods that look and smell good to you.

- If red meat (such as beef) tastes or smells strange, use chicken, turkey, eggs, dairy products, or fish that doesn't have a strong smell instead.

- Help the flavor of meat, chicken, or fish by marinating it in sweet fruit juices, sweet wine, Italian dressing, or sweet-and-sour sauce.

- Try using small amounts of flavorful seasonings such as basil, oregano, or rosemary.

- Try tart foods such as oranges or lemonade that may have more taste. A tart lemon custard might taste good and will also provide needed protein and calories. (Do not try this if you have a sore mouth or throat.)

- Serve foods at room temperature.

- Try using bacon, ham, or onion to add flavor to vegetables.

- Stop eating foods that cause an unpleasant taste.

- Visit your dentist to rule out dental problems that may affect the taste or smell of food.

- Ask your dentist about special mouthwashes and good mouth care.

Dry Mouth

Chemotherapy and radiation therapy in the head or neck area can reduce the flow of saliva and often cause dry mouth. When this happens, foods are harder to chew and swallow. Dry mouth also can change the way foods taste. The suggestions below may be helpful in dealing with dry mouth. Also try some of the ideas for dealing with a sore mouth or throat, which can make foods easier to swallow.

- Try very sweet or tart foods and beverages such as lemonade; these foods may help your mouth produce more saliva. (Do not try this if you also have a tender mouth or sore throat.)
- Suck on sugar-free, hard candy or popsicles or chew sugar-free gum. These can help produce more saliva.
- Use soft and pureed foods, which may be easier to swallow.
- Keep your lips moist with lip salves.
- Eat foods with sauces, gravies, and salad dressings to make them moist and easier to swallow.
- Have a sip of water every few minutes to help you swallow and talk more easily.
- If your dry mouth problem is severe, ask your doctor or dentist about products that coat and protect your mouth and throat.

Nausea

Nausea, with or without vomiting, is a common side effect of surgery, chemotherapy, radiation therapy, and biological therapy. The disease itself, or other conditions unrelated to your cancer or treatment, also may cause nausea.

Whatever the cause, nausea can keep you from getting enough food and needed nutrients. Here are some ideas that may be helpful:

- Ask your doctor about medicine to help control nausea and vomiting. These drugs are called antiemetics.
- Try toast and crackers, yogurt, sherbet, pretzels, angel food cake, oatmeal, skinned chicken (baked or broiled, not fried), fruits and vegetables that are soft or bland (such as canned peaches), clear liquids (sipped slowly), and ice chips.

- Avoid fatty, greasy, fried, spicy, or hot food with strong odors; and sweets such as candy, cookies, or cake.

- Eat small amounts often and slowly.

- Avoid eating in a room that's stuffy, too warm, or has cooking odors that might disagree with you.

- Drink fewer liquids with meals. Drinking liquids can cause a full, bloated feeling.

- Drink or sip liquids throughout the day, except at mealtimes. Using a straw may help.

- Drink beverages cool or chilled. Try freezing favorite beverages in ice cube trays.

- Eat foods at room temperature or cooler; hot foods may add to nausea.

- Don't force yourself to eat favorite foods when you feel nauseated. This may cause a permanent dislike of those foods.

- Rest after meals, because activity may slow digestion. It's best to rest sitting up for about an hour after meals.

- If nausea is a problem in the morning, try eating dry toast or crackers before getting up.

- Wear loose-fitting clothes.

- Avoid eating for 1 to 2 hours before treatment if nausea occurs during radiation therapy or chemotherapy.

- Try to keep track of when your nausea occurs and what causes it (specific foods, events, surroundings). If possible, make appropriate changes in your diet or schedule. Share the information with your doctor or nurse.

Vomiting

Vomiting may follow nausea and may be brought on by treatment, food odors, gas in the stomach or bowel, or motion. In some people, certain surroundings, such as the hospital, may cause vomiting.

If vomiting is severe or lasts for more than a few days, contact your doctor.

Very often, if you can control nausea, you can prevent vomiting. At times, though, you may not be able to prevent either nausea or vomiting. You may find some relief by using relaxation exercises or meditation. These usually involve deep rhythmic breathing and quiet concentration and can be done almost anywhere. If vomiting occurs, try these hints to prevent further episodes.

- Ask your doctor about medicine to control nausea and vomiting (antiemetics).

- Do not drink or eat until you have the vomiting under control.

- Once you have controlled vomiting, try small amounts of clear liquids (see Clear Liquid Diet). Begin with 1 teaspoonful every 10 minutes, gradually increase the amount to 1 tablespoonful every 20 minutes, and finally try 2 tablespoonfuls every 30 minutes.

- When you are able to keep down clear liquids, try a full-liquid diet (see Full Liquid Diet). Continue taking small amounts as often as you can keep them down. If you feel okay on a full-liquid diet, gradually work up to your regular diet. If you have a hard time digesting milk, you may want to try a soft diet instead of a full-liquid diet. When you feel okay on the soft diet, gradually add more foods to return to your regular diet.(You can find information about these and other diets under "Special Diets for Special Needs.")

Diarrhea

Diarrhea may have several causes, including chemotherapy, radiation therapy to the abdomen, infection, food sensitivity, and emotional upset.

Long-term or severe diarrhea may cause other problems. During diarrhea, food passes quickly through the bowel before the body absorbs enough vitamins, minerals, and water. This may cause dehydration and increase the risk of infection. Contact your doctor if the diarrhea is severe or lasts for more than a couple of days. Here are some ideas for coping with diarrhea:

- Drink plenty of liquids during the day. Drinking fluids is important because your body may not get enough water when you have diarrhea.

- Eat small amounts of food throughout the day instead of three large meals.

- Eat plenty of foods and liquids that contain sodium (salt) and potassium. These minerals are often lost during diarrhea. Good liquid choices include bouillon or fat-free broth. Foods high in potassium that don't cause diarrhea include bananas, peach and apricot nectar, and boiled or mashed potatoes.

- Try these nutritious low-fiber foods: yogurt, rice or noodles, grape juice, farina or cream of wheat, eggs (cooked until the whites are solid, not fried), ripe bananas, smooth peanut butter, white bread, skinned chicken or turkey, lean beef, or fish (boiled or baked, not fried), cottage cheese, cream cheese.

- Eliminate greasy, fatty, or fried foods, raw vegetables and fruits; high-fiber vegetables such as broccoli, corn, beans, cabbage, peas, and cauliflower; strong spices, such as hot pepper, curry, and Cajun spice mix.

- Drink liquids that are at room temperature.

- Avoid very hot or very cold foods and beverages.

- Limit foods and beverages that contain caffeine, including coffee, strong tea, some sodas, and chocolate.

- Be careful when using milk and milk products because diarrhea may be caused by lactose intolerance. (If you think you have this problem, see "Low-Lactose Diet.") Ask your doctor or registered dietitian for advice.

- After sudden, short-term attacks of diarrhea (acute diarrhea), try a clear-liquid diet during the first 12 to 14 hours. This lets the bowel rest while replacing the important body fluids lost during diarrhea (see Clear-Liquid Diet.)

Constipation

Some anticancer drugs and other drugs, such as pain medicines, may cause constipation. This problem also may occur if your diet lacks enough fluid or bulk or if you have been bedridden.

Here are some suggestions to prevent and treat constipation:

- Drink plenty of liquids—at least eight 8-ounce glasses every day. This will help to keep your stools soft.

- Take a hot drink about one-half hour before your usual time for a bowel movement.

- Eat high-fiber foods, such as whole-grain breads, cereals, and pastas; fresh fruits and vegetables dried beans and peas; and whole-grain products such as barley or brown rice. Eat the skin on fruits and potatoes.

- Get exercise, such as walking, every day. Talk to your doctor or a physical therapist about the amount and type of exercise that is right for you.

- Add unprocessed wheat bran to foods such as cereals, casseroles, and homemade breads.

If these suggestions don't work, ask your doctor about medicine to ease constipation. Be sure to check with your doctor before taking any laxatives or stool softeners.

Weight Gain

Sometimes patients gain excess weight during treatment without eating extra calories. For example, certain anticancer drugs, such as prednisone, can cause the body to hold on to fluid, causing weight gain; this condition is known as edema. The extra weight is in the form of water and does not mean you are eating too much.

It is important not to go on a diet if you notice weight gain. Instead, tell your doctor so you can find out what may be causing this change. If anticancer drugs are causing your body to retain water, your doctor may ask you to speak with a registered dietitian. The registered dietitian can teach you how to limit the amount of salt you eat, which is important because salt causes your body to hold extra water. Drugs called diuretics also may be prescribed to get rid of extra fluid.

Tooth Decay

Cancer and cancer treatment can cause tooth decay and other problems for your teeth and gums. Changes in eating habits also may add to the problem. If you eat frequently or consume a lot of sweets, you may need to brush your teeth more often. Brushing after each meal or snack is a good idea.

Here are some ideas for preventing dental problems:

- Be sure to see your dentist regularly. Patients who are receiving treatment that affects the mouth (e.g., radiation to the head and neck) may need to see the dentist more often than usual.

- Use a soft toothbrush. Ask your doctor, nurse, or dentist to suggest a special kind of toothbrush and/or toothpaste if your gums are very sensitive.

- Rinse your mouth with warm water when your gums and mouth are sore.

- If you are not having trouble with poor appetite or weight loss, limit the amount of sugar in your diet.

- Avoid eating foods that stick to the teeth, such as caramels or chewy candy bars.

Lactose Intolerance

Lactose intolerance means that your body can't digest or absorb the milk sugar called lactose. Milk, other dairy products, and foods to which milk has been added contain lactose.

Lactose intolerance may occur after treatment with some antibiotics, radiation to the stomach, or any treatment that affects the digestive tract. The part of your intestines that breaks down lactose may not work properly during treatment. For some people, symptoms of lactose intolerance (gas, cramping, diarrhea) disappear a few weeks or months after the treatments end or when the intestine heals. For others a permanent change in eating habits may be needed.

If you have this problem, your doctor may advise you to follow a diet that is low in foods that contain lactose (see "Low-Lactose Diet.") If milk had been a main source of protein in your diet, it will be important to get enough protein from other foods. Products such as soybean and aged cheeses are good sources of protein and other nutrients. You also may want to try low-lactose milk or liquid drops or caplets that help break down the lactose in milk and other dairy products.

Saving Time and Energy

Your body needs both rest and nourishment during and after treatment for cancer. If you are usually the cook, here are some suggestions for saving time and energy in preparing meals.

- Let someone else do the cooking when possible.

- If you know that your recovery time from treatment or surgery is going to be longer than 1 or 2 days, prepare a helper list. Decide who can help you shop, cook, set the table, and clean up. Write it down, discuss it, and post it where it can easily be seen. If children help, plan a small reward for them.

- Write out menus. Choose things that you or your family can put together easily. Casseroles, TV dinners, hot dogs, hamburgers, and meals that you have prepared and frozen ahead are all good ideas. Cook larger batches to be frozen so you will have them for future use. Add instructions so that other people can help you.

- Use shopping lists. Keep them handy so that they can be used as guides either by you or other people.

- When making casseroles for freezing, only partially cook rice and macaroni products. They will cook further in the reheating process. Add ½ cup liquid to refrigerated or frozen casseroles when reheating because they can get dry during refrigeration. Remember that frozen casseroles take a long time to heat completely—at least 45 minutes in deep dishes in the oven.

- Don't be shy about accepting gifts of food and offers of help from family and friends. Let them know what you like and offer your recipes. If people bring food you can't use right away, freeze it. That home cooked meal can break the monotony of quickie suppers. It also can save time when you're on a tight schedule. Date the food when you put it in the refrigerator or freezer.

- Have as few dishes, pots, and pans to wash as possible. Cook in dishes and pans that can also make attractive servers. Use paper napkins and disposable dishes, especially for dessert. Paper cups are fine for kids and for medicines. Disposable pans are a great time-saver—foil containers from frozen foods make good disposable pans. Soak dirty dishes to cut down washing time.

- When you are preparing soft dishes, choose foods that the whole family can eat, such as omelets, scrambled eggs, macaroni and cheese, meatloaf, tuna salad sandwiches, or tuna casseroles. Set aside enough food to be pureed in the blender or food processor for yourself.

- Use mixes, frozen ready-to-eat main dishes, and takeout foods whenever possible. The less time spent cooking and cleaning up, the more time for relaxation and the family.

- If someone is cooking for you, share this information with them for ideas for food selection and preparation. They will also get a better sense of your special needs.

Improving Your Nutrition

There are many ways to improve your nutrition to lessen the side effects of your treatment and to keep eating as well as you can when your treatment or illness is causing side effects. Table 29.1 provides a list of snacks you may want to try. Table 29.2 offers ideas for increasing protein in your diet, and Table 29.3 shows ways of increasing calories.

When side effects of treatment occur, they usually go away after treatment ends. Long-term treatment, however, may necessitate long-term changes in your diet to help you handle side effects and keep up your strength.

The ideas and suggestions listed here have worked for other cancer patients during their treatment. Each person is different, though, and you will have to find out what works best for you.

Table 29.1. Snacks

Have these on hand for quick and easy nibbles:

- Applesauce
- Bread products, including muffins and crackers
- Buttered popcorn
- Cakes and cookies made with whole-grains, fruits, nuts, wheat germ, or granola
- Cereal
- Cheese, hard or semisoft
- Cheesecake
- Chocolate milk
- Cottage cheese
- Cream cheese and other soft cheese
- Cream soups
- Dips made with cheese, beans, or sour cream
- Dried fruits, such as raisins, prunes, or apricots
- Fruits (fresh or canned)
- Gelatin salads and desserts
- Granola
- Hard-boiled and deviled eggs
- Ice cream, frozen yogurt, popsicles
- Juices
- Milkshakes, instant breakfast drinks
- Nuts
- Peanut butter
- Pizza
- Puddings and custards
- Quesadillas
- Sandwiches
- Vegetables (raw or cooked)
- Yogurt (regular or frozen)

Table 29.2. How to Increase Protein (continued on next page)

Hard or Semisoft Cheese
- Melt on sandwiches, bread, muffins, tortillas, hamburgers, hot dogs, other meats or fish, vegetables, eggs, or desserts, such as stewed fruit or pies.
- Grate and add to soups, sauces, casseroles, vegetable dishes, mashed potatoes, rice, noodles, or meatloaf

Cottage Cheese/ Ricotta Cheese
- Mix with or use to stuff fruits and vegetables.
- Add to casseroles, spaghetti, noodles, and egg dishes, such as omelets, scrambled eggs, and soufflés.
- Use in gelatin, pudding-type desserts, cheesecake, and pancake batter.
- Use to stuff crepes and pasta shells or manicotti.

Milk
- Use milk in beverages and in cooking when possible.
- Use in preparing hot cereal, soups, cocoa, and pudding.
- Add cream sauces to vegetable and other dishes.

Powdered Milk
- Add to regular milk and milk drinks, such as pasteurized eggnog and milkshakes.
- Use in casseroles, meatloaf, breads, muffins, sauces, cream soups, mashed potatoes, puddings and custards, and milk-based desserts.

Commercial Products
- See the section below on "Commercial Products to Improve Nutrition."
- Use instant breakfast powder in milk drinks and desserts.
- Mix with ice cream, milk, and fruit or flavorings for a high-protein milkshake.

Ice Cream, Yogurt, and Frozen Yogurt
- Add to carbonated beverages, such as ginger ale; add to milk drinks, such as milkshakes.
- Add to cereals, fruits, gelatin desserts, and pies; blend or whip with soft or cooked fruits.
- Sandwich ice cream or frozen yogurt between enriched cake slices, cookies, or graham crackers.

Table 29.2. How to Increase Protein (continued from previous page)

Eggs

- Add chopped, hard-cooked eggs to salads and dressings, vegetables, casseroles, and creamed meats.
- Add extra eggs or egg whites to quiches and to pancake and French toast batter. Add extra egg whites to scrambled eggs and omelets.
- Make a rich custard with eggs, high-protein milk, and sugar.
- Add extra hard-cooked yolks to deviled-egg filling and sandwich spreads.
- *Avoid raw eggs, which may contain harmful bacteria, because your treatment may make you susceptible to infection.* Make sure all eggs you eat are well cooked or baked; avoid eggs that are "runny."

Nuts, Seeds, and Wheat Germ

- Add to casseroles, breads, muffins, pancakes, cookies, and waffles.
- Sprinkle on fruit, cereal, ice cream, yogurt, vegetables, salads, and toast as a crunchy topping; use in place of bread crumbs.
- Blend with parsley or spinach, herbs, and cream for a noodle, pasta, or vegetable sauce.
- Roll banana in chopped nuts.

Peanut Butter

- Spread on sandwiches, toast, muffins, crackers, waffles, pancakes, and fruit slices.
- Use as a dip for raw vegetables such as carrots, cauliflower, and celery.
- Blend with milk drinks and beverages.
- Swirl through soft ice cream and yogurt.

Meat and Fish

- Add chopped, cooked meat or fish to vegetables, salads, casseroles, soups, sauces, and biscuit dough.
- Use in omelets, soufflés, quiches, sandwich fillings, and chicken and turkey stuffings.
- Wrap in pie crust or biscuit dough as turnovers.
- Add to stuffed baked potatoes.

Beans/Legumes

- Cook and use dried peas, legumes, beans, and bean curd (tofu) in soups or add to casseroles, pastas, and grain dishes that also contain cheese or meat. Mash with cheese and milk.

Table 29.3. How to Increase Calories (continued on next page)

Butter and Margarine

- Add to soups, mashed and baked potatoes, hot cereals, grits, rice, noodles, and cooked vegetables.
- Stir into cream soups, sauces, and gravies.
- Combine with herbs and seasonings, and spread on cooked meats, hamburgers, and fish and egg dishes.
- Use melted butter or margarine as a dip for raw vegetables and seafoods, such as shrimp, scallops, crab, and lobster.

Whipped Cream

- Use sweetened on hot chocolate, desserts, gelatin, puddings, fruits, pancakes, and waffles.
- Fold unsweetened into mashed potatoes or vegetable purees.

Table Cream

- Use in cream soups, sauces, egg dishes, batters, puddings, and custards.
- Put on hot or cold cereal.
- Mix with noodles, pasta, rice, and mashed potatoes.
- Pour on chicken and fish while baking.
- Use as a binder in hamburgers, meatloaf, and croquettes.
- Add to milk in recipes.
- Make hot chocolate with cream and add marshmallows.

Cream Cheese

- Spread on breads, muffins, fruit slices, and crackers.
- Add to vegetables.
- Roll into balls and coat with chopped nuts, wheat germ, or granola.

Sour Cream

- Add to cream soups, baked potatoes, macaroni and cheese, vegetables, sauces, salad dressings, stews, baked meat, and fish.
- Use as a topping for cakes, fruit, gelatin desserts, breads, and muffins.
- Use as a dip for fresh fruits and vegetables.
- For a good dessert, scoop it on fresh fruit, add brown sugar, and let it sit in the refrigerator for a while.

Salad Dressings and Mayonnaise

- Spread on sandwiches and crackers.
- Combine with meat, fish, and egg or vegetable salads.

Table 29.3. How to Increase Calories (continued from previous page)

- Use as a binder in croquettes.
- Use in sauces and gelatin dishes.

Honey, Jam, and Sugar
- Add to bread, cereal, milk drinks, and fruit and yogurt desserts.
- Use as a glaze for meats, such as chicken.

Granola
- Use in cookie, muffin, and bread batters.
- Sprinkle on vegetables, yogurt, ice cream, pudding, custard, and fruit.
- Layer with fruits and bake.
- Mix with dry fruits and nuts for a snack.
- Substitute for bread or rice in pudding recipes.

Dried Fruits
- Cook and serve for breakfast or as a dessert or snack.
- Add to muffins, cookies, breads, cakes, rice and grain dishes, cereals, puddings, and stuffings.
- Bake in pies and turnovers.
- Combine with cooked vegetables, such as carrots, sweet potatoes, yams, and acorn and butternut squash.
- Combine with nuts or granola for snacks.

Eggs
- Add chopped, hard-cooked eggs to salads and dressings, vegetables, casseroles, and creamed meats.
- Make a rich custard with eggs, milk, and sugar.
- Add extra, hard-cooked yolks to deviled-egg filling and sandwich spread.
- Beat eggs into mashed potatoes, vegetable purees, and sauces. (Be sure to keep cooking these dishes after adding the eggs because raw eggs may contain harmful bacteria.)
- Add extra eggs or egg whites to custards, puddings, quiches, scrambled eggs, omelets, and to pancake and French toast batter before cooking.

Food Preparation
- Bread meats and vegetables.
- Sauté and fry foods when possible, because these cooking methods add more calories than baking or broiling.
- Add sauces or gravies.

Special Diets For Special Needs

When you have special needs because of your illness or treatment, your doctor or registered dietitian may prescribe a special diet. They also may suggest a commercial product to help you meet your nutritional needs. In this section, you will find guidelines for several special diets used during cancer treatment. You also will learn about products that can boost nutrition. Remember that special diets and products to improve nutrition should be used only as recommended by your doctor or registered dietitian.

Special diets are an important tool for correcting nutritional problems that occur during cancer treatment. For example, a soft diet may be best if your mouth, throat, esophagus, or stomach is sore. Or, if your treatment makes it difficult for you to digest dairy products, you may need to follow a low-lactose diet. Some diets are well balanced and can be followed for long periods of time. However, some special diets should be followed for only a few days because they may not provide enough nutrients for the long term.

Only your doctor or registered dietitian should decide whether you need a special diet and for how long. If you are already following a special diet for another health problem, such as diabetes or high cholesterol, you and your doctor and registered dietitian should work together to develop your new plan.

Guidelines for common special diets appear in this section, including:

- Clear-liquid diet.
- Full-liquid diet.
- Soft diet.
- Fiber-restricted diet.
- Low-lactose diet.

For each diet, you will find a brief explanation of when the diet usually is recommended, the major foods it includes, and a suggested meal pattern. This information will help you follow the diet recommended by your doctor or registered dietitian. If you think you need a special diet, talk with your doctor or registered dietitian.

Clear-Liquid Diet

Clear-liquid diets are useful if the body can't handle the softest foods or heavy or thick liquids. Patients usually follow this type of diet after surgery or before stomach or bowel surgery. Patients with severe nausea and vomiting may also have this diet. A clear-liquid diet often lasts 1 to 2 days or until you can drink or eat other beverages and foods. It cannot meet the daily servings suggested (except for fruit juices), but it helps ensure that your body doesn't lose too much fluid as you recover and become ready for a regular diet.

Clear-Liquid Diet Suggested Meal Pattern

Breakfast
1 cup juice
1 cup clear broth
½ cup gelatin dessert
Coffee or tea* with sugar

Snack
1 cup fruit juice or soft drink
½ cup gelatin dessert

Lunch
1 cup juice
1 cup clear broth
½ cup gelatin dessert
Coffee or tea* with sugar

Snack
1 cup fruit juice or soft drink
½ cup gelatin dessert

Dinner
1 cup juice
1 cup clear broth
½ cup gelatin dessert
Coffee or tea* with sugar

Snack
1 cup fruit juice or soft drink
½ cup gelatin dessert

*Your doctor may recommend decaffeinated coffee or tea.
**Check with your doctor about alcohol. Alcohol cannot be used safely with some medicines.

Table 29.4. Clear-Liquid Diet

Type of Food	Allowed Items	Excluded Items
Beverages	Water; carbonated beverages; cereal beverages; coffee, tea;* fruit-flavored drinks; strained lemonade, limeade, and fruit punches	Milk, milk drinks, all others**
Breads Cereals Flours	None	All
Cheeses	None	All
Desserts	Plain gelatin desserts, fruit ices without milk or pieces of fruit, popsicles	All others
Eggs	None	All
Fats	None	All
Fruits Fruit Juices	Apple, cranberry, and grape juice; strained citrus juices if tolerated	All others
Meat Poultry Fish Legumes	None	All
Milk Milk Products	None	All
Potatoes Rice Pasta	None	All
Soup	Bouillon, clear fat-free broths, consommé	All others
Sweets	Honey, jelly, syrups, plain sugar candy in small amounts	All others
Vegetables	Strained vegetable broth	All others
Miscellaneous	Salt	All others

*Your doctor may recommend decaffeinated coffee or tea.
**Check with your doctor about alcohol. Alcohol cannot be used safely with some medicines.

Full-Liquid Diet

You may follow a full-liquid diet when your body can digest all liquids but can't handle solid food yet. Your doctor or registered dietitian may recommend this diet after surgery or when you can't chew and swallow food. All liquids served at room or body temperature are part of this diet. This diet can include most of the recommended food groups except meat. Extra milk has been included to ensure adequate protein. When planned properly, this diet can be used for long periods. In these instances, your doctor may prescribe a commercial supplement and/or certain vitamins. However, you should only take these if your doctor or registered dietitian recommends them.

If you must follow a full-liquid diet over a long period, you can increase the protein and calorie content of the diet by following some of the suggestions in Table 29.2 and Table 29.3.

Full-Liquid Diet Suggested Meal Pattern

Breakfast
1 cup fruit juice
1 cup strained cereal
1 cup milk
Coffee or tea* with sugar

Snack
1 cup fruit juice

Lunch
1 cup strained soup, (made with vegetable purée)
1 cup strained cereal
½ cup allowed dessert
1 cup fruit juice
1 cup milk or yogurt

Coffee or tea* with sugar
Snack
1 cup milk or eggnog

Dinner
1 cup strained cream soup (with a small amount of strained meat)
1 cup milk
1 cup strained cereal
½ cup allowed dessert
1 cup vegetable juice
Coffee or tea* with sugar

Snack
1 cup milk or yogurt

*Your doctor may recommend decaffeinated coffee or tea.
**Check with your doctor before drinking alcohol. Alcohol cannot be used safely with some medicines.

Table 29.5. Full-Liquid Diet

Type of Food	Allowed Items	Excluded Items
Beverages	Cereal beverages; coffee, tea*; fruit drinks; strained lemonade, limeade, or fruit punches; water	None**
Breads Cereals Flours	Refined or strained cooked cereal	Breads and cereals in solid form
Cheeses	Cheese soup	All others
Desserts	Plain gelatin desserts, junket, soft or baked custards, sherbets, plain cornstarch pudding, fresh or frozen yogurt, ice milk, smooth ice cream	All others, particularly those with fruits or seeds
Eggs	Pasteurized eggnog	All others
Fats	Butter, cream, oils, margarine	All others
Fruits Fruit Juices	All juices and nectars, thin fruit purees	All others
Meat Poultry Fish Legumes	Small amounts of strained meat in broth or gelatin	All others
Milk Milk Products	Buttermilk and chocolate, skim, and whole milk; ice milk; milkshakes; plain yogurt	All others, yogurt with pieces of fruit
Potatoes Rice Pasta	Potatoes pureed in soup	All others
Soups	Bouillon, broth, clear cream soups, any strained or blenderized soup	All others
Sweets	Honey, jelly, syrups in small amounts	All others
Vegetables	Tomato puree for cream soups; tomato, vegetable juices	All others
Miscellaneous	Flavoring extracts, salt	All others

*Your doctor may recommend decaffeinated coffee or tea.
**Check with your doctor before drinking alcohol. Alcohol cannot be used safely with some medicines.

Soft Diet

A soft diet is useful when your body is ready for more than liquids but still unable to handle a regular solid diet. Soft food is easier to eat than regular food when the mouth, throat, esophagus, and/or stomach are sore. This soreness can occur to these parts of the body during and after radiation therapy or during chemotherapy. A soft diet can be used for long periods because it contains all needed nutrients. The diet consists of bland, lower fat foods that you soften by cooking, mashing, pureeing, or blending.

The table lists foods included in a soft diet as well as foods you should try to avoid. Keep in mind, however, that you may be able to eat some of the "excluded" foods without any discomfort or problems. In general, though, it is probably best to avoid fried or greasy foods and foods that may cause gas.

Soft Diet Suggested Meal Pattern

Breakfast

½ cup fruit or juice
2 eggs, scrambled
1 slice toast
1 tsp. butter or margarine
Jelly
Sugar and cream
Beverage

Snack

½ to 1 cup cereal
1 cup milk
Sugar

Lunch

½ cup fruit juice
2 oz. meat, fish, or poultry
½ cup vegetable
2 slices bread
1 tsp. butter or margarine

1 cup milk

Snack

Banana
2 tbsp. creamy peanut butter

Dinner

4 oz. meat, fish, or poultry
1 cup potato
½ cup vegetable
1 slice bread or roll
1 tsp. butter or margarine
1 serving fruit or allowed dessert
Beverage

Snack

½ cup fruit or allowed dessert
1 cup milk, milkshake, or pasteurized eggnog

**Check with your doctor before drinking alcohol. Alcohol cannot be used safely with some medicines.

Table 29.6. Soft Diet (continued on next page)

Type of Food	Allowed Items	Excluded Items
Beverages	All	None**
Breads	French, Vienna, Italian, seedless rye, white, refined whole wheat, cornbread, or any except whole-grain; if tolerated, muffins, French toast, crackers, biscuits, rolls, pancakes, waffles	Brown, cracked wheat, pumpernickel, raisin,rye with seeds, buckwheat; whole-grain crackers; rolls with coconut, raisins, nuts,or whole grains; tortillas
Cereals	Refined, cooked, or ready-to eat, such as cream of wheat, farina, hominy grits, corn-meal, oatmeal, puffed rice	Whole-grain or bran
Flours	All except those excluded	Whole-grain, bran, or wheat
Cheeses	All except those excluded	Sharp or strongly fla-vored cheeses; those containing whole seeds and spices
Desserts	Ice milk, ice cream, sherbet, ices, custards, gelatins, or others with allowed fruits	Desserts made with excluded fruits, nuts, coconut
Eggs	All except those excluded	Raw, fried
Fats	Butter, cream, cream substi-tutes, vegetable shortening and oils, margarine, mayonnaise,sour cream, commercial French dressing	Other salad dressings; salt pork; fried foods
Fruits Fruit Juices	All juices and nectars; avocado, banana, canned or cooked apples, apricots, cherries, grapefruit and orange sections without membrane, peaches, pears, seedless grapes, tomatoes; soft melons, such as water-melon, if tolerated	All raw fruit except avocado and banana; all dried fruit; berries, crabapples,coconut, figs, grapes, pine-apples, plums, rhubarb
Meat	Tender beef, lamb, veal, or liver that is baked, broiled, creamed, roasted, or stewed; roasted or stewed pork	Fried, salted, and smoked meats;chitter-lings; corned beef, sausage; cold cuts

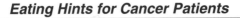

Table 29.6. Soft Diet (continued from previous page)

Type of Food	Allowed Items	Excluded Items
Poultry	Chicken, Cornish game hen, turkey, chicken livers	Duck, goose; fried poultry
Fish	Cooked, fresh, or frozen fish without bones; tuna, salmon	Fried fish, shellfish, anchovies, caviar, herring, sardines, snails, skate
Legumes Nuts	Creamy peanut butter	All other legumes, nuts, and seed kernels
Milk Milk Products	All	None
Potatoes Rice Pasta	Baked, boiled, creamed, scalloped, mashed, au gratin; mashed sweet potatoes; dumplings; noodles; brown or white rice; spaghetti	French fries, hashbrowns, potato salad, whole sweet potatoes or yams; bread stuffing; fritters; chow mein noodles; wild rice; barley
Soups	Bouillon, broth, consommé, strained cream and vegetable	Bean, split pea, onion; bisques; gumbos; unstrained chowders
Sweets	Apple butter, butterscotch candy, caramels, chocolate, fondant, plain fudge, lollipops, marshmallows, mints, honey, jelly, syrups, sugars in small amounts	Candied fruits, nut brittle, jams, preserves, marmalade, marzipan, fruit sauces with prohibited fruits
Vegetables	Canned or cooked asparagus, carrots, beets, eggplant, mushrooms, parsley, pumpkin, spinach, squash, vegetable juice cocktail, raw lettuce if tolerated	All raw vegetables except lettuce; all canned or cooked vegetables not specifically listed as allowed
Miscellaneous	Aspic, catsup, gelatin, gravy, pretzels, soy sauce, vinegar; brown, cheese, cream, tomato, and white sauces; all finely chopped or ground leaf herbs and spices	Garlic, horseradish; olives, pickles; popcorn, potato chips; relishes; chili, a-la-king, Creole, barbecue, cocktail, sweet-and-sour, Newburg, and Worcestershire sauces; whole and seed herbs and spices

**Check with your doctor before drinking alcohol. Alcohol cannot be used safely with some medicines.

Fiber Restricted Diet

Your doctor or registered dietitian may recommend a fiber-restricted diet if your gastrointestinal (GI) tract cannot digest fiber in foods. This type of diet is often used after GI surgery before patients return to their regular diet. A fiber-restricted diet also may be needed when treatment, such as radiation, damages the bowel or when the GI tract becomes irritated.

A fiber-restricted diet limits the amount of vegetables, fruits, cereals, and grains that you can eat. It also limits to two cups per day the amount of milk and milk products, such as cream, yogurt, and cheese, that you can eat. Milk does not contain fiber, but it leaves a residue in the GI tract that can irritate the bowel and cause diarrhea and cramping. The diet also is helpful for the many cancer patients who have a hard time digesting the milk sugar, lactose. (See also "Low Lactose Diet".) A fiber-restricted diet can be changed easily, depending on how you feel after eating certain foods. Use the diet in this chapter as a guide and discuss any changes with your doctor or registered dietitian.

There may be times when a low-residue diet, which is more limited than a fiber-restricted diet, is needed. On the low-residue diet, you may be able to eat most strained vegetables and fruit juices, such as white potatoes without skin, and tomato juice. All other forms of vegetables and fruits may be excluded from the diet. The low-residue diet also limits the amount of fat and dairy products you can eat. Your doctor or registered dietitian will let you know if you need to follow a low residue diet.

Your registered dietitian may gradually increase fiber and milk products in your diet according to how well you handle them.

Low-Lactose Diet

All milk products contain lactose (or milk sugar). The doctor or registered dietitian may recommend a low-lactose diet after radiation therapy to the intestines, which often makes lactose hard to digest for a time. Fermented milk products, such as buttermilk, acidophilus milk, sour cream, and yogurt, usually are easier to handle than whole milk. You also can buy low-lactose milk or use liquid drops or caplets that help break down the lactose in milk and other dairy products. Lactose is often used as a filler in many products such as instant coffee and some medicines. Carefully read labels on commercial foods to see if they contain lactose or any milk products or milk solids.

Fiber-Restricted Diet Suggested Meal Pattern

Breakfast
½ cup strained fruit juice*
1 egg
1 slice white toast
3 tsp. butter or margarine
Jelly

Snack
1 cup milk**
1 serving allowed cereal
Sugar

Lunch
½ cup soup***
2 oz. meat, poultry, or fish
½ cup allowed vegetable
2 slices white bread or roll
1 serving allowed dessert

Snack
2 slices white toast
2 tsp. butter or margarine
Jelly or honey

Dinner
5 oz. meat, poultry, or fish
1 cup milk**
3 tsp. butter or margarine
1 baked potato, without skin
1 serving allowed dessert
½ cup vegetable juice

Snack
½ cup strained fruit juice*
3 plain cookies

* 2 servings of fruit/juices allowed per day.
** 2 servings of milk allowed per day.
*** Count as ½ cup milk if made with milk.

Table 29.7. Fiber-Restricted Diet (continued on next page)

Type of Food	Allowed Items	Excluded Items
Beverages	Fruit-flavored drinks; carbonated beverages, coffee, tea;* milk drinks and milk used in cooking (2 cups milk or milk products allowed per day, if tolerated); all others except excluded items, no limitations	Prune juice, pear nectar**
Breads	French, Vienna, Italian, refined wheat, white, and rye breads without seeds; crackers; biscuits; French toast; plain hard crust; zwieback rolls	Breads, crackers, rolls, or cereals containing whole grain or graham flour; bran, seeds, nuts, or raisins; cornbread
Cereals	All refined, cooked, or dry cereals, such as cream of wheat or rice and flaked or puffed cereals	All whole-grain cereals made from prohibited flours or other foods; oatmeal; granola
Cheeses	Cottage, cream, American, Swiss, Muenster, or other mild cheese; 1 oz. may be substituted for 1 cup milk	All others
Desserts	Custards, gelatin puddings, plain cookies and cakes, sherbets; ½ cup ice cream (may be substituted as ½ cup milk allowance), pastries made with allowed ingredients	All desserts containing seeds, nuts, coconut, or raisins; tough-skinned fruits
Eggs	All except raw	Raw
Fats	Butter, oils, cream, dry cream substitutes, margarine, mayonnaise, shortenings, smooth salad dressings, sour cream	Salad dressing made with excluded foods; tartar sauce
Fruits	Canned or cooked fruits without seeds, skins, or membranes— apples, applesauce, cherries, grapefruit, oranges, tangerine, peaches, pineapple, pears, fruit cocktail; raw—ripe bananas, melon, grapefruit, oranges, tangerine; juice—all except prune juice and pear nectar (2 servings allowed per day)	All other fruits; dried fruits; berries; figs; grapes with seeds; stewed prunes, prune purée; plums; pear nectar

Table 29.7. Fiber-Restricted Diet (continued from previous page)

Type of Food	Allowed Items	Excluded Items
Meat Poultry	Tender beef, ham, lamb, liver, poultry, or veal that is baked, broiled, or stewed; lean or low-fat cold cuts and frankfurters	Fried meats and poultry, smoked or cured meats, cold cuts, corned beef, frankfurters, pastrami, sausage
Fish	Fresh or frozen fish without bones, canned tuna or salmon, cooked shellfish	All fried or smoked fish, sardines, herring
Legumes Nuts	None	All dried legumes, lima beans, peas, nuts
Milk Milk Products	Buttermilk and chocolate, skim, low-fat, and whole milk if tolerated; yogurt, plain, custard-style, with allowed fruits and without nuts (2 cups, including that used in cooking, allowed per day)	Yogurt containing fruits
Potatoes Rice Pasta	Boiled, creamed, mashed, and scalloped potatoes without skin; macaroni, noodles, white rice, spaghetti (1 serving potato allowed per day; all others, no limitation)	Potato skin, potato cakes, french fries, hash browns, potato salad, sweet potato, brown and wild rice, barley, hominy
Soups	Cream and broth-based soups made with allowed foods	All others
Sweets	Honey, jelly, syrup, plain hard candy, molasses, marsh-mallows, gumdrops	Jams, preserves, candies with fruits, coconut, raisins, nuts, candied fruits
Vegetables	Canned or cooked asparagus tips, green or wax beans, mushrooms, peas, pumpkin, raw lettuce, if tolerated (no limitation on vegetable juices; 1 serving whole vegetables allowed per day)	All raw vegetables except lettuce; canned or cooked vegetables not specifically allowed, such as the high-fiber vegetables: beans, carrots, peas, spinach and other greens, beets
Miscellaneous	Ground or finely chopped herbs and spices, salt, flavor-ing extracts, catsup, chocolate, mild gravy, white sauce, soy sauce, vinegar	All other spices and condiments, olives, pickles, potato chips, popcorn

*Your doctor may recommend decaffeinated coffee or tea.
**Check with your doctor before drinking alcohol. Alcohol cannot be used safely with some medicines.

Lactose tolerance varies from person to person. Ask your doctor or registered dietitian about choosing allowed foods and about low-lactose dairy products that you can buy at the grocery store.

Low-Lactose Diet Suggested Meal Pattern

Breakfast
½ cup fruit juice
1 serving cereal
1 slice toast
1 tsp. margarine*
Jelly
1 cup acidophilus or low-lactose milk
Sugar
Salt and pepper
Beverage

Snack
Crackers*
2 tbsp. peanut butter
Jelly or honey

Lunch
3 oz. meat or substitute
½ cup vegetable and/or salad
2 slices bread or roll
2 tsp. margarine*
1 serving fruit
Salt and pepper
Beverage

Snack
Broth-based soup
1 slice bread or roll
1 tsp. margarine*

Dinner
1 serving salad
3 oz. meat or substitute
½ cup rice
½ cup vegetable
1 serving fruit or dessert
1 cup acidophilus or low-lactose milk
Salt and pepper

Snack
½ cup juice
Popcorn or pretzels*

* Should not contain milk solids.

*Your doctor may recommend decaffeinated coffee or tea.
**Check with your doctor before drinking alcohol. Alcohol cannot be used safely with some medicines.

Table 29.8. Low-Lactose Diet (continued on next page)

Type of Food	Allowed Items	Excluded Items
Beverages	Water, lactose-free carbonated beverages, fruit-flavored drinks, fruit punches, lemonade, limeade, nondairy product drinks, low-lactose milk, acidophilus milk, coffee, and tea*	Artificial fruit drinks containing lactose, all beverages and nutritional supplements made with milk and milk products with the exception of buttermilk, low-lactose milk, and yogurt**
Bread	All	None
Cereals	Any cooked or dry cereal not containing lactose	Instant hot cereals, high-protein cereals, all cereals with added milk or lactose
Flours	All	None
Cheeses	Fermented cheeses (cheddar and any cheese aged with bacteria)	All others
Desserts	Fruit ices; gelatins; angel food cake; desserts made with nondairy products, buttermilk, or sour cream	Ice cream, puddings, and other desserts containing milk or milk products
Eggs	All except raw eggs and eggs prepared with milk or milk products	Creamed, scrambled, omelets, or other eggs prepared with milk; raw eggs
Fats	Margarine not containing milk solids, vegetable oils, mayonnaise, shortening	All others: cream, half-and-half, table and whipping cream, butter
Fruits Fruit Juices	All fresh, canned, or frozen fruit juices; fruits not processed with lactose	Any canned or frozen fruits and fruit juices processed with lactose
Meat Poultry Fish Legumes Nuts	Any except those specifically excluded	Creamed or breaded fish, poultry, meat; cold cuts, hot dogs, liver, sausage, or other processed meats containing milk or lactose; gravies made with milk

Table 29.8. Low-Lactose Diet (continued from previous page)

Type of Food	Allowed Items	Excluded Items
Milk Milk Products	Fermented milk products such as acidophilus milk, buttermilk, yogurt, and sour cream; low-lactose products; "lactose-digesting" pills or caplets	All milk, milk products except those allowed
Potatoes Rice Pasta	White or sweet potatoes, macaroni, noodles, spaghetti or other pasta, rice	Any prepared with milk, such as commercially prepared creamed or scalloped potato products containing dried milk
Soups	Broth-based soups	Cream soups, chowders, commercially prepared soups that contain milk or milk products
Sweets	Honey, jams, preserves,	Candy containing lactose, syrups, molasses milk, or cocoa; butter-scotch candies; caramels; chocolates (Read all labels carefully)
Vegetables	All vegetables except those prepared with milk	Any prepared with milk, such as creamed, scalloped, or any processed vegetables containing lactose
Miscellaneous	Catsup, chili sauce, horseradish, olives, pickles, vinegar, gravies prepared without milk, mustard, all herbs and spices, peanut butter, unbuttered popcorn	Chocolate, cocoa, milk gravies, cream sauces, chewing gum, instant coffee, powdered soft drinks, artificial juices containing milk or lactose

*Your doctor may recommend decaffeinated coffee or tea.
**Check with your doctor before drinking alcohol. Alcohol cannot be used safely with some medicines.

Commercial Products to Improve Nutrition

If you cannot get enough calories and protein from your diet, commercial nutrition supplements, such as formulas and instant breakfast powders, maybe helpful. There also are products that can be added to any food or beverage to boost calorie content. These supplements are high in protein and calories and have extra vitamins and minerals. They come in liquid, pudding, and powder forms. Prepackaged blenderized diets made from whole foods also are available. These are a convenient and inexpensive alternative to homemade preparations. Most commercial nutrition supplements contain little or no lactose. However, it is important to check the label if you are sensitive to lactose.

These products need no refrigeration until you open them. Thus, you can carry nutrition supplements with you and take them whenever you feel hungry or thirsty. They are good chilled as between-meal and bedtime snacks. You may want to take a can or two with you when you go for treatments or other times when long waits may tire you. Ask your registered dietitian which supplements would be best for you.

Many supermarkets and drugstores carry a variety of commercial nutrition supplements. If you don't see these products on the shelf, ask the store manager if they can be ordered. You also may want to ask your doctor or registered dietitian for information about products for special patients. Be sure to ask for manufacturers' names, and, as mentioned above, be sure to read the label to see if any of the products contains lactose.

Chapter 30

Nutrition Intervention in the Treatment of Eating Disorders

Onset of an eating disorder typically follows a period of restrictive dieting; however, only a minority of people who diet develop eating disorders. Those who do are emotionally and psychologically vulnerable when they develop the self-destructive behaviors characteristic of an eating disorder (e.g., practicing unsafe dieting techniques, taking unproven diet products, and maintaining arbitrary standards of weight). As purveyors of food, nutrition, and health information, registered dietitians should identify and inform health professionals and the lay public of the dangers of fad diets and diet products and should educate the public regarding healthful weight ranges and weight stabilization methods. Dietitians should also discuss risk factors for developing an eating disorder. Such interventions may play an important part in the treatment and prevention of eating disorders.[1-3]

Diagnostic criteria for anorexia nervosa and bulimia nervosa are stated in the fourth edition of the *Diagnostic and Statistical Manual of Mental Disorders (DSM-IV)*.[4] Although considered to be mental disorders, eating disorders are remarkable for their nutrition-related problems. In anorexia nervosa, nutrition-related problems include refusal to maintain a minimally healthy body weight (i.e., 85% of that

Dan W. Reiff, MPH, RD and Kathleen Kim Lampson Reiff, PhD, "Position of The American Dietetic Association: Nutrition intervention in the Treatment of Anorexia Nervosa, Bulimia Nervosa, and Binge Eating," Copyright 1987 The American Dietetic Association (ADA). Reprinted by permission. This ADA Position was adopted by the House of Delegates on October 18, 1987, and reaffirmed on September 12, 1992. The update will be in effect until October 1999.

expected), dramatic weight loss, fear of gaining weight even though underweight, preoccupation with food, and abnormal food-consumption patterns.[4] In bulimia nervosa, problems include recurrent episodes of binge eating, a sense of lack of control over eating, compensatory behavior after binge eating to prevent weight gain (e.g., self-induced vomiting, abuse of laxatives or diuretics, fasting).[4] For a person with either diagnosis to recover fully, issues concerning food-intake patterns, food- and weight-related behaviors, body image, and weight regulation must be resolved.[5,6] The registered dietitian is the logical member of the treatment team to address these issues with people recovering from anorexia nervosa and bulimia nervosa.

Eating disorders are complex disorders involving two sets of issues and behaviors: those directly relating to food and weight and those involving the relationships with oneself and with others. The name "eating disorder" is somewhat misleading in that it implies that the essence of the problem is disordered eating and suggests that the solution is to learn to eat normally again. If changes in food- and weight-related behavior alone are the focus of treatment, interventions are likely to be counterproductive rather than therapeutic. Thus, registered dietitians who treat persons with eating disorders should be cognizant of the psychological and nutritional aspects of eating disorders throughout the recovery process. Health care professionals who work with patients throughout their recovery process will benefit from familiarizing themselves with the process of nutrition care.

Position Statement

It is the position of The American Dietetic Association (ADA) that nutrition education and nutrition intervention be integrated into the team treatment of patients with anorexia nervosa, bulimia nervosa, and binge eating during the assessment and treatment phases of outpatient and/or inpatient therapy.

Medical Nutrition Therapy

Medical nutrition therapy, as defined by ADA, is the use of specific nutrition services to treat an illness, injury, or condition. It involves: (a) assessment of the patient's nutritional status, and (b) treatment, which includes diet therapy, counseling, or use of specialized nutrition supplements. Medical nutrition therapy for eating disorders is a collaborative process in which the registered dietitian and the recovering person work together to change the patient's food- and weight-related behaviors. Typically, this is a lengthy process because emotional and psychological issues may make these changes extremely difficult.[6]

The process of medical nutrition therapy has two phases with regard to treating eating disorders: the education phase and the experimental phase.[6] All registered dietitians have the qualifications to provide nutrition care during the education phase. However, only registered dietitians with additional training and experience in the treatment of eating disorders are qualified to do the nutrition interventions of the experimental phase.

The primary focus of the education phase is to provide nutrition information to the person with the eating disorder. The interactions between the registered dietitian and patient are often brief and factual in nature; thus, a very limited relationship develops in which it would be inappropriate to discuss subjects such as the emotions generated by attempts to change body weight.

In the experimental phase, the registered dietitian has a special interest in long-term, relationship-based counseling and is a member of a multidisciplinary treatment team.[6] In addition to formal education in dietetics, the dietitian involved in this phase should have been trained in basic counseling skills through a combination of course work and/or supervision by a psychotherapist. This approach could be called "psychonutritional." Ongoing supervision by and communication with a psychotherapist who may be part of the treatment team are strongly advised if the registered dietitian is to discuss emotional issues related to behavior change or weight. In some work settings, the registered dietitian may be called a "nutrition therapist."[6]

The Education Phase

The focus of the education phase is to provide a foundation of information that will make it possible for the patient to make notable changes in food- and weight-related behaviors during the experimental phase. The education phase has the following five primary objectives.

Collect Relevant Information. Nutrition assessment of this heterogeneous population should include a comprehensive history of weight changes, eating and exercise patterns, and purging behaviors. A detailed history helps the dietitian quantify behaviors and nutrient intake patterns, identify the effect of behavior on patient lifestyle, and direct treatment plans and goals.[6-11]

Establish a Collaborative Relationship between the Person with the Eating Disorder and the Registered Dietitian. Nutrition intervention involves forming a therapeutic alliance with the patient that will enable her or him to talk about and later resolve food fears and to develop realistic goals for weight and behavior change. The initial nutrition interview and history itself can be a therapeutic experience as it allows the patient to discuss secretive behaviors and food fears openly with a supportive and understanding health care provider. The interview should be performed in a nonjudgmental manner to help establish trust and collaboration with the patient.[6,7,12,13]

Define and Discuss Relevant Principles and Concepts of Food, Nutrition, and Weight Regulation. Understanding why and how the body responds to starvation, binge eating, purging, and/or restriction is typically necessary before a person will risk making behavioral changes.[9] Bodily responses to starvation include: symptoms of starvation, the effects of starvation and partial starvation on metabolic rate, ability to differentiate hydration shifts from muscle and fat weight shifts, abnormal and normal hunger, a healthy weight range for the individual, the way in which food- and weight-related behaviors change during the process of recovery, minimum food intake needed to stabilize weight and metabolic rate, optimal food intake for health, and the concept of and/or a carefully estimated set-point for weight.

Present Examples of Hunger Patterns, Typical Food Intake Patterns, and the Total Caloric Intake of a Person Who Has Recovered from an Eating Disorder. This technique is an additional means of helping the person with the eating disorder think about the changes she or he will eventually need to make to recover fully.[6]

Educate the Family. Involving family members in the recovery process will increase their understanding of the eating disorder and their support for treatment. The registered dietitian can help decrease family frustration at mealtimes by relieving the family of the responsibility for monitoring food intake or changing food-related behaviors. Concrete suggestions on meal planning, nutrient needs, and strategies for dealing with inappropriate food- and weight-related behaviors should be offered cautiously in conjunction with therapy. That allows the family to work toward a supportive rather than a confrontational environment around food. The dietetics practitioner plays an important role in educating the family and significant others on the nutrition needs of the patient and the effect of starvation on patient behavior.[6,14,15]

The Experimental Phase

During the experimental phase the recovering person makes changes in food- and weight-related behaviors. Nutrition intervention sessions are intended to be the forum for planning strategies for food- and weight-related behavior change, thus freeing psychotherapy sessions for exploration of psychological issues. By this time, the patient should already have established a supportive relationship with a psychotherapist in which feelings that may arise during therapy can be processed. Likewise, a patient's ability to make changes in food intake, weight, and behaviors may decrease substantially when emotionally painful issues surface during the course of therapy. If the registered dietitian has been supportive during the assessment phase, then a patient can be comfortable about stopping and resuming medical nutrition therapy, if appropriate, because of changing medical needs and/or progress in therapy.

The experimental phase has the following primary objectives for the patient:

Separate Food- and Weight-Related Behaviors from Feelings and Psychological Issues.[6] This process involves helping the person separate her or his identity, feelings, and unresolved issues from the focus on food, hunger, and weight so that the two problems can be worked on separately. The registered dietitian can facilitate this process by helping patients understand that their drive to be thin and their behaviors are symptoms of underlying issues and by discussing the ephemeral nature of societal expectations about weight and body issues. The underlying issues themselves will be addressed in psychotherapy.[6]

Change Food Behaviors in an Incremental Fashion until Food Intake Patterns Are Normalized. When working with persons with eating disorders, it is important to remember that each person's recovery process is unique; thus, treatment plans need to be highly individualized. No one approach to behavior change works for everyone. The key to nutrition intervention for outpatients is a very gradual change in food intake patterns and food- and weight-related behaviors. In most cases, patients should be discouraged from attempting sudden major changes in behavior.

The registered dietitian can help the patient avoid oversimplifying what constitutes recovery by increasing awareness of the complexities of an eating disorder. In this way, the patient is less likely to interpret a notable change in behavior, such as being "purge-free" for several months, to mean recovery. In addition, the registered dietitian can educate the patient that setbacks are normal and should be considered opportunities to learn about unresolved issues that need to be addressed in psychotherapy and to evaluate and alter approaches to behavior change. Providing and discussing a list of indicators of recovery that includes indicators related to food, weight, and activity as well as to psychological, rational, and emotional state may help the recovering person better understand what needs to be addressed, changed, and/or resolved in order to recover fully.[6]

Self-monitoring techniques may be effective with some patients to quantify progress, identify problems, and help the patient maintain a sense of control over the behavior change process. Commonly used monitoring techniques include keeping food and/or behavior records, noting the quantity and frequency of laxative use during a specified period, recording the frequency of binge/purge episodes, and charting weight gain or fluctuations in weight and associated factors (e.g., hydration shift because of increased sodium intake). Completing food and behavior contracts are also ways of monitoring patient progress and identifying problems.[10] With patients for whom these methods are ineffective or counterproductive, such as those who become obsessive or over involved in the record-keeping process, less structured supportive methods may work well. Because behavior change is often easier for less entrenched behaviors, an example of possible intervention would be to help patients with anorexia nervosa gradually add back to their daily food intakes the foods they had most recently omitted from their diets.

Nutrition intervention strategies that are designed to correct specific medical concerns, especially those in which results are seen fairly readily, are effective in that the patient has an increased sense of control over her or his body and is able to see that there is a direct relationship between food intake and health.

Behavior-change efforts are most effective when coupled with education intervention. For example, the registered dietitian may explain to the patient why laxatives have limited value in weight loss and what to expect while decreasing laxative use (e.g., bloating, hydration shifts). The patient and dietitian then work together to develop a plan to decrease the use of laxatives by a specified amount while increasing fiber and fluid intake. Or, dietitian can explain not only how much energy the body needs but why it needs a certain amount of energy (e.g., basal metabolic rate, growth, digesting and absorbing food) before developing a plan to increase caloric intake.[9]

Slowly Increase or Decrease Weight. Proceeding too quickly with nutrition change may cause the patient to become defensive, withdraw from medical psychotherapy, and discredit the value of nutrition intervention. Requesting too many changes too quickly reinforces the patient's perceived inability to control her or his environment, which is likely to undermine self-esteem further. For example, patients with anorexia nervosa may be overwhelmed by rapid diet changes and experience their ultimate fear of uncontrolled weight gain.[2]

Learn to Maintain a Weight That Is Healthful for That Individual without Using Abnormal Food- and Weight-Related Behaviors. Providing nutrition education to patients about nutrient needs for growth and weight control and helping patients make appropriate food choices will promote recovery. Encouraging regular mealtimes, variety and moderation of intake, and the gradual reintroduction of feared foods will increase patient confidence in food selection and weight control.[6,7,10-16] In addition to individual nutrition counseling, education and/or support groups in which these issues are explored can be very effective in helping recovering people make changes.

Learn to Be Comfortable in Social Eating Situations. Persons who develop an eating disorder tend to avoid social aspects of eating or only participate on their terms. Some changes in social eating patterns are attributable to food and weight issues, however, equally as many are directly related to difficulties in relationships with people, which are communicated indirectly through changes in social eating (e.g., refusing to eat what the rest of the family eats as a means of being in control). One indicator of recovery is that persons with an eating disorder are able to eat with others without calling attention to themselves through abnormal eating; are flexible enough to eat with others without controlling what is eaten, when meals are served, or where meals are eaten; and do not focus on food as a way to deal with anxiety about interpersonal situations. Because the patient must make many cognitive changes concerning her or his relationship with food and weight as well as concerning their relationships with people before this can happen, most people are not ready to confront social eating issues until the later stages of treatment.[6]

The Multidisciplinary Team

Research regarding the most effective treatment modalities for patients with anorexia nervosa and bulimia nervosa continues to be reported in the literature. Because of the complex etiology of eating disorders, a multidisciplinary approach appears to be the most effective method of treating patients with anorexia nervosa and bulimia nervosa.[1,5,6,7,14,16-20]

The advantages of the team treatment method include pooled knowledge, which provides a sound basis for differential diagnosis and treatment planning; team support; shared responsibility for patient care; and provision of a model of collaborative relationships for the patient.[1,6,17,18] The challenges of the treatment method are to maintain open lines of communication; avoid replication of family dynamics; recognize the strengths and limitations of individual team members; and avoid power struggles with patients, their families, or within the team that limit collaborative treatment. For treatment to be effective, the team needs to function as a cohesive treatment network with a consistent, well-defined, mutually agreed upon concept of what an eating disorder is, how treatment evolves, and what constitutes recovery.[2,6,10,11,18] It is important for the registered dietitian to explain the conceptual framework regarding the treatment of eating disorders (e.g., the question of whether people can fully recover, the medical risks involved, the roles of the team members, conditions for hospitalization, estimated length of treatment) to treatment team members, referring professionals, family members, and patients.

Having a list of recovery indicators that includes food-, weight-, and activity-related behaviors to use as a guideline for patients, their families, and members of the treatment team may help clarify goals and progress in treatment.[6] In addition, having patients focus on team treatment goals rather than on one aspect of care helps them understand how psychological and medical concerns relate to their food- and weight-related behaviors.

The registered dietitian is a key member of the treatment team. Ideally, the team should include professionals who specialize in the treatment of persons with eating disorders and who can address the medical, psychiatric, dental, psychological, and medical nutrition needs of the patient.[1,6,8,14,20] In addition to education and nutrition intervention, the registered dietitian is involved in clinically monitoring the patient's health status. Because persons with eating disorders are sometimes not regularly monitored by a physician, the dietetics practitioner can be instrumental in recognizing potential medical problems and communicating them to the team physician. For example, as a result of clinical observation and/or reports from the patient, the dietitian may refer the patient back to the physician for further laboratory work or a physical examination.

Models of Collaboration between the Registered Dietitian and the Psychotherapist

Within the team context, a psychonutritional approach to the treatment of persons with eating disorders is recommended in which psychotherapy and medical nutrition therapy are considered very important throughout the entire recovery process.[6] Of all the team members, the registered dietitian typically works most closely with the psychotherapist. Following are five possible models of collaboration between the dietitian and the psychotherapist members of the team.[6]

The Continuous Contact Model. Both the dietitian and the psychotherapist work with the person with the eating disorder throughout the recovery process, although each focuses on a different aspect of treatment. This model requires the registered dietitian to have supervised training in counseling skills.

The Food Plan-Only Model. The registered dietitian does a one- or two-session consultation in which an individualized food plan is designed for the patient and specific questions are answered.

The Education-Only Model. The person with the eating disorder meets with the registered dietitian for a six- to ten-session consultation in which nutrition topics relevant to eating disorders are discussed.

The Education/Behavioral Change-Only Model. The therapist refers the person with the eating disorder to the registered dietitian (in this case, a dietitian with additional training and experience in the treatment of eating disorders is qualified to do the nutrition intervention) for education about nutrition concepts relevant to eating disorders early in treatment. The person then stops medical nutrition therapy to return at a later time when she or he is ready to work intensively on changing food- and weight-related behaviors.

The Intermittent Contact Model. The person with the eating disorder has intermittent contact with the registered dietitian (in this case, a dietitian with additional training and experience in the treatment of eating disorders is qualified to do the nutrition intervention) throughout her or his recovery as the patient and the psychotherapist deem it necessary.

The registered dietitian should present these five alternatives to team members, new referring professionals, patients, and their families as appropriate. The health care team will select the model of collaboration to be used.

Hospitalization/Residential Treatment

Under certain circumstances, the treatment team will recommend hospitalization or residential treatment. The qualified dietetics professional plays an integral role whether treatment is outpatient or inpatient.

Outpatient treatment alone is sufficient for the recovery of most persons with eating disorders; however, for some persons, especially those with anorexia nervosa, hospitalization or residential treatment becomes necessary. The decision to hospitalize a patient for treatment of an eating disorder should be made on a case by case basis. Medical and psychiatric factors considered include amount of weight lost, body mass index (weight [kg]/height [m^2]), rapidity of progressive weight loss (1 to 2 lb/week in spite of competent psychotherapy), severe metabolic disturbances, certain cardiac dysfunctions, syncope, psychomotor retardation, severe depression or suicide risk, severe bingeing and purging (with risk of aspiration), psychosis, family crisis, inability to perform activities of daily living, or lack of response to outpatient treatment programs.[1,6,21-23] It appears that most severely underweight patients (less than 20% below average weight for height) and those who are physiologically unstable will need the comprehensive treatment, support, and medical management available only in a hospital or residential setting. Most people with bulimia nervosa do not require inpatient treatment.[20]

Upon admission of a patient, the registered dietitian may find it useful to obtain a detailed history of diet, weight, and food- and weight-related behavior. Such information can be used to individualize treatment goals and help staff anticipate problems with compliance to inpatient protocols. The initial interview should be performed in a supportive and nonjudgmental manner to establish an alliance with the patient.

A hospital or residential setting can provide a safe, controlled environment for initiating or reestablishing medical, psychological, and nutritional rehabilitation.[2,6,21,24,25] A defined nutrition care plan for each patient with an eating disorder should specify parameters of nutritional rehabilitation. The care plan may outline daily caloric intake, rate of weight gain, weight-range goal for discharge, any limitations of food choices, and whether the patient should be supervised during meals and immediately after. In addition, limits on activity may be useful in ensuring weight gain in patients with low body weights.[23,26]

Nutrition-repletion methods, such as nasogastric tube feedings and peripheral intravenous feeding, carry increased medical and psychological risks. Most clinicians believe they are only needed in life-threatening situations.[21] When using these techniques, the rate of refeeding must be carefully monitored. Use should be limited to stabilizing the health status of medically precarious patients who are unable to consume sufficient energy orally.[23,24,26] The medical risks associated with the more aggressive forms of nutrition repletion in very underweight patients include fluid retention, electrolyte changes, and hypophosphatemia.[27] The psychological risks may include the patient's perceived loss of control, loss of identity, increased body distortion, and mistrust of the treatment team. Both feeding methods may be potentially lifesaving medical treatments but should not be used as punishment for recalcitrant patients.[28,29]

The treatment team should involve the patient's family throughout the inpatient stay to help the family understand treatment goals and to learn about the eating disorder and the functions it serves for both patient and family.[6,30] It is essential that no one be blamed for the disorder but that the family learn to communicate verbally rather than through food.[6,31] The extent of involvement of family members should be assessed by the therapist and discussed with the patient.

The inpatient setting provides an excellent opportunity for the registered dietitian to work with groups of people recovering from eating disorders. Nutrition education groups in which patients can learn about food- and weight-related issues together and be taught how to support each other in making changes can be very effective.

For persons recovering from anorexia nervosa, a cooking group in which patients practice planning, cooking, and eating meals under the supervision of a dietetics practitioner and then discuss their reactions in the context of an actual dining experience is one way to help patients resume control over selecting and eating food before discharge.[32]

Arranging for outpatient follow-up is essential because the transition from a structured program in a hospital or residential treatment setting to outpatient care with its choices and responsibilities can be difficult and frightening. It is extremely important that the patient be referred to and have an appointment scheduled with an outpatient registered dietitian before leaving treatment so that progress in food- and weight-related behavior change can be sustained and continued without interruption.

New Thinking Regarding Compulsive Eating/Binge Eating

During the past 4 years, there has been substantial debate among eating disorders experts about the appropriateness of diagnosing people as having an eating disorder if their primary symptom is recurrent episodes of binge eating without the regular use of inappropriate compensatory behaviors (e.g., self-induced vomiting, fasting). The outcome of this debate is that Binge Eating Disorder is included in the *DSM-IV*[4] under the category of Eating Disorder Not Otherwise Specified, which is reserved for disorders of eating that do not meet the criteria for anorexia nervosa or bulimia nervosa. Recurrent binge eating behaviors are not a new phenomenon—they were referred to as compulsive eating in the past—but it was not until 1994 that persons who binge eat were considered to have a mental disorder.

Many people who seek help for weight loss from a health professional will see a registered dietitian first. In such cases, the registered dietitian is responsible for making the initial evaluation, diagnosis, and, when appropriate, recommendations or referrals for psychotherapy and more complex nutrition care. A notable number of persons who want to lose weight meet the diagnostic criteria for binge eating disorder. Some of these individuals may initially be resistant to seeking psychotherapy because they do not understand that there is a relationship between underlying emotional or psychological issues and the inability to cease binge eating. The dietitian's role in the treatment of binge eating disorder is that same as for anorexia nervosa and bulimia nervosa.

Regardless of whether a person who seeks weight loss treatment has binge eating disorder, the dietitian should explain the new thinking regarding weight loss. First, the vast majority of people who lose weight by dieting are unable to maintain the lower body weight because their set-point may be such that it is genetically impossible for her or him to lose a substantial amount of weight and maintain the loss without dramatically restricting caloric intake and/or increasing exercise for the rest of their lives.[6,33] However, it appears that some people can lose limited amounts of weight by decreasing fat intake, using certain medications (e.g., fenfluramine), or increasing exercise. Second, a patient may have psychological issues underlying overeating behaviors that need to be resolved in psychotherapy before addressing the issue of whether substantial weight loss is possible.

In addition, new research indicates that health risks do not substantially increase for many people at higher weights, but may increase with weight cycling or very-low-calorie diets.[34] "Epidemiological studies reveal the ill effects of obesity occur at much higher weight thresholds than had been thought. As you move into 50 or 60% overweight, your risk of dying goes up mildly, say 1.5%," explained Stunkard.[34] "At 100% it goes up more steeply, but the view that fatness, in general, is bad for you has probably been exaggerated." It has also been found that distribution of body fat influences health. People with upper-body (visceral) obesity, usually men, suffer most of the medical complications of obesity (e.g., hypertension, diabetes) whereas people with lower-body (hip and thigh) obesity, usually women, are at very low medical risk. Consequently, only those with upper-body obesity need medical attention and need to lose weight. Fortunately, it appears that modest weight loss (10 or 15 lb) appears to be adequate to reverse a large number of the metabolic ill effects of obesity for most people. Alternatively, most women may benefit more from counseling about body image issues and about how to stop the pursuit of thinness than from weight loss itself.[34]

The dietitian should consider three categories of risk in determining whether weight loss should be a treatment option: (a) the risk of increased morbidity or mortality as a result of being at a higher weight, (b) the risk incurred by weight cycling, and (c) the psychological risk of telling a person that it is possible to lose a substantial amount of weight and maintain the loss when, in fact, this may not be possible for most people because of the biological impasse known as the set-point for weight. If the dietitian determines that weight loss is not an option to pursue, it may be appropriate to discuss why losing weight is important to the patient and to suggest that accepting oneself at or near the present body weight, learning how to prevent future weight gain, and ceasing binge eating may be healthier and more realistic options than attempting to lose a substantial amount of weight.

Conclusion

Registered dietitians are becoming increasingly recognized as integral members of the multidisciplinary team of health professionals who treat persons with anorexia nervosa and bulimia nervosa. The registered dietitian provides nutrition education or medical nutrition and has the essential expertise to facilitate the highly individualized changes in food- and weight-related behaviors that are necessary for full recovery from an eating disorder.

Future recommendations for registered dietitians interested in working with persons with eating disorders include the following: become increasingly involved in national movements that emphasize prevention of eating disorders; promote discussion and research of the apparent physiologically limited ability to lose weight and maintain weight loss; publish articles about innovative methods of practice and case studies that will educate other professionals regarding nutrition interventions; provide opportunities for advanced training in medical nutrition therapy at the graduate level; become more involved in research regarding the treatment of eating disorders; and develop a protocol for treating persons with binge eating disorder. Following these recommendations will not only increase the visibility of registered dietitians who treat persons with eating disorders, but will further establish their credibility as essential members of the treatment process.

References

1. Herzog DB, Copeland PM. Eating disorders. *N Engl J Med.* 1985; 313: 295-303.

2. Garrow JS. Dietary management of obesity and anorexia nervosa. *J Hum Nutr.* 1980; 34:131-138.

3. Kirkley BG. Bulimia: clinical characteristics, development, and etiology. *J Am Diet Assoc.* 1986; 86: 468-472.

4. *Diagnostic and Statistical Manual of Mental Disorders. 4th ed.* Washington, DC: American Psychiatric Association; 1994.

5. Rock C, Yager J. Nutrition and eating disorders: a primer for clinicians. *Int J Eating Disorders*. 1987;6: 267-280.

6. Reiff D, Reiff KL. *Eating Disorders: Nutrition Therapy in the Recovery Process*. Gaithersburg, Md: Aspen Publishers; 1992.

7. Story M. Nutrition management and the dietary treatment of bulimia. *J Am Diet Assoc*. 1986;86: 517-519.

8. Kahm A. Nutritional counseling for anorexic and bulimic patients. In: Lemberg R, ed. *Controlling Eating Disorders with Facts, Advice, and Resources*. Phoenix, Ariz: Oryx Press; 1992: 113-120.

9. Huse DM, Lucas AR. Dieting patterns in anorexia nervosa. *Am J Clin Nutr*. 1984;40: 251-254.

10. Willard SG, Anding RH, Winstead DK. Nutritional counseling as an adjunct to psychotherapy in bulimia treatment. *Psychosomatics*. 1983; 24: 545-551.

11. Huse DM, Lucas AR. Dietary treatment of anorexia nervosa. *J Am Diet Assoc*. 1983; 83: 687-690.

12. Gannon MA, Mitchell JE. Subjective evaluation of treatment methods by patients treated for bulimia. *J Am Diet Assoc*. 1986;86: 520-521.

13. Johnson C, Connors M. *The Etiology and Treatment of Bulimia Nervosa*. New York, NY: Basic Books; 1987.

14. Garner DM, Rockett W, Olmsted MP, Johnson C, Cosina DV. Psychoeducational principles in the treatment of bulimia and anorexia nervosa. In: Garner DM, Garfinkel PE, eds. *Anorexia Nervosa and Bulimia*. New York, NY: Guilford Press; 1985: 513-572.

15. Beaumont PJV, Chambers TL, Rouse L, Abraham F. The diet composition and nutritional knowledge of patients with anorexia nervosa. *J Hum Nutr*. 1981; 35: 265-273.

16. Health and Public Policy Committee, American College of Physicians. Position paper on eating disorders: anorexia nervosa and bulimia. *Ann Intern Med*. 1986; 105:790-794.

17. Reiff D. Nutrition therapy in treatment of anorexia nervosa and bulimia nervosa. Presented at the Anorexia/Bulimia Nervosa Symposium on Theories of Treatment; February 1984; Bergen, Norway. Universitetsforlaget As 1985.

18. Kaluce R, *et al*. The evolution of a multitherapy orientation. In: Garner D, Garfinkel PE, eds. *Anorexia Nervosa and Bulimia*. New York, NY: Guilford Press; 1984: 458-490.

19. Anderson A, *et al*. A multidisciplinary team treatment for patients with anorexia nervosa and their families. *Int J Eating Disorders*. 1983; 2 (3):181-192.

20. American Psychiatric Association practice guidelines for eating disorders. *Am J Psychiatry*. 1993;150: 207-228.

21. Anderson AE, Morse C, Santmyer K. In-patient treatment for anorexia nervosa. In: Garner DM, Garfinkel PE, eds. *Anorexia Nervosa and Bulimia*. New York, NY: Guilford Press; 1985: 311-343.

22. Hodges W. Medical factors in eating disorders. In: Reiff D, Reiff KL. *Eating Disorders: Nutrition Therapy in the Recovery Process*. Gaithersburg, Md: Aspen Publishers; 1992: 441-456.

23. Tolstrup K. The treatment of anorexia nervosa in childhood and adolescence. *J Child Psychol Psychiatry*. 1975;16: 75-78.

24. Gwirstsman HE, George DT, Kay H, Ebert MH. Constructing an in-patient treatment program for bulimia. In: Kay WH, Gwirstsman HE, eds. *A Comprehensive Approach to the Treatment of Normal Weight Bulimia*. Washington, DC: American Psychiatric Press; 1985.

25. Garfinkel PE, Garner DM. *Anorexia Nervosa: A Multidimensional Perspective*. New York, NY: Brunner/Mazel; 1982.

26. Krause MV, Mahan LK. *Food, Nutrition and Diet Therapy. 8th ed*. Philadelphia, Pa: WB Saunders Co; 1992.

27. Claggett MS. Anorexia nervosa: a behavioral approach. *Am J Nurs*. 1980; 80:1471-1472.

28. Maloney MJ, Farrell MK. Tubefeeding for very low weight anorectic patients. *Am J Psychiatry*. 1980;137: 310-314. Letter.

29. Garfinkel PE, Garner DM, Kennedy S. Special problems of in-patient management. In: Garner DM, Garfinkel PE, eds. *Anorexia Nervosa and Bulimia*. New York, NY: Guilford Press;1985: 344-362.

30. Bayer LM, Bauers CM, Kapp SR. Psychosocial aspects of nutritional support. *Nurs Clin North Am*. 1983;18: 119-128.

31. Sparnon J, Hornyak L. Structured eating experiences in the inpatient treatment of anorexia nervosa. In: Hornyak L, Baker E, eds. *Experiential Therapies for Eating Disorders*. New York, NY: Guilford Press; 1989: 207-233.

32. Keesey R. A set-point theory of obesity. In: Brownell K, Foreyt J, eds. *Handbook of Eating Disorders*. New York, NY: Basic Books; 1986: 63-87.

33. Berg F. Health risks of weight loss. *Healthy Weight J*. 1994;8: 81-84.

34. Miller J. New findings on obesity presented. *Psychiatric Times Med Behav*. 1992; 38.

For More Information

The American Dietetic Association
216 West Jackson Boulevard
Chicago, Illinois 60606-6995
(312) 899-0040
(312) 899-1979 fax
Website: www.eatright.org

Chapter 31

Medical Foods

What Is a Medical Food?

A medical food is prescribed by a physician when a patient has special nutrient needs in order to manage a disease or health condition, and the patient is under the physician's ongoing care. The label must clearly state that the product is intended to be used to manage a specific medical disorder or condition. An example of a medical food is a food for use by persons with phenylketonuria, i.e., foods formulated to be free of the amino acid phenylalanine.

Medical foods are not meant to be used by the general public and may not be available in stores or supermarkets. Medical foods are not those foods included within a healthy diet intended to decrease the risk of disease, such as reduced-fat foods or low-sodium foods, nor are they weight loss products.

How Does FDA Oversee Medical Foods?

Until recently, medical foods received little attention. But the number and types of foods marketed as medical foods are increasing. While FDA is working to more clearly define and regulate medical foods, specific requirements for the safety or appropriate use of medical foods have not yet been established. Medical foods do not have to include nutrition information on their labels, and their claims do not need to meet specific standards.

U. S. Food and Drug Administration, Center for Food Safety and Applied Nutrition, Office of Special Nutritionals, May 1997.

Currently, FDA is exploring ways to more specifically regulate medical foods. This might include safety evaluations, standards for claims, and requiring specific information on the labels. In order to do this, FDA must first propose rules for medical foods. After publication of such a proposal, a public comment period would occur during which individuals and organizations write to offer their comments for changes to the proposed rules.

Where Can I Get More Information about FDA's Role in Overseeing Medical Foods?

In November of 1996, FDA published a type of document known as an "advanced notice of proposed rulemaking" (ANPR). This document contains FDA's current thinking about how to best develop rules for medical foods.

For more information, contact the FDA at:

U.S. Food and Drug Administration
Center for Food Safety and Applied Nutrition
5600 Fishers Lane
Rockville, MD 20847
(301) 443-9767
Website: www.fda.gov

Part Four

Weight Control

Chapter 32

Losing Weight Safely

Americans trying to lose weight have plenty of company. According to a 1995 report from the Institute of Medicine (IOM), tens of millions of Americans are dieting at any given time, spending more than $33 billion yearly on weight-reduction products, such as diet foods and drinks.

Yet, studies over the last two decades by the National Center for Health Statistics show that obesity in the United States is actually on the rise. Today, approximately 35 percent of women and 31 percent of men age 20 and older are considered obese, up from approximately 30 percent and 25 percent, respectively, in 1980.

The words obesity and overweight are generally used interchangeably. However, according to the IOM report, their technical meanings are not identical. Overweight refers to an excess of body weight that includes all tissues, such as fat, bone and muscle. Obesity refers specifically to an excess of body fat. It is possible to be overweight without being obese, as in the case of a body builder who has a substantial amount of muscle mass. It is possible to be obese without being overweight, as in the case of a very sedentary person who is within the desirable weight range but who nevertheless has an excess of body fat. However, most overweight people are also obese and vice versa. Men with more than 25 percent and women with more than 30 percent body fat are considered obese.

Many people who diet fail to lose weight—or, if they do lose, fail to maintain the lower weight over the long term. As the IOM report,

FDA Consumer, January-February 1996.

"Weighing The Options: Criteria for Evaluating Weight-Management Programs," points out, obesity is "a complex, multifactorial disease of appetite regulation and energy metabolism."

Because many factors affect how much or how little food a person eats and how that food is metabolized, or processed, by the body, losing weight is not simple. For example, recent studies suggest a role for genetic makeup in obesity. This area is still controversial, and more studies will be needed before scientists can say with certainty that a person's genes may set limits on how much weight can be lost and maintained.

Yet many people persist in seeking simple cures to this complex health problem. Lured by fad diets or pills that promise a quick and easy path to thinness, they end up disappointed when they regain lost weight.

"When it comes to weight loss, if something sounds too good—or too easy, or too delicious—to be true, it probably is," says Victor Herbert, M.D., J.D., professor of medicine and director of the Nutrition Center at the Mount Sinai School of Medicine and Bronx VA Medical Centers in New York City, and member of the board of directors of the National Council Against Health Fraud. "If a weight loss claim is sensational, it is not true; if it is true, it is not sensational."

No Shortcuts

"There are no shortcuts—no magic pills," adds Lori Love of the Food and Drug Administration's Center for Food Safety and Applied Nutrition. Losing weight sensibly and safely requires a multifaceted approach that includes setting reasonable weight-loss goals, changing eating habits, and getting adequate exercise. Appetite suppressants (diet pills) or other products may help some people over the short term, but they are not a substitute for adopting healthful eating habits over the long term.

The first step in losing weight safely is to determine a realistic weight goal. Two types of tables are commonly used as guidelines. One is the weight-for-height table developed in 1990 by the U.S. Department of Agriculture and the Department of Health and Human Services. This table offers a range of suggested weights for adults based on height and age.

Another table uses body mass index (BMI), a mathematical formula that correlates weight with body fat. In 1993, the National Institute of Diabetes and Digestive and Kidney Diseases developed a table that correlates height, weight and BMI.

A physician or other health provider can help you set a reasonable goal with these tables. To reach the goal safely, plan to lose 1 to 2 pounds weekly by consuming approximately 300 to 500 fewer calories daily than usual (women and inactive men generally need to consume approximately 2,000 calories to maintain weight; men and very active women may consume up to 2,500 calories daily).

Moderation, Variety and Balance

After determining a reasonable goal weight, devise an eating plan based on the cornerstones of healthful eating—moderation, variety and balance, suggests Herbert.

"Moderation means not eating too much or too little of any particular food or nutrient; variety means eating as wide a variety as possible from each, and within each, of the five basic food groups; and balance refers to the balance achieved by following moderation and variety, as well as the balance of calories consumed versus calories expended," he explains. To lose weight, fewer calories should be consumed than expended; to maintain weight loss, the number of calories consumed and expended should be about the same.

The five basic food groups and the recommended number of servings from each are incorporated into the Food Guide Pyramid developed by USDA and HHS. These groups are (1) bread, cereal, pasta, and rice; (2) vegetables; (3) fruits; (4) milk, yogurt and cheese; and (5) meat, poultry, fish, dry beans, eggs, and nuts. A sixth group (fats, oils and sweets) consists mainly of items that are pleasing to the palate but high in fat and/or calories; these should be eaten in moderation.

Using the Food Label

To help consumers plan a healthful diet, FDA and USDA have revamped food labels. By law, most food labels now must display a Nutrition Facts panel containing information about how the food can fit into an overall daily diet. Nutrition Facts state how much saturated fat, cholesterol, fiber, and certain nutrients are contained in each serving. Serving sizes must now be based on standards set for similar kinds of food, so the nutritional value of similar products may be compared.

On the food label, percent Daily Value shows what percentage of a given nutrient is provided in one portion for daily diets of 2,000 and 2,500 calories.

Whether or not a given food fits into a weight-loss diet depends on what other foods you eat that day. For most people, the goal is to select a variety of foods that together add up to approximately 100 percent of the Daily Value for total carbohydrate, dietary fiber, vitamins, and minerals; total fat, cholesterol and sodium each may add up to less than 100 percent.

This system permits a good deal of flexibility. No food is inherently "bad"; it is the total diet for the day that counts. You may compensate for an occasional rich dessert or serving of fried food by eating foods that are low in fat, oil or sugar for the rest of the day. However, high-fat foods should be limited, because they can quickly use up a day's supply of calories without providing high percentages of vital nutrients.

Simple modifications in food selection and preparation allow you to include traditional favorites and snacks within the context of a healthful weight-loss diet; for example, select 1 percent or skim milk products instead of those made with whole milk, lean cuts of meat and poultry, and nonfat frozen yogurt instead of ice cream. Low-fat plain yogurt may be substituted for sour cream in dips, dressings or spreads; reduced-fat cheeses may be used instead of those made from whole milk. Broil, roast or steam foods instead of frying.

Look on the nutrition label for words such as "low," "light" or "reduced" to describe the calorie and fat content per serving. These foods must have significantly fewer calories or significantly less fat than similar products that do not make these claims. Foods that are advertised as "low in cholesterol" also must be low in saturated fat.

Foods that claim to contain fewer calories or less fat than similar servings of similar products must show the difference on the label. For example, on a container of low-fat cottage cheese, the label would show that a serving of the low-fat product contains 80 calories and 1.5 grams of fat while regular cottage cheese contains 120 calories and 5 grams of fat per serving.

Include small portions of desserts or high-fat snacks rather than attempting to cut them out altogether. Eliminating favorite foods may result in cravings that can lead to binge eating and weight gain.

Avoid low-calorie fad diets that exclude whole categories of food such as carbohydrates (bread and pasta) or proteins (meat and poultry). These diets may be harmful because they generally do not include all nutrients necessary for good health. "Every fad diet that demands an unusual eating pattern, such as emphasizing only a few types of foods, deviates from one or more of the guidelines of moderation, variety and balance," says Herbert. "The greater the deviation, the more harmful the diet is likely to be."

Exercise

Regular exercise is important for overall health as well as for losing and maintaining weight. There is evidence to suggest that body fat distribution affects health risks. For example, excess fat in the abdominal area (as opposed to hips and thighs) is associated with greater risk for high blood pressure, diabetes, early heart disease, and certain types of cancer. Vigorous exercise can reduce abdominal fat and thus lower the risk of these diseases.

A half hour of brisk walking or other aerobic activity three times weekly can help the body use up calories consumed daily as well as excess calories stored as fat. Weight-bearing exercises also help tone muscles and may reduce the risk of osteoporosis.

Diet Pills

The 1991/1992 Weight Loss Practices Survey, sponsored by FDA and the National Heart, Lung, and Blood Institute, found that 5 percent of women and 2 percent of men trying to lose weight use diet pills. Products considered by FDA to be over-the-counter weight control drugs are primarily those containing the active ingredient phenylpropanolamine (PPA), such as Dexatrim and Acutrim. PPA is available OTC for weight control in a 75-mg controlled-release dosage form, when combined with a restricted diet and exercise.

Using diet pills containing PPA will not make a big difference in the rate of weight loss, says Robert Sherman of FDA's Office of OTC Drug Evaluation. "Even the best studies show only about a half pound greater weight loss per week using PPA combined with diet and exercise," he adds. Sherman cautions that the recommended dosage of these pills should not be exceeded because of the risk of possible adverse effects, such as elevated blood pressure and heart palpitations.

Since PPA is also used as a nasal decongestant in over-the-counter cough and cold products, consumers should read the labels of OTC decongestants to see if they contain PPA. They should not take PPA in two products labeled for different uses.

Sherman notes that FDA has received a small number of reports indicating that PPA use might be associated with an increased risk of stroke. A large-scale safety study was begun in September 1994 to explore the possibility. Based on available data, the agency does not believe that an increased risk of stroke is a concern when PPA is used at recommended dosages.

Weight-Loss Programs

Many people turn to weight-loss programs for help in planning a daily diet and changing lifestyle habits. The IOM report provides guidelines for evaluating the potential effectiveness of such programs.

"To improve their chances for success, consumers should choose programs that focus on long-term weight management; provide instruction in healthful eating, increasing activity, and improving self-esteem; and explain thoroughly the potential health risks from weight loss," according to the report. Consumers should also demand evidence of success. If it is absent or consists primarily of testimonials or other anecdotal evidence, "the program should be viewed with suspicion."

IOM recommends that potential clients be given a truthful, unambiguous, non-misleading statement about the program's approaches and goals, and a full disclosure of costs. The cost breakdown should include initial and ongoing costs, as well as the cost of extra products.

The basic tenet of weight loss—to eat fewer calories than you burn and to stay active—is easy to say but, like most lifestyle changes, not so easy to do. With realistic goals, and a commitment to losing weight slowly, safely and sensibly, the chances of long-term success improve dramatically.

Obesity a Disease

Obesity is now considered a disease—not a moral failing. According to a new report from the Institute of Medicine, "obesity is a heterogeneous disease in which genetic, environmental, psychological, and other factors are involved. It occurs when energy intake exceeds the amount of energy expended over time. Only in a small minority of cases is obesity caused by such illnesses as hypothyroidism or the result of taking medications, such as steroids, that can cause weight gain."

Public health concerns about this disease relate to its link to numerous other diseases that can lead to premature illness or death. The report notes that overweight individuals who lose even relatively small amounts of weight are likely to:

- lower their blood pressure (and thereby the risk of heart attack and stroke)

- reduce abnormally high levels of blood glucose (associated with diabetes)

- bring blood levels of cholesterol and triglycerides (associated with cardiovascular disease) down to more desirable levels

- reduce sleep apnea, or irregular breathing during sleep

- decrease the risk of osteoarthritis of the weight-bearing joints

- decrease depression

- increase self-esteem.

Of course, losing excess weight is also likely to improve appearance, which is a strong motivation for many people.

To order a copy of the IOM report, call (1-800) 624-6242 (in Washington, D.C., call 202-334-3313). The cost is $30 plus $4 shipping and handling.

—by Marilynn Larkin

Marilynn Larkin is a writer in New York City.

Chapter 33

Helping Your Overweight Child

In the United States at least one child in five is overweight and the number of overweight children continues to grow. Over the last 2 decades, this number has increased by more than 50 percent, and the number of "extremely" overweight children has nearly doubled (*Arch Pediatr Adolesc Med*. 1995: 149:1085-91). A doctor determines if children are overweight by measuring their height and weight. Although children have fewer weight-related health problems than adults, overweight children are at high risk of becoming overweight adolescents and adults. Overweight adults are at risk for a number of health problems including heart disease, diabetes, high blood pressure stroke, and some forms of cancer.

What Causes Children to Become Overweight?

Children become overweight for a variety of reasons. The most common causes are genetic factors, lack of physical activity, unhealthy eating patterns, or a combination of these factors. In rare cases, a medical problem, such as an endocrine disorder, may cause a child to become overweight. Your physician can perform a careful physical exam and some blood tests, if necessary, to rule out this type of problem.

Genetic Factors

Children whose parents or brothers or sisters are overweight may be at an increased risk of becoming overweight themselves. Although

National Institute of Diabetes and Digestive and Kidney Diseases (NIDDK), NIH Pub. No. 97-4096, January 1997, last updated February 1998.

weight problems run in families, not all children with a family history of obesity will be overweight. Genetic factors play a role in increasing the likelihood that a child will be overweight, but shared family behaviors such as eating and activity habits also influence body weight.

Lifestyle

A child's total diet and his or her activity level both play an important role in determining a child's weight. The increasing popularity of television and computer and video games contributes to children's inactive lifestyles. The average American child spends approximately 24 hours each week watching television—time that could be spent in some sort of physical activity.

Is My Child Overweight?

If you think that your child is overweight, it is important to talk with your child's doctor. A doctor is the best person to determine whether your child has a weight problem. Physicians will measure your child's weight and height to determine if your child's weight is within a healthy range. A physician will also consider your child's age and growth patterns to determine whether your child is overweight. Assessing overweight in children is difficult because children grow in unpredictable spurts.

For example, it is normal for boys to have a growth spurt in weight and catch up in height later. It is best to let your child's doctor determine whether your child will "grow into" a normal weight. If your doctor finds that your child is overweight, he or she may ask you to make some changes in your family's eating and activity habits.

How Can I Help My Overweight Child?

Be Supportive

One of the most important things you can do to help overweight children is to let them know that they are okay whatever their weight. Children's feelings about themselves often are based on their parents' feelings about them. If you accept your children at any weight, they will be more likely to accept and feel good about themselves. It is also important to talk to your children about weight, allowing them to share their concerns with you. Your child probably knows better than anyone else that he or she has a weight problem. For this reason, overweight children need support, acceptance, and encouragement from their parents.

Focus on the Family

Parents should try not to set children apart because of their weight, but focus on gradually changing their family's physical activity and eating habits. Family involvement helps to teach everyone healthful habits and does not single out the overweight child.

Increase your family's physical activity. Regular physical activity, combined with healthy eating habits, is the most efficient and healthful way to control your weight. It is also an important part of a healthy lifestyle. Some simple ways to increase your family's physical activity include the following:

- Be a role model for your children. If your children see that you are physically active and have fun, they are more likely to be active and stay active for the rest of their lives.

- Plan family activities that provide everyone with exercise and enjoyment, like walking, dancing, biking, or swimming. For example, schedule a walk with your family after dinner instead of watching TV. Make sure that you plan activities that can be done in a safe environment.

- Be sensitive to your child's needs. Overweight children may feel uncomfortable about participating in certain activities. It is important to help your child find physical activities that they enjoy and that aren't embarrassing or too difficult.

- Reduce the amount of time you and your family spend in sedentary activities, such as watching TV or playing video games.

- Become more active throughout your day and encourage your family to do so as well. For example, walkup the stairs instead of taking the elevator, or do some activity during a work or school break—get up and stretch or walk around.

The point is not to make physical activity an unwelcome chore, but to make the most of the opportunities you and your family have to be active.

Teach your family healthy eating habits. Teaching healthy eating practices early will help children approach eating with the right attitude—that food should be enjoyed and is necessary for growth, development, and for energy to keep the body running. The best way to begin is to learn more about children's nutritional needs by reading or talking with a health professional and then to offer them some healthy options, allowing your children to choose what and how much they eat. The pamphlet "Dietary Guidelines for Americans" is a good source of dietary advice for healthy Americans ages 2 years and older. This pamphlet is available from WIN (the address is given at the end of this chapter).

Here Are Some Ways to Help Your Child Develop Good Attitudes about Eating

Don't place your child on a restrictive diet. Children should never be placed on a restrictive diet to lose weight, unless a doctor supervises one for medical reasons. Limiting what children eat may be harmful to their health and interfere with their growth and development.

To promote proper growth and development and prevent overweight, parents should offer the whole family a wide variety of foods from each of the food groups displayed in the Food Guide Pyramid. The Food Guide Pyramid applies to healthy people ages 2 years and older.

The Food Guide Pyramid illustrates the importance of balance among food groups in a daily eating pattern. Select most of your daily servings of food from the food groups that are the largest in the picture and closest to the bottom of the Pyramid. A range of servings is given for each food group. The smaller number is for children who consume about 1,300 calories a day, such as 2-4 years of age. The larger number is for those who consume about 3,000 calories a day, such as boys 15-18 years of age.

- Most of the foods in your diet should come from the grain products group (6-11 servings), the vegetable group (3-5 servings), and the fruit group (2-4 servings). (See Table 33.1. for suggested serving sizes.)

- Your diet should include moderate amounts of foods from the milk group (2-3 servings) and the meat and beans group (2-3 servings).

- Foods that provide few nutrients and are high in fat and sugars should be used sparingly. Fat should not be restricted in the diets of children younger than 2 years of age.

If you are unsure about how to select and prepare a variety of foods for your family, consult a physician or registered dietitian for nutrition counseling. You may also want to refer to the readings and organizations listed at the end of this fact sheet for more information on healthy eating.

Carefully cut down on the amount of fat in your family's diet. Reducing fat is a good way to cut calories without depriving your child of nutrients. Simple ways to cut the fat in your family's diet include eating lowfat or nonfat dairy products, poultry without skin and lean meats, and lowfat or fat-free breads and cereals. Making small changes to the amount of fat in your family's diet is a good way to prevent excess weight gain in children: however, major efforts to change your child's diet should be supervised by a health professional. In addition, fat should not be restricted in the diets of children younger than 2 years of age. After that age, children should gradually adopt a diet that contains no more than 30 percent of calories from fat by the time the child is about 5 years old.

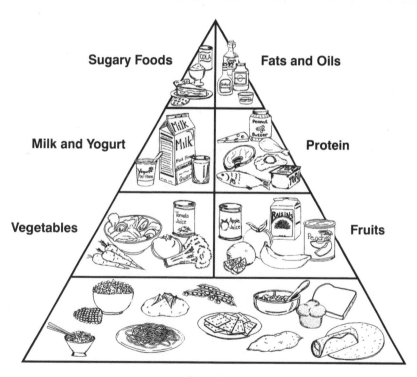

Figure 33.1. The Food Pyramid.

Don't overly restrict sweets or treats. While it is important to be aware of the fat, salt, and sugar content of the foods you serve, all foods-even those that are high in fat or sugar-have a place in the diet, in moderation.

Guide your family's choices rather than dictate foods. Make a wide variety of healthful foods available in the house. This practice will help your children learn how to make healthy food choices.

Encourage your child to eat slowly. A child can detect hunger and fullness better when eating slowly. Eat meals together as a family as often as possible.

Table 33.2. Suggested Serving Sizes

One Serving Equals (Serving sizes are for children and adults ages 2 years and older.)

Bread, Cereal, Rice, and Pasta Group
- 1 slice of bread
- 1 ounce of ready to eat cereal
- 1 1/2 cup of cooked cereal, rice, or pasta

Milk, Yogurt, and Cheese Group
- 1 cup of milk or yogurt
- 1 1/2 ounces of natural cheese
- 2 ounces of processed cheese

Vegetable Group
- 1 cup of raw vegetables or 1/2 cup of frozen leafy vegetables (cooked)
- 1/2 cup of other vegetables - cooked or chopped raw
- 3/4 cup of vegetable juice

Meat, Poultry, Fish, Dry Beans, and Nuts Group
- 2-3 ounces of cooked lean meat, poultry, or fish
- 1/2 cup of cooked dry beans or 1 egg counts as 1 ounce of lean meat
- 2 tablespoons of peanut butter or 1/3 cup of nuts count as 1 ounce of meat

Fruit Group
- 1 medium apple, banana, or orange
- 1/2 cup of chopped, cooked, or canned fruit
- 3/4 cup of fruit juice

Try to make mealtimes pleasant with conversation and sharing, not a time for scolding or arguing. If mealtimes are unpleasant, children may try to eat faster to leave the table as soon as possible. They then may learn to associate eating with stress.

Involve children in food shopping and preparing meals. These activities offer parents hints about children's food preferences, teach children about nutrition, and provide children with a feeling of accomplishment. In addition, children may be more willing to eat or try foods that they help prepare.

Plan for snacks. Continuous snacking may lead to overeating, but snacks that are planned at specific times during the day can be part of a nutritious diet, without spoiling a child's appetite at mealtimes. You should make snacks as nutritious as possible, without depriving your child of occasional chips or cookies, especially at parties or other social events. Below are some ideas for healthy snacks.

- Fresh, frozen, or canned vegetables and fruit served either plain or with lowfat or fat-free cheese or yogurt

- Dried fruit, served with nuts or sunflower or pumpkin seeds

- Breads and crackers made with enriched flour and whole grains, served with fruit spread or fat-free cheese

- Frozen desserts, such as nonfat or lowfat ice cream, frozen yogurt, fruit sorbet, popsicles, water ice, and fruit juice bars

Children of preschool age can easily choke on foods that are hard to chew, small and round, or sticky, such as hard vegetables, whole grapes, hard chunks of cheese, raisins, nuts, and seeds, and popcorn. Its important to carefully select snacks for children in this age group.

Discourage eating meals or snacks while watching TV. Try to eat only in designated areas of your home, such as the dining room or kitchen. Eating in front of the TV may make it difficult to pay attention to feelings of fullness, and may lead to overeating.

Try not to use food to punish or reward your child. Withholding food as a punishment may lead children to worry that they will not get enough food. For example, sending children to bed without any dinner may cause them to worry that they will go hungry. As a result, children may try to eat whenever they get a chance. Similarly, when foods, such as sweets, are used as a reward, children may assume that these foods are better or more valuable than other foods. For example, telling children that they will get dessert if they eat all of there vegetables sends the wrong message about vegetables.

Make sure your child's meals outside the home are balanced. Find out more about your school lunch program, or pack your child's lunch to include a variety of foods. Also select healthier items when dining at restaurants.

Set a good example. Children are good learners, and they learn best by example. Setting a good example for your kids by eating a variety of foods and being physically active will teach your children healthy lifestyle habits that they can follow for the rest of their lives.

Is Additional Help Available?

If you need to make changes to your family's eating and exercise habits, but are finding it difficult, a registered dietitian (RD) may be able to help. Your physician may be able to refer you to an RD, or you can call the National Center for Nutrition and Dietetics of The American Dietetic Association at 800-366-1655 and ask for the name of an RD in your area.

If your efforts at home are unsuccessful in helping your child reach a healthy weight and your physician determines that your child's health is at risk unless he or she loses weight steadily, you may want to consider a formal treatment program. To locate a weight-control program for your child, you may want to contact a local university-based medical center. The Weight-control Information Network (WIN), described at the end of this chapter, maintains a list of nationwide university-based medical centers.

Look for the following characteristics when choosing a weight-control program for your child. The program should:

- Be staffed with a variety of health professionals. The best programs may include RDs, exercise physiologists, pediatricians or family physicians, and psychiatrists or psychologists.

- Perform a medical evaluation of the child. Before being enrolled in a program, your child's weight, growth, and health should be reviewed by a physician. During enrollment, your child's weight, growth, and health should be monitored by a health professional at regular intervals.

- Focus on the whole family, not just the overweight child.

- Be adapted to the specific age and capabilities of the child. Programs for 4-year-olds are different from those developed for children 8 or 12 years of age in terms of degree of responsibility of the child and parents.

- Focus on behavioral changes.

- Teach the child how to select a variety of foods in appropriate portions.

- Encourage daily activity and limit sedentary activity, such as watching TV.

- Include a maintenance program and other support and referral resources to reinforce the new behaviors and to deal with underlying issues that contributed to overweight.

The overall goal of a successful treatment program should be to help the whole family focus on making healthy changes to their eating and activity habits that they will be able to maintain throughout life.

Additional Reading

Epstein, L.H. and Squires, S. *The Stoplight Diet for Children: An Eight-Week Program for Parents and Children.* Boston: Little, Brown and Company, 1988. Available in public libraries.

Ikeda, J. *If My Child is Too Fat, What Should I Do About It?* Publication # 21455, 1990. Available from the Cooperative Extension, University of California, Division of Agriculture and Natural Resources; tel. 415-642-2431.

Satter, E. *How To Get Your Kids To Eat ... But Not Too Much.* Palo Alto, CA: Bull Publishing Co., 1987. Available in public libraries.

Resources

The American Academy of Pediatrics (Marketing Division)
Northwest Point Boulevard
Elk Grove Village, IL 60009
(708) 228-5005

Food and Nutrition Information Center
United States Department of Agriculture
Website: http://www.nal.usda.gov/fnic

The National Center for Nutrition and Dietetics
The American Dietetic Association
216 West Jackson Boulevard
Chicago, IL 60606-6995
Consumer Nutrition Hotline: (800) 366-1655.

National Heart, Lung, and Blood Institute Information Center
P.O. Box 30105
Bethesda, MD 20824-0105
(301) 251-1222

President's Council on Physical Fitness and Sports
701 Pennsylvania Avenue, NW, Suite 250
Washington, DC 20004
(202) 272-3421

Weight-control Information Network

The Weight-control Information Network (WIN) is a service of the National Institute of Diabetes and Digestive and Kidney Diseases (NIDDK), part of the National Institutes of Health, under the U.S. Public Health Service. Authorized by Congress(Public Law 103-43), WIN assembles and disseminates to health professionals and the public information on weight control, obesity, and nutritional disorders. WIN responds to requests for information; develops, reviews, and distributes publications; and develops communications strategies to encourage individuals to achieve and maintain a healthy weight.

Publications produced by the clearinghouse are reviewed carefully for scientific accuracy, content, and readability.

Weight-control Information Network
1 Win Way
Bethesda, MD 20892-3665
Phone: (301) 984-7378 or 1-800-WIN-8098
Fax: (301) 984-7196
E-mail: win@info.niddk.nih.gov

Chapter 34

Understanding Adult Obesity

What Is Obesity?

"Obesity" is one of those words that has one meaning to the public and a more precise one to the medical world. To most people, to be obese means to be very overweight. To doctors and scientists, however, a person can be considered obese even if the degree of overweight is not very great.

"Overweight" refers to an excess amount of body weight that includes all tissues—muscle, bone, and fat—as well as water.

"Obesity" refers specifically to having excess body fat. One can be overweight without being obese: a body builder who has a lot of muscle, for example. For practical purposes, however, most people who are overweight are also obese.

Many Americans are at increased health risk because they are obese. The U.S. Surgeon General, in a 1988 report on nutrition and health, estimated that one-fourth of adult Americans are overweight. Obesity is a known risk factor for chronic diseases including heart disease, diabetes, high blood pressure, stroke, and some forms of cancer.

This chapter provides basic information about obesity: what it is, what causes it, how to measure it.

National Institute of Diabetes and Digestive and Kidney Diseases (NIDDK), NIH Pub. No. 94-3680, November 1993.

How Is Obesity Measured?

Everyone needs a certain amount of body fat for stored energy, heat insulation, shock absorption, and other functions. As a rule, women have more fat than men. Doctors generally agree that men with more than 25 percent body fat and women with more than 30 percent body fat are obese. Precisely measuring a person's body fat, however, is not easy. The most accurate method is to weigh a person underwater—a procedure limited to laboratories with sophisticated equipment.

There are two simpler methods for estimating body fat, but they can yield inaccurate results if done by an inexperienced person or if done on someone with severe obesity. One is to measure skinfold thickness in several parts of the body. The second involves sending a harmless amount of electric current through a person's body (bioelectric impedance analysis). Both methods are commonly used in health clubs and in commercial weight-loss programs, but results should be viewed skeptically.

Because measuring a person's body fat is tricky, doctors often rely on other means to diagnose obesity. Two widely used measurements are weight-for-height tables and body mass index. While both measurements have their limitations, they are reliable indicators that someone may have a weight problem. They are easy to calculate and require no special equipment.

Weight-for-Height Tables

Most people are familiar with weight-for-height tables. Doctors have used these tables for decades to determine whether a person is overweight. The tables usually have a range of acceptable weights for a person of a given height.

One problem with using weight-for-height tables is that doctors disagree over which is the best table to use. Many versions are available, all with different weight ranges. Some tables take a person's frame size, age, and sex into account; others do not. A limitation of all weight-for-height tables is that they do not distinguish excess fat from muscle. A very muscular person may appear obese, according to the tables, when he or she is not. Still, weight-for-height tables can be used as general guidelines.

The table printed here is from the 1990 edition of *Dietary Guidelines for Americans*, a pamphlet printed jointly by the U.S. Departments of Agriculture and Health and Human Services. This table has a wide range for what the pamphlet calls "healthy" or "suggested" weights.

In this table, the higher weights generally apply to men, who tend to have more muscle and bone. The lower weights more often apply to women, who have less muscle and bone. The table also shows higher weights for people age 35 and older, which some experts question.

Table 34.1. Suggested Weights for Adults

Height[1]	Weight in pounds[2]	
	19 to 34 years	35 years and over
5'0"	97-128	108-138
5'1"	101-132	111-143
5'2"	104-137	115-148
5'3"	107-141	119-152
5'4"	111-146	122-157
5'5"	114-150	126-162
5'6"	118-155	130-167
5'7"	121-160	134-172
5'8"	125-164	138-178
5'9"	129-169	142-183
5'10"	132-174	146-188
5'11"	136-179	151-194
6'0"	140-184	155-199
6'1"	144-189	159-205
6'2"	148-195	164-210
6'3"	152-200	168-216
6'4"	156-205	173-222
6'5"	160-211	177-228
6'6"	164-216	182-234

[1]*Without shoes.*
[2]*Without clothes.*
[3]*The higher weights in the ranges generally apply to men, who tend to have more muscle and bone; the lower weights more often apply to women, who have less muscle and bone.*

Body Mass Index (BMI)

Body mass index, or BMI, is a new term to most people. However, it is the measurement of choice for many physicians and researchers studying obesity. BMI uses a mathematical formula that takes into account both a person's height and weight. BMI equals a person's

Table 34.2. Body Weights in Pounds According to Height and Body Mass Index*

| Height (in.) | Body Mass Index (kg/m²) | | | | | | | | | | | | | |
	19	20	21	22	23	24	25	26	27	28	29	30	35	40
	Body Weight (lb.)													
58	91	96	100	105	110	115	119	124	129	134	138	143	167	191
59	94	99	104	109	114	119	124	128	133	138	143	148	173	198
60	97	102	107	112	118	123	128	133	138	143	148	153	179	204
61	100	106	111	116	122	127	132	137	143	148	153	158	185	211
62	104	109	115	120	126	131	136	142	147	153	158	164	191	218
63	107	113	118	124	130	135	141	146	152	158	163	169	197	225
64	110	116	122	128	134	140	145	151	157	163	169	174	204	232
65	114	120	126	132	138	144	150	156	162	168	174	180	210	240
66	118	124	130	136	142	148	155	161	167	173	179	186	216	247
67	121	127	134	140	146	153	159	166	172	178	185	191	223	255
68	125	131	138	144	151	158	164	171	177	184	190	197	230	262
69	128	135	142	149	155	162	169	176	182	189	196	203	236	270
70	132	139	146	153	160	167	174	181	188	195	202	207	243	278
71	136	143	150	157	165	172	179	186	193	200	208	215	250	286
72	140	147	154	162	169	177	184	191	199	206	213	221	258	294
73	144	151	159	166	174	182	189	197	204	212	219	227	265	302
74	148	155	163	171	179	186	194	202	210	218	225	233	272	311
75	152	160	168	176	184	192	200	208	216	224	232	240	279	319
76	156	164	172	180	189	197	205	213	221	230	238	246	287	328

Each entry gives the body weight in pounds (lb.) for a person of a given height and body mass index. Pounds have been rounded off. To use the table, find the appropriate height in the left-hand column. Move across the row to a given weight. The number a the top of the column is the body mass index for the height and weight.

Adapted with permission from Bray, B.A., Gray, D.S. Obesity, Part I. Pathogenesis. Western Journal Medicine. 1998;149:429-41.

weight in kilograms divided by height in meters squared (BMI = kg/ m^2). The table printed here has already done the math and metric conversions. To use the table, find the appropriate height in the left-hand column. Move across the row to the given weight. The number at the top of the column is the BMI for that height and weight.

In general, a person age 35 or older is obese if he or she has a BMI of 27 or more. For people age 34 or younger, a BMI of 25 or more indicates obesity. A BMI of more than 30 usually is considered a sign of moderate to severe obesity.

The BMI measurement poses some of the same problems as the weight-for-height tables. Doctors don't agree on the cut-off points for "healthy" versus "unhealthy" BMI ranges. BMI also does not provide information on a person's percentage of body fat. However, like the weight-for-height table, BMI is a useful general guideline.

Body Fat Distribution: 'Pears' vs. 'Apples'

Doctors are concerned with not only how much fat a person has but where the fat is on the body.

Women typically collect fat in their hips and buttocks, giving their figures a "pear" shape. Men, on the other hand, usually build up fat around their bellies, giving them more of an "apple" shape. This is not a hard and fast rule, though. Some men are pear-shaped and some women become apple-shaped, especially after menopause.

People whose fat is concentrated mostly in the abdomen are more likely to develop many of the health problems associated with obesity.

Doctors have developed a simple way to measure whether someone is an apple or a pear. The measurement is called waist-to-hip ratio.

Waist-to-Hip Ratio

To find out someone's waist-to-hip ratio, measure the waist at its narrowest point, then measure the hips at the widest point. Divide the waist measurement by the hip measurement.

A woman with a 35-inch waist and 46-inch hips would do the following calculation:

$$35 \div 46 = 0.76$$

Women with waist-to-hip ratios of more than 0.8 or men with waist-to-hip ratios of more than 1.0 are "apples." They are at increased health risk because of their fat distribution.

What Causes Obesity?

In scientific terms, obesity occurs when a person's calorie intake exceeds the amount of energy he or she burns. What causes this imbalance between consuming and burning calories is unclear. Evidence suggests that obesity often has more than one cause. Genetic, environmental, psychological, and other factors all may play a part.

Genetic Factors

Obesity tends to run in families, suggesting that it may have a genetic cause. However, family members share not only genes but also diet and lifestyle habits that may contribute to obesity. Separating these lifestyle factors from genetic ones is often difficult. Still, growing evidence points to heredity as a strong determining factor of obesity. In one study of adults who were adopted as children, researchers found that the subjects' adult weights were closer to their biological parents' weights than their adoptive parents' weights. The environment provided by the adoptive family apparently had less influence on the development of obesity than the person's genetic makeup.

Nevertheless, people who feel that their genes have doomed them to a lifetime of obesity should take heart. As discussed in the next section, many people genetically predisposed to obesity do not become obese or manage to lose weight and keep it off.

Environmental Factors

Although genes are an important factor in many cases of obesity, a person's environment also plays a significant part. Environment includes lifestyle behaviors such as what a person eats and how active he or she is.

Americans tend to have high-fat diets, often putting taste and convenience ahead of nutritional content when choosing meals. Most Americans also don't get enough exercise.

People can't change their genetic makeup, of course, but they can change what they eat and how active they are. Some people have been able to lose weight and keep it off by:

- Learning how to choose more nutritious meals that are lower in fat.

- Learning to recognize environmental cues (such as enticing smells) that may make them want to eat when they are not hungry.

- Becoming more physically active.

Psychological Factors

Psychological factors also may influence eating habits. Many people eat in response to negative emotions such as boredom, sadness, or anger.

While most overweight people have no more psychological disturbance than normal weight people, about 30 percent of the people who seek treatment for serious weight problems have difficulties with binge eating. During a binge eating episode, people eat large amounts of food while feeling they can't control how much they are eating. Those with the most severe binge eating problems are considered to have binge eating disorder. These people may have more difficulty losing weight and keeping the weight off than people without binge eating problems. Some will need special help, such as counseling or medication, to control their binge eating before they can successfully manage their weight.

Other Causes of Obesity

Some rare illnesses can cause obesity. These include hypothyroidism, Cushing's syndrome, depression, and certain neurologic problems that can lead to overeating. Certain drugs, such as steroids and some antidepressants, may cause excessive weight gain. A doctor can determine if a patient has any of these conditions, which are believed to be responsible for only about 1 percent of all cases of obesity.

What Are the Consequences of Obesity?

Health Risks

Obesity is not just a cosmetic problem. It's a health hazard. Someone who is 40 percent overweight is twice as likely to die prematurely as an average-weight person. (This effect is seen after 10 to 30 years of being obese.) Obesity has been linked to several serious medical conditions, including diabetes, heart disease, high blood pressure, and stroke. It is also associated with higher rates of certain types of cancer. Obese men are more likely than nonobese men to die from cancer of the colon, rectum, and prostate. Obese women are more likely than nonobese women to die from cancer of the gallbladder, breast, uterus, cervix, and ovaries.

Other diseases and health problems linked to obesity include:

- Gallbladder disease and gallstones.

- Osteoarthritis, a disease in which the joints deteriorate, possibly as a result of excess weight on the joints.

- Gout, another disease affecting the joints.

- Pulmonary (breathing) problems, including sleep apnea, in which a person can stop breathing for a short time during sleep.

Doctors generally agree that the more obese a person is, the more likely he or she is to have health problems.

Psychological and Social Effects

One of the most painful aspects of obesity may be the emotional suffering it causes. American society places great emphasis on physical appearance, often equating attractiveness with slimness, especially in women. The messages, intended or not, make overweight people feel unattractive. Many people assume that obese people are gluttonous, lazy, or both. However, more and more evidence contradicts this assumption.

Obese people often face prejudice or discrimination at work, at school, while looking for a job, and in social situations. Feelings of rejection, shame, or depression are common.

Who Should Lose Weight?

Doctors generally agree that people who are 20 percent or more overweight, especially the severely obese person, can gain significant health benefits from weight loss.

Many obesity experts believe that people who are less than 20 percent above their healthy weight should try to lose weight if they have any of the following risk factors.

Risk Factors

- Family history of certain chronic diseases. People with close relatives who have had heart disease or diabetes are more likely to develop these problems if they are obese.

- Pre-existing medical conditions. High blood pressure, high cholesterol levels, or high blood sugar levels are all warning signs of some obesity-associated diseases.

- "Apple" shape. People whose weight is concentrated around their abdomens may be at greater risk of heart disease, diabetes, or cancer than people of the same weight who are pear-shaped.

Fortunately, even a modest weight loss of 10 to 20 pounds can bring significant health improvements, such as lowering one's blood pressure and cholesterol levels.

How Is Obesity Treated?

The method of treatment will depend on how obese a person is. Factors such as an individual's overall health and motivation to lose weight are also important considerations. Treatment may include a combination of diet, exercise, and behavior modification. In some cases of severe obesity, gastrointestinal surgery may be recommended.

Research on Obesity

The National Institute of Diabetes and Digestive and Kidney Diseases (NIDDK) is the part of the National Institutes of Health chiefly responsible for obesity research. NIDDK supports the study of obesity in its own labs and clinics and at universities, hospitals, and research centers across the United States. NIDDK-funded research has helped scientists learn more about the role of genes and metabolism in obesity. Other NIDDK-supported studies have examined the relationship between obesity and various medical conditions. On-going NIDDK research efforts include better ways to define and treat the various types of obesity and understanding how the body stores and uses fat.

NIDDK also oversees the National Task Force on Prevention and Treatment of Obesity. The task force comprises leading obesity and nutrition experts who gather and assess the latest information on obesity treatment and prevention. The task force also helps guide basic and clinical research on obesity. Scientific papers and general-interest brochures and pamphlets approved by the task force are available from the NIDDK's Obesity Resource Information Center.

In addition to NIDDK, other sections of the NIH sponsor obesity research. They include: the National Heart, Lung, and Blood Institute (NHLBI); the National Center for Research Resources (NCRR); the National Institute of Child Health and Human Development (NICHD); the National Institute on Mental Health (NIMH); the National Cancer Institute (NCI); the National Institute on Aging (NIA); the National Institute of Nursing Research (NINR); the National

Institute of Arthritis and Musculoskeletal and Skin Diseases (NIAMS); the National Institute of Neurological Diseases and Stroke (NINDS); and the National Institute of Environmental and Health Sciences (NIEHS).

Additional Reading on Obesity

"Are You Eating Right?" *Consumer Reports*, October 1992. This article summarizes advice from 68 nutrition experts, including a discussion on weight control and health risks of obesity. Available in public libraries.

Bray, G.A. "Pathophysiology of Obesity." *American Journal of Clinical Nutrition*. 1992; Supplement to Vol. 55 (2): 488S-494S. This article comes from the proceedings of an NIH Consensus Development Conference on Gastrointestinal Surgery for Severe Obesity. Written for health professionals in technical language. Available in medical libraries.

"Dietary Guidelines for Americans." Fourth Edition, 1995. Home and Garden Bulletin No. 232. This pamphlet, issued by the U.S. Agriculture and Health and Human Services Departments, contains information about maintaining a healthy weight, as well as dietary and nutrition recommendations. Available through the Government Printing Office, Publication No. 1996-402-519.

"Exercise and Weight Control." The President's Council on Physical Fitness and Sports, Department of Health and Human Services. This brochure discusses the difference between being "overweight" and "overfat" and the role diet and exercise can play in a weight loss program. Copies can be obtained from the President's Council on Physical Fitness and Sports, Dept. No. 176, 701 Pennsylvania Ave. NW, Washington, DC 20004.

"The Facts About Weight Loss Products and Programs." This brochure, produced by the Federal Trade Commission in conjunction with the Food and Drug Administration and the National Association of Attorneys General, has tips on evaluating diet claims and weight loss programs. Copies can be obtained from the FTC, Public Affairs Branch, Room 130, Sixth St. and Pennsylvania Ave. NW, Washington, DC 20580.

"Getting Slim." *U.S. News & World Report*, May 14, 1990. This article, written for the general public, discusses definitions of obesity, the role of genes, body mass index, and apple/pear weight distribution patterns. Available in public libraries.

Long, P. "The Great Weight Debate." *Health*. February/March, 1992, pp. 42-47. This article, written for the general public, discusses the controversy over which weight-for-height table is best to use. It also provides some simple guidelines for determining whether someone needs to lose weight. Available in public libraries.

"Methods for Voluntary Weight Loss and Control." National Institutes of Health Technology Assessment Conference Statement, March 30-April 1, 1992. This publication, written for health professionals, summarizes findings of a conference discussing success rates of various methods of weight loss, short-term and long-term effects of losing weight, and related topics. Copies are available from the Office of Medical Applications Research, National Institutes of Health, Federal Building, Room 618, Bethesda, MD 20892.

Yanovski. S.Z. "A Practical Approach to Treatment of the Obese Patient." *Archives of Family Medicine*. 1993; Vol. 2, No. 3, pp 309-316. Written for health professionals, this article provides guidance on evaluating overweight patients and developing plans for treatment.

Chapter 35

Federal Clinical Practice Guidelines for Obesity

The first Federal guidelines on the identification, evaluation, and treatment of overweight and obesity in adults were released today by the National Heart, Lung, and Blood Institute (NHLBI), in cooperation with the National Institute of Diabetes and Digestive and Kidney Diseases (NIDDK).

These clinical practice guidelines are designed to help physicians in their care of overweight and obesity, a growing public health problem that affects 97 million American adults—55 percent of the population.

These individuals are at increased risk of illness from hypertension, lipid disorders, type 2 diabetes, coronary heart disease, stroke, gallbladder disease, osteoarthritis, sleep apnea and respiratory problems, and certain cancers. The total costs attributable to obesity-related disease approaches $100 billion annually.

"Overweight and obesity pose a major public health challenge. The development of these guidelines was a pioneering achievement since they were the first ever developed by the Institute using an evidence-based model and methodology," said NHLBI Director Dr. Claude Lenfant. "This report will be an invaluable clinical tool for any health care professional who works with overweight or obese patients," he added.

The guidelines are based on the most extensive review of the scientific evidence on overweight and obesity conducted to date. The

National Heart, Lung, and Blood Institute (NHLBI), NIH News Release, June 17, 1998.

review involved a systematic analysis of the published scientific literature to address 35 key clinical questions on how different treatment strategies affect weight loss and how weight control affects the major risk factors for heart disease and stroke as well as other chronic diseases and conditions.

The guidelines present a new approach for the assessment of overweight and obesity and establish principles of safe and effective weight loss. According to the guidelines, assessment of overweight involves evaluation of three key measures—body mass index (BMI), waist circumference, and a patient's risk factors for diseases and conditions associated with obesity.

The guidelines' definition of overweight is based on research which relates body mass index to risk of death and illness. The 24-member expert panel that developed the guidelines identified overweight as a BMI of 25 to 29.9 and obesity as a BMI of 30 and above, which is consistent with the definitions used in many other countries, and supports the *Dietary Guidelines for Americans* issued in 1995. BMI describes body weight relative to height and is strongly correlated with total body fat content in adults. According to the guidelines, a BMI of 30 is about 30 pounds overweight and is equivalent to 221 pounds in a 6' person and to 186 pounds in someone who is 5'6". The BMI numbers apply to both men and women. Some very muscular people may have a high BMI without health risks.

The panel recommends that BMI be determined in all adults. People of normal weight should have their BMI reassessed in 2 years.

"The evidence is solid that the risk for various cardiovascular and other diseases rises significantly when someone's BMI is over 25 and that risk of death increases as the body mass index reaches and surpasses 30," said Dr. F. Xavier Pi Sunyer, chairman of the expert panel and director of the Obesity Research Center, St. Luke's/Roosevelt Hospital Center in New York City.

"The guidelines tell the truth about the risks associated with unhealthy weight. We hope that physicians and the public will take the message seriously and use the guidelines to begin to deal effectively with a difficult problem," asserted Dr. Pi-Sunyer.

According to a new analysis of the National Health and Nutrition Examination Survey (NHANES III), as BMI levels rise, average blood pressure and total cholesterol levels increase and average HDL or good cholesterol levels decrease. Men in the highest obesity category have more than twice the risk of hypertension, high blood cholesterol, or both compared to men of normal weight. Women in the highest obesity category have four times the risk of either or both of these risk factors.

The guidelines recommend weight loss to lower high blood pressure, to lower high total cholesterol and to raise low levels of HDL or good cholesterol, and to lower elevated blood glucose in overweight persons with two or more risk factors and in obese persons. Overweight patients without risk factors should prevent further weight gain, advise the guidelines.

In addition to measuring BMI, health care professionals should evaluate a patient's risk factors, such as elevations in blood pressure or blood cholesterol, or family history of obesity-related disease. At a given level of overweight or obesity, patients with additional risk factors are considered to be at higher risk for health problems, requiring more intensive therapy and modification of any risk factors.

Physicians are also advised to determine waist circumference, which is strongly associated with abdominal fat. Excess abdominal fat is an independent predictor of disease risk. A waist circumference of over 40 inches in men and over 35 inches in women signifies increased risk in those who have a BMI of 25 to 34.9.

According to the guidelines, the most successful strategies for weight loss include calorie reduction, increased physical activity, and behavior therapy designed to improve eating and physical activity habits. Other recommendations include:

- Patients should engage in moderate physical activity, progressing to 30 minutes or more on most or preferably all days of the week.

- Reducing dietary fat alone—without reducing calories—will not produce weight loss. Cutting back on dietary fat can help reduce calories and is heart-healthy.

- The initial goal of treatment should be to reduce body weight by about 10 percent from baseline, an amount that reduces obesity-related risk factors. With success, and if warranted, further weight loss can be attempted.

- A reasonable time line for a 10 percent reduction in body weight is six months of treatment, with a weight loss of 1 to 2 pounds per week.

- Weight-maintenance should be a priority after the first 6 months of weight-loss therapy.

- Physicians should have their patients try lifestyle therapy for at least 6 months before embarking on physician-prescribed drug therapy. Weight loss drugs approved by the FDA for long-term use may be tried as part of a comprehensive weight loss program that includes dietary therapy and physical activity in carefully selected patients (BMI of 30 or more without additional risk factors, BMI of 27 or more with two or more risk factors) who have been unable to lose weight or maintain weight loss with conventional nondrug therapies. Drug therapy may also be used during the weight maintenance phase of treatment. However, drug safety and effectiveness beyond one year of total treatment have not been established.

- Weight loss surgery is an option for carefully selected patients with clinically severe obesity—BMI of 40 or more or BMI of 35 or more with coexisting conditions when less invasive methods have failed and the patient is at high risk for obesity-associated illness. Lifelong medical surveillance after surgery is a necessity.

- Overweight and obese patients who do not wish to lose weight, or are otherwise not candidates for weight loss treatment, should be counseled on strategies to avoid further weight gain.

- Age alone should not preclude weight loss treatment in older adults. A careful evaluation of potential risks and benefits in the individual patient should guide management.

According to NHANES III, the trend in the prevalence of overweight and obesity is upward. The guidelines note that from 1960 to 1994, the prevalence of obesity in adults (BMI 30 or more) increased from nearly 13 percent to 22.5 percent of the U.S. population, with most of the increase occurring in the 1990s.

"There are several possible reasons for the increase," asserted Karen Donato, coordinator of the Obesity Education Initiative. "When people read labels, they're more likely to notice what's lowfat and healthy but may not be looking at calories. Also, more people are eating out and portion sizes have increased. Another issue is decreased physical activity. So people are consuming more calories and are less active. It doesn't take much to tip the energy balance," she said.

The upward trend in adult obesity has also been observed in children, notes the report. Since treatment issues surrounding overweight children and adolescents are quite different from the treatment of adults, the panel called for a separate guideline for youth as soon as possible. However, a healthy eating plan and increased physical activity is an important goal for all family members.

With that in mind, the guidelines contain practical information on healthy eating. Based on this material, the NHLBI has developed consumer tips on shopping, eating, and dining out.

The guidelines have been reviewed by 115 health experts at major medical and professional societies. They have been endorsed by the coordinating committees of the National Cholesterol Education Program and the National High Blood Pressure Education Program, the North American Association for the Study of Obesity, the NIDDK Task force on the Prevention and Treatment of Obesity, and the American Heart Association. These groups represent 54 professional societies, government agencies, and consumer organizations. *Clinical Guidelines on the Identification, Evaluation, and Treatment of Overweight and Obesity in Adults* will be distributed to primary care physicians in the U.S. as well as to other interested health care practitioners. It is available on the NHLBI Website (at www.nhlbi.nih.gov). Single free copies of the consumer tips referred to above are available by writing to the NHLBI Information Center, P.O. Box 30105, Bethesda, MD 20824-0105.

Chapter 36

Prescription Medications for the Treatment of Obesity

Obesity is a chronic disease that affects many people and often requires long-term treatment to promote and sustain weight loss. As in other chronic conditions, such as diabetes or high blood pressure, long-term use of prescription medications may be appropriate for some individuals. While most side effects of prescription medications for obesity are mild, serious complications have been reported. Valvular heart disease has recently been reported to occur in association with the use of certain appetite suppressant medications. As a result of these reports, the manufacturer has voluntarily withdrawn two medications, fenfluramine (Pondimin) and dexfenfluramine (Redux) from the market. There are few long-term studies evaluating the safety or effectiveness of other currently approved appetite suppressant medications. In particular, the safety and effectiveness of combining more than one appetite suppressant medication or combining appetite suppressant medications with other medications for the purpose of weight loss is unknown. Appetite suppressant medications should be used only by patients who are at increased medical risk because of their obesity and should not be used for "cosmetic" weight loss.

Medications That Promote Weight Loss

The medications most often used in the management of obesity are commonly known as "appetite suppressant" medications. Appetite

National Institute of Diabetes and Digestive and Kidney Diseases (NIDDK), NIH Publication No. 97-4191, December 1996, updated February 1998.

suppressant medications promote weight loss by decreasing appetite or increasing the feeling of being full. These medications decrease appetite by increasing serotonin or catecholamine—two brain chemicals that affect mood and appetite.

Most currently available appetite suppressant medications are approved by the U.S. Food and Drug Administration (FDA) for short-term use, meaning a few weeks or months. Sibutramine is the only appetite suppressant medication approved for longer-term use in significantly obese patients, although the safety and effectiveness have not been established for use beyond one year. (See Table 36.1 for the generic and trade names of prescription appetite suppressant medications.) While the FDA regulates how a medication can be advertised or promoted by the manufacturer, these regulations do not restrict a doctor's ability to prescribe the medication for different conditions, in different doses, or for different lengths of time. The practice of prescribing medication for periods of time or for conditions not approved is known as "off-label" use. While such use often occurs in the treatment of many conditions, you should feel comfortable about asking your doctor if he or she is using a medication or combination of medications in a manner that is not approved by the FDA. The use of more than one appetite suppressant medication at a time (combined drug treatment) is an example of an off-label use. Using currently approved appetite suppressant medication for more than a short period of time (i.e., more than "a few weeks" is also considered off-label use.

Single Drug Treatment

Several appetite suppressant medications are available to treat obesity. In general, these medications are modestly effective, leading

Table 36.1. Prescription Appetite Suppressant Medications

Generic Name	Trade Name(s)
Dexfenfluramine	Redux (Withdrawn)
Diethylpropion	Tenuate, Tenuate dospan
Fenfluramine	Pondimin (Withdrawn)
Mazindol	Sanorex, Mazanor
Phendimetrazine	Bontril, Plegine, Prelu-2, X-Trozine
Phentermine	Adipex-P, Fastin, Ionamin, Oby-trim
Sibutramine	Meridia

to an average weight loss of 5 to 22 pounds above that expected with non-drug obesity treatments. People respond differently to appetite suppressant medications, and some people experience more weight loss than others. Some obese patients using medication lose more than 10 percent of their starting body weight—an amount of weight loss that may reduce risk factors for obesity-related diseases, such as high blood pressure or diabetes. Maximum weight loss usually occurs within 6 months of starting medication treatment. Weight then tends to level off or increase during the remainder of treatment. Studies suggest that if a patient does not lose at least 4 pounds over 4 weeks on a particular medication, then that medication is unlikely to help the patient achieve significant weight loss. Few studies have looked at how safe or effective these medications are when taken for more than 1 year.

Some antidepressant medications have been studied as appetite suppressant medications. While these medications are FDA approved for the treatment of depression, their use in weight loss is an "off-label" use. Studies of these medications generally have found that patients lost modest amounts of weight for up to 6 months. However, most studies have found that patients who lost weight while taking antidepressant medications tended to regain weight while they were still on the drug treatment.

NOTE: Amphetamines and closely-related compounds are not recommended for use in the treatment of obesity due to their potential for abuse and dependence.

Combined Drug Treatment

Combined drug treatment using fenfluramine and phentermine ("fen/phen") is no longer available due to the withdrawal of fenfluramine from the market. Little information is available about the safety or effectiveness of other drug combinations for weight loss, including fluoxetine/phentermine, phendimetrazine/phentermine, herbal combinations, or others. Until more information on their safety or effectiveness is available, using combinations of medications for weight loss is not recommended except as part of a research study.

Potential Benefits of Medication Treatment

Over the short term, weight loss in obese individuals may reduce a number of health risks. Studies looking at the effects of appetite suppressant medication treatment on obesity-related health risks have found that some agents lower blood pressure, blood cholesterol, triglycerides (fats) and decrease insulin resistance (the body's inability to use blood sugar) over the short term. However, long-term studies are needed to determine if weight loss from appetite suppressant medications can improve health.

Potential Risks and Areas of Concern When Considering Medication Treatment

When considering long-term appetite suppressant medication treatment for obesity, you should consider the following areas of concern and potential risks.

Potential for Abuse or Dependence

Currently, all prescription medications to treat obesity are controlled substances, meaning doctors need to follow certain restrictions when prescribing appetite suppressant medications. Although abuse and dependence are not common with non-amphetamine appetite suppressant medications, doctors should be cautious when they prescribe these medications for patients with a history of alcohol or other drug abuse.

Development of Tolerance

Most studies of appetite suppressant medications show that a patient's weight tends to level off after 4 to 6 months while still on medication treatment. While some patients and physicians may be concerned that this shows tolerance to the medications, the leveling off may mean that the medication has reached its limit of effectiveness. Based on the currently available studies, it is not clear if weight gain with continuing treatment is due to drug tolerance.

Reluctance to View Obesity As a Chronic Disease

Obesity often is viewed as the result of a lack of willpower, weakness, or a lifestyle "choice"—the choice to overeat and under-exercise. The belief that persons choose to be obese adds to the hesitation of health professionals and patients to accept the use of long-term appetite suppressant medication treatment to manage obesity. Obesity, however, is more appropriately considered a chronic disease than a lifestyle choice. Other chronic diseases, such as diabetes and high blood pressure, are managed by long-term drug treatment, even though these diseases also improve with changes in lifestyle, such as diet and exercise. Although this issue may concern physicians and patients, social views on obesity should not prevent patients from seeking medical treatment to prevent health risks that can cause serious illness and death. Appetite suppressant medications are not "magic bullets," or a one-shot fix. They cannot take the place of improving one's diet and becoming more physically active. The major role of medications appears to be to help a person stay on a diet and exercise plan to lose weight and keep it off.

Side Effects

Because appetite suppressant medications are used to treat a condition that affects millions of people, many of whom are basically healthy, their potential for side effects is of great concern. Most side effects of these medications are mild and usually improve with continued treatment. Rarely, serious and even fatal outcomes have been reported. Two approved appetite suppressant medications that affect serotonin release and reuptake have been withdrawn from the market (fenfluramine, dexfenfluramine). Medications that affect catecholamine levels (such as phentermine, diethylpropion, and mazindol) may cause symptoms of sleeplessness, nervousness, and euphoria (feeling of well-being). Sibutramine acts on both the serotonin and catecholamine systems, but unlike fenfluramine and dexfenfluramine, sibutramine does not cause release of serotonin from cells. The primary known side-effects of concern with sibutramine are elevations in blood pressure and pulse, which are usually small, but which may be significant in some patients. People with poorly controlled high blood pressure, heart disease, irregular heart beat, or history of stroke should not take sibutramine, and all patients taking the medication should have their blood pressure monitored on a regular basis.

Primary pulmonary hypertension (PPH) is a rare but potentially fatal disorder that affects the blood vessels in the lungs and results in death within 4 years in 45 percent of its victims. Patients who use appetite suppressant medications for more than 3 months have a greater risk for developing this condition, estimated at 1 in 22,000 to 1 in 44,000 patients per year. While the risk of developing PPH is very small, physicians and patients should be aware of this possible complication when considering the risks and benefits of using appetite suppressant medications in the long-term treatment of obesity. Patients taking appetite suppressant medications should contact their doctors if they experience any symptoms such as shortness of breath, chest pain, faintness, or swelling in lower legs and ankles. It should be noted that the vast majority of cases of PPH have occurred in patients who were taking fenfluramine or dexfenfluramine, either alone or in combination. There have been only a few case reports of PPH in patients taking phentermine alone, although the possibility that phentermine alone may be associated with PPH cannot be ruled-out. No cases of PPH have been reported with sibutramine, but because of the low incidence of this disease in the underlying population, it is not know whether or not sibutramine may cause this disease.

Some animal studies have suggested that appetite suppressant medications affecting the serotonin system, such as fenfluramine and dexfenfluramine, can lead to damage to the central nervous system. Damage to the central nervous system has not been reported in humans. Some patients have reported depression or memory loss when using some appetite suppressant medications or combinations of medications, but it is not known if these problems are caused by the medication or by other factors.

In July, 1997, researchers at the Mayo Clinic reported a case series of 24 women who developed an unusual form of disease of the heart valves. All 24 women were using the combination of fenfluramine and phentermine. The disease primarily affected the left side of the heart, and five patients required valve replacement. In cases where samples of valve tissue were obtained, there was an unusual appearance of the heart valves generally only seen with a serotonin-producing tumor called carcinoid or with excessive amounts of medications containing ergot. Following these initial case reports, the Food and Drug Administration (FDA) has continued to receive a number of reports of similar valve disease from physicians. Some of these cases involved patients who were taking fenfluramine or dexfenfluramine alone. No cases were reported in patients taking phentermine alone. In addition, physicians at five sites provided information to the FDA regarding patients, most of whom did not have signs or symptoms of valve disease. About 30% of patients at these sites showed some evidence of damaged valves, usually mild or moderate. While this was not a controlled study, and further studies are needed to determine how common the problem is in treated patients compared to the general population of overweight people, the findings were of enough concern to prompt the FDA to ask the manufacturers of fenfluramine and dexfenfluramine to voluntarily recall the drugs. This withdrawal took place on September 15, 1997. Patients who were on fenfluramine or dexfenfluramine have been advised to discontinue the drug, and to contact their physicians for an evaluation to look for signs and symptoms of heart disease and to determine the need for an echocardiogram. For more information about the withdrawal of fenfluramine and dexfenfluramine, you can access the FDA website on Questions and Answers about Withdrawal of Fenfluramine (Pondimin) and Dexfenfluramine (Redux) at http://www.fda.gov/cder/news/fenphenqa2.htm. Two small studies looking at relationships between sibutramine and valvular heart disease did not find any increase in valve lesions in patients taking sibutramine compared with placebo.

Commonly Asked Questions about Appetite Suppressant Medication Treatment

Q: Can medications replace physical activity or changes in eating habits as a way to lose weight?

A: No. The use of appetite suppressant medications to treat obesity should be combined with physical activity and improved diet to lose and maintain weight successfully over the long term.

Q: Will I regain some weight after I stop taking appetite suppressant medications?

A: Probably. Most studies show that the majority of patients who stop taking appetite suppressant medications regain the weight they had lost. Maintaining healthy eating and physical activity habits will increase your likelihood of keeping weight off.

Q: How long will I need to take appetite suppressant medications to treat obesity?

A: The answer depends upon whether the medication helps you to lose and maintain weight and whether you have any side effects. Because obesity is a chronic disease, any treatment, whether drug or nondrug, may need to be continued for years, and perhaps a lifetime, to improve health and maintain a healthy weight. There is little information on how safe and effective appetite suppressant medications are for more than 1 year of use.

Q: What dosage of appetite suppressant medication would be right for me?

A: There is no one correct dose for appetite suppressant medications. Your doctor will decide what works best for you based on his or her evaluation of your medical condition and response to treatment.

Q: I only need to lose 10 pounds. Are appetite suppressant medications appropriate for me?

A: Appetite suppressant medications may be appropriate for carefully selected patients who are at significant medical risk because of their obesity. They are not recommended for use by people who are only mildly overweight unless they have health problems that are made worse by their weight. These medications should not be used only to improve appearance.

What to Discuss with Your Doctor Before Choosing Appetite Suppressant Medication Treatment

Before choosing appetite suppressant medication treatment for the long-term management of obesity, you should talk to your doctor about any concerns you may have. In addition, it is important that you discuss the following issues with your doctor.

How will I be evaluated to determine if I am an appropriate candidate for appetite suppressant medication treatment?

Your physician will look at a number of factors to determine if you are a good candidate for prescription appetite suppressant medication treatment of obesity. He or she will determine how overweight you are and where your body fat is distributed. Your doctor may do the following:

- Take a careful medical history and perform a physical examination.

- Look at your personal weight history.

- Ask whether you have relatives with illnesses related to overweight, such as noninsulin-dependent diabetes mellitus (NIDDM) or heart disease.

- Discuss the methods you have used to lose weight in the past.

- Evaluate your risk for obesity-related health problems by measuring your blood pressure and doing blood tests.

If your doctor determines that you have obesity-related health problems or are at high risk for such problems, and if you have been unable to lose weight or maintain weight loss with nondrug treatment, he or she may recommend that you use prescription appetite suppressant medications. Appetite suppressant medications may be appropriate for carefully selected patients who are at significant medical risk because of their obesity. They are not recommended for people who are only mildly overweight unless they have health problems that are made worse by their weight. These medications should not be used only to improve appearance.

What other medical conditions or medications might influence my decision to take an appetite suppressant medication?

It is important that you notify your physician if you have any of the following medical conditions:

- Pregnancy or breast-feeding
- History of drug or alcohol abuse
- History of an eating disorder
- History of depression or manic depressive disorder
- Use of monoamine oxidase (MAO) inhibitors or antidepressant medications
- Migraine headaches requiring medication
- Glaucoma
- Diabetes
- Heart disease or heart condition, such as an irregular heart beat
- High blood pressure
- Planning on surgery that requires general anesthesia

What type of program will be provided along with the medication to help me improve my eating and physical activity habits?

Studies show that appetite suppressant medications work best when combined with a weight-management program that helps you improve your eating and physical activity habits. Ask your doctor any questions or concerns that you may have about good nutrition and physical activity.

Appropriate Treatment Goals for Using Prescription Appetite Suppressant Medications

If you and your doctor believe that the use of appetite suppressant medications may be helpful for you, it is important to discuss the goals of treatment. Improving your health and reducing your risk for disease should be the primary goals. For most severely obese people, achieving an "ideal body weight" is both unrealistic and unnecessary to improve their health and reduce their risk for disease. Most patients should not expect to reach an ideal body weight using the currently available medications. Even a modest weight loss of 5 to 10 percent of your starting body weight can improve your health and reduce your risk factors for disease. Use of appetite suppressant medications for cosmetic purposes is not appropriate.

Appetite suppressant medications should be used with a program of behavioral treatment and nutritional counseling, designed to help you make long-term changes in your diet and physical activity. You should see your physician regularly so that he or she can monitor how you are responding to the medication, not only in terms of weight loss, but how it effects your overall health. Again, if you experience any serious symptoms, such as chest pains or shortness of breath, contact your doctor immediately.

Long-term use of prescription appetite suppressant medications may be helpful for carefully selected individuals, but little information is available on the safety and effectiveness of these medications when used for more than 1 year. By evaluating your risk of experiencing obesity-related health problems, you and your physician can make an informed choice as to whether medication can be a useful part of your weight-management program.

End note: This text is a modified version of a review article on the long-term use of appetite suppressant medications to manage obesity, appearing in a 1996 issue of the *Journal of the American Medical Association*. Both the review article and this fact sheet were developed with the advice of the National Task Force on Prevention and Treatment of Obesity, a working group of leading obesity and nutrition researchers from across the country. This text was revised in October, 1997, in response to additional information reported regarding an association between valvular heart disease and certain appetite suppressant medications, and in February, 1998 in response to the approval of sibutramine.

Weight-control Information Network

The Weight-control Information Network (WIN) is a service of the National Institute of Diabetes and Digestive and Kidney Diseases (NIDDK), part of the National Institutes of Health, under the U.S. Public Health Service. Authorized by Congress (Public Law 103-43),

WIN assembles and disseminates to health professionals and the public information on weight control, obesity, and nutritional disorders. WIN responds to requests for information; develops, reviews, and distributes publications; and develops communications strategies to encourage individuals to achieve and maintain a healthy weight.

Publications produced by the clearinghouse are reviewed carefully for scientific accuracy, content, and readability.

Weight-control Information Network
1 Win Way
Bethesda, MD 20892-3665
Phone: (301) 984-7378 or 1-800-WIN-8098
Fax: (301) 984-7196
E-mail: win@info.niddk.nih.gov

Chapter 37

FDA Warns against Drug Promotion of "Herbal Fen-Phen"

The FDA has become aware of the increasing promotion of various dietary supplement-type products as "natural" herbal alternatives to the prescription drug combination commonly known as "fen-phen."

So-called "herbal fen-phen" products are being marketed over the internet and through weight loss clinics, print ads and retail outlets as natural alternatives to the prescription drugs phentermine and fenfluramine (commonly referred to as "fen-phen"). FDA considers these products to be unapproved drugs because their names reflect that they are intended for the same use as the anti-obesity drugs, fenfluramine and phentermine. The agency is warning consumers that these unapproved drugs have not been shown to be safe or effective and may contain ingredients that have been associated with injuries.

Two anti-obesity drugs, fenfluramine (brand name Pondimin) and dexfenfluramine (brand name Redux), have been withdrawn from the marketplace because of safety concerns. FDA believes the use of unapproved alternative products may increase as a result of the withdrawal. Herbal fen-phen products contain none of these prescription drugs.

The main ingredient of most herbal fen-phen products is ephedra, commonly known as Ma Huang. Ephedra is an amphetamine-like

FDA Talk Paper, Food and Drug Administration U.S. Department of Health and Human Services Public Health Service, 5600 Fishers Lane, Rockville, MD 20857, November 6, 1997. *FDA Talk Papers* are prepared by the Press Office to guide FDA personnel in responding with consistency and accuracy to questions from the public on subjects of current interest. Talk Papers are subject to change as more information becomes available.

compound with potentially powerful stimulant effects on the nervous system and heart. FDA has received and investigated more than 800 reports of adverse events associated with the use of ephedrine alkaloid-containing products since 1994. These events ranged from episodes of high blood pressure, heart rate irregularities, insomnia, nervousness, tremors and headaches to seizures, heart attacks, strokes and death.

Many ephedra-containing herbal fen-phen products also contain *Hypericum perforatum*, an herb commonly known as St. John's Wort and sometimes referred to as "herbal Prozac." The actions and possible side effects of St. John's Wort have not been studied under carefully controlled trials either alone or in combination with ephedra.

Other herbal fen-phen products contain 5-hydroxy-tryptophan, a compound closely related to L-tryptophan, a dietary supplement widely used in this country until 1990. Used primarily as a sleep aid, L-tryptophan was pulled from the market after it was found to be linked to more than 1,500 cases, including about 38 deaths, of a rare blood disorder known as eosinophilia myalgia syndrome.

FDA regards any over-the-counter product commercially promoted as an alternative to prescription anti-obesity drugs (such as phentermine and fenfluramine) to be a drug. The agency is taking appropriate regulatory action to remove such products from the market.

More Information

For more information, contact FDA's Consumer Hotline: 800-532-4440.

Chapter 38

Very Low-Calorie Diets

Obesity affects up to one-fourth of adult Americans, increasing risk of death from diseases like diabetes, high blood pressure, and heart disease. Traditional weight loss methods include low-calorie diets between 800 to 1,500 calories a day and regular exercise. An alternative method sometimes considered for bringing about significant short-term weight loss in moderately to severely obese people is the very low-calorie diet (VLCD).

What Is a Very Low-Calorie Diet (VLCD)?

VLCDs are commercially prepared formulas of 800 calories or less that replace all usual food intake. VLCDs are not the same as over-the-counter meal replacements, which are meant to be substituted for one or two meals a day. VLCDs, when used under proper medical supervision, effectively produce significant short-term weight loss in moderately to severely obese patients.

Who Should Use a VLCD?

VLCDs are generally safe when used under proper medical supervision in patients with a body mass index (BMI) greater than 30. BMI is a mathematical formula that takes into account both a person's height and weight. To calculate BMI, a person's weight in kilograms

National Institute of Diabetes and Digestive and Kidney Diseases (NIDDK), NIH Publication No. 95-3894, March 1995; e-text last updated February 9, 1998.

is divided by height in meters squared. Use of VLCDs in patients with a BMI of 27 to 30 should be reserved for those who have medical complications resulting from their obesity. VLCDs are not recommended for pregnant women or breastfeeding women. VLCDs are not appropriate for children or adolescents, except in specialized treatment programs.

Very little information exists regarding the usage of VLCDs in older individuals. Because individuals over 50 already experience normal depletion of lean body mass, use of a VLCD may not be warranted. Additionally, persons over 50 may not tolerate the side effects associated with VLCDs because of preexisting medical conditions or need for other medications. Therefore, a physician, on a case by case basis, must evaluate increased risks and potential benefits of drastic weight loss in older individuals. Additionally, people with significant medical problems or who are on medications may be able to use a VLCD, but this too must be determined on an individual basis by a physician.

Health Benefits Associated with a VLCD

A VLCD may allow a severely to moderately obese patient to lose about 3 to 5 pounds per week, for an average total weight loss of 44 pounds over 12 weeks. Such a weight loss can improve obesity-related medical conditions, including diabetes, high blood pressure, and high cholesterol. Combining a VLCD with behavioral therapy and exercise may also increase weight loss and may slow weight regain. However, VLCDs are no more effective than more modest dietary restrictions in the long-term maintenance of reduced weight.

Adverse Effects Associated with a VLCD

Many patients on a VLCD for 4 to 16 weeks report minor side effects such as fatigue, constipation, nausea, and diarrhea, but these conditions usually improve within a few weeks and rarely prevent patients from completing the program. The most common serious side effect seen with VLCDs is gallstone formation. Gallstones, which often develop in obese people, anyway, (especially women), are even more common during rapid weight loss. Some research indicates that rapid weight loss appears to decrease the gallbladder's ability to contract bile. But, it is unclear whether VLCDs directly cause gallstones or whether the amount of weight loss is responsible for the formation of gallstones.

Conclusion

For most obese individuals, obesity is a long-term condition that requires a lifetime of attention even after a formal weight loss treatment ends. Although VLCDs are efficient for short-term weight loss, they are no more effective than other dietary treatments in the long-term maintenance of reduced weight. Therefore, obese patients should be encouraged to commit to a long-term treatment program that includes permanent lifestyle changes of healthier eating, regular physical activity, and an improved outlook about food because without a long-term commitment, their body weights will drift back up the scale.

Endnote: This text is a modified version of a previously published review article on very low-calorie diets, appearing in the August 25, 1993, issue of the *Journal of the American Medical Association*. Both the review article and this text were developed with the advice of the National Task Force on the Prevention and Treatment of Obesity, a subcommittee of the National Digestive Diseases Advisory Board.

For More Information

The Weight-Control Information Network (WIN) is a service of the National Institute of Diabetes and Digestive and Kidney Diseases (NIDDK), part of the National Institutes of Health, under the U.S. Public Health Service. Authorized by Congress(Public Law 103-43), WIN assembles and disseminates to health professionals and the public information on weight control, obesity, and nutritional disorders. WIN responds to requests for information; develops, reviews, and distributes publications; and develops communications strategies to encourage individuals to achieve and maintain a healthy weight.

Weight-Control Information Network
1 Win Way
Bethesda, MD 20892-3665
(301) 984-7378
1-800-WIN-8098
(301) 984-7196 Fax
E-mail: win@info.niddk.nih.gov

Chapter 39

Weight Cycling

What Is Weight Cycling?

Weight cycling is the repeated loss and regain of body weight. When weight cycling is the result of dieting, it is often called "yo-yo" dieting. A weight cycle can range from small weight losses and gains (5 to 10 lbs. per cycle) to large changes in weight (50 lbs. or more per cycle).

You may have heard stories in the press claiming that weight cycling may be harmful to your health. You also may have heard that staying at one weight is better for you than weight cycling, even if you are obese. However, no convincing evidence supports these claims, and most obesity researchers believe that obese individuals should continue to try to control their body weight.

If I Regain Lost Weight, Won't Losing It Again Be Even Harder?

People who repeatedly lose and regain weight should not experience more difficulty losing weight each time they diet. Most studies have shown that weight cycling does not affect one's metabolic rate. Metabolic rate is the rate at which food is burned for energy. Based on these findings, weight cycling should not affect the success of future weight-loss efforts. However, everyone, whether they have dieted

National Institute of Diabetes and Digestive and Kidney Diseases (NIDDK), Weight-Control Information Network (WIN), NIH Pub. No. 95-3901, March 1995.

or not, experiences a slowing of the metabolism as they age. In addition, older people are often less physically active than when they were younger. Therefore, people often find it more difficult to lose weight as they get older.

Will Weight Cycling Leave Me with More Fat and Less Lean Tissue Than If I Had Not Dieted at All?

Weight cycling has not been proven to increase the amount of fat tissue in people who lose and regain weight. Researchers have found that after a weight cycle people have the same amount of fat and lean tissue as they did prior to weight cycling.

Some people are concerned that weight cycling can cause more fat to collect in the abdominal area. People who tend to carry their excess fat in the abdominal area (apple-shaped), instead of in the hips and buttocks (pear-shaped), are more likely to develop the health problems associated with obesity. However, studies have not found that after a weight cycle people have more abdominal fat than they did before weight cycling.

Is Weight Cycling Harmful to My Health?

A number of studies have suggested that weight cycling (and weight loss) may be associated with an increase in mortality. Unfortunately, these studies were not designed to answer the question of how intentional weight loss by an obese person affects health. Most of the studies did not distinguish between those who lost and regained weight through dieting from those whose change in weight may have been due to other reasons, such as unsuspected illness or stress. In addition, most of the people followed in these studies were not obese. In fact, some evidence shows that if weight cycling does have any negative effects on health, they are seen mostly in people of low or normal weight. Some studies have looked at the relationship between weight cycling and risk factors for illness, such as high blood pressure, high blood cholesterol, or high blood sugar. Most of these studies have not found an association between weight cycling and harmful changes in risk factors.

Is Remaining Overweight Healthier than Weight Cycling?

At this time, no conclusive studies have shown that weight cycling is harmful to the health of an obese person. On the other hand, the health risks of obesity are well known. The costs of obesity-related illnesses are more than $39 billion each year. Obesity is linked to serious medical conditions such as:

- High blood pressure
- Heart disease
- Stroke
- Diabetes
- Certain types of cancer
- Gout, and
- Gallbladder disease.

Not everyone who is obese has the same risk for these conditions—a person's sex, amount of fat, location of fat, and family history of disease all play a role in determining an individual's risk of obesity-related problems. However, experts agree that even a modest weight loss can improve the health of an obese person.

Conclusions

Further research on the effects of weight cycling is needed. In the meantime, if you are obese, don't let fear of weight cycling stop you from achieving a modest weight loss. Although health problems associated with weight cycling have not been proven, the health-related problems of obesity are well known.

If you are not obese and have no risk factors for obesity-related illness, focus on preventing further weight gain by increasing your exercise and eating healthy foods, rather than trying to lose weight. If you do need to lose weight, you should be ready to commit to life-long changes in your eating behaviors, diet, and physical activity.

For Further Reading

Weight Cycling. By the National Task Force on the Prevention and Treatment of Obesity, this article reprint from the October 19, 1994, issue of *JAMA* addresses concerns about the effects of weight cycling and provides guidance on the risk-to-benefit ratio of attempts at weight loss, given current scientific knowledge.

Dietary Guidelines for Americans. Fourth Edition, 1995. Home and Garden Bulletin No. 232. This pamphlet, issued by the U.S. Agriculture and Health and Human Services Departments, contains information about maintaining a healthy weight, as well as dietary and nutrition recommendations.

Weight-Control Information Network

The Weight-Control Information Network (WIN) is a service of the National Institute of Diabetes and Digestive and Kidney Diseases (NIDDK), part of the National Institutes of Health, under the U.S. Public Health Service. Authorized by Congress (Public Law 103-43), WIN assembles and disseminates to health professionals and the general public information on weight control, obesity, and nutritional disorders. WIN responds to requests for information; develops, reviews, and distributes publications; and develops communication strategies to encourage individuals to achieve and maintain a healthy weight.

Publications produced by WIN are reviewed carefully for scientific accuracy, content, and readability. Materials produced by other sources are also reviewed for scientific accuracy and are distributed, along with WIN publications, to answer requests.

Weight-Control Information Network
1 WIN Way
Bethesda, MD 20892-3665
(301) 984-7378
(800) WIN-8098
(301) 984-7196 fax
E-mail: WIN@matthewgroup.com

Chapter 40

Beyond Dieting: Physical Activity and Weight Control

Regular physical activity is an important part of effective weight loss and weight maintenance. It also can help prevent several diseases and improve your overall health. It does not matter what type of physical activity you perform—sports, planned exercise, household chores, yard work, or work-related tasks—all are beneficial. Studies show that even the most inactive people can gain significant health benefits if they accumulate 30 minutes or more of physical activity per day. Based on these findings, the U.S. Public Health Service has identified increased physical activity as a priority in Healthy People 2000, our national objectives to improve the health of Americans by the year 2000.

Research consistently shows that regular physical activity, combined with healthy eating habits, is the most efficient and healthful way to control your weight. Whether you are trying to lose weight or maintain it, you should understand the important role of physical activity and include it in your lifestyle.

How Can Physical Activity Help Control My Weight?

Physical activity helps to control your weight by using excess calories that otherwise would be stored as fat. Your body weight is regulated by the number of calories you eat and use each day. Everything you eat contains calories, and everything you do uses calories, including

National Institute of Diabetes and Digestive and Kidney Diseases (NIDDK), Weight-Control Information Network (WIN), NIH Pub. No. 96-4031, April 1996.

sleeping, breathing, and digesting food. Any physical activity in addition to what you normally do will use extra calories.

Balancing the calories you use through physical activity with the calories you eat will help you achieve your desired weight. When you eat more calories than you need to perform your day's activities, your body stores the extra calories and you gain weight (a; *see* Figure 40.1.). When you eat fewer calories than you use, your body uses the stored calories and you lose weight (b). When you eat the same amount of calories as your body uses, your weight stays the same (c).

Any type of physical activity you choose to do—strenuous activities such as running or aerobic dancing or moderate-intensity activities such as walking or household work—will increase the number of calories your body uses. The key to successful weight control and improved overall health is making physical activity a part of your daily routine.

What Are the Health Benefits of Physical Activity?

In addition to helping to control your weight, research shows that regular physical activity can reduce your risk for several diseases and conditions and improve your overall quality of life. Regular physical activity can help protect you from the following health problems.

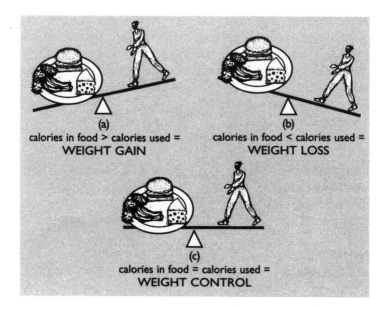

Figure 40.1. The relationship between physical activity and body weight.

- **Heart Disease and Stroke.** Daily physical activity can help prevent heart disease and stroke by strengthening your heart muscle, lowering your blood pressure, raising your high-density lipoprotein (HDL) levels (good cholesterol) and lowering low-density lipoprotein (LDL) levels (bad cholesterol), improving blood flow, and increasing your heart's working capacity.

- **High Blood Pressure.** Regular physical activity can reduce blood pressure in those with high blood pressure levels. Physical activity also reduces body fatness, which is associated with high blood pressure.

- **Non-insulin Dependent Diabetes.** By reducing body fatness, physical activity can help to prevent and control this type of diabetes.

- **Obesity.** Physical activity helps to reduce body fat by building or preserving muscle mass and improving the body's ability to use calories. When physical activity is combined with proper nutrition, it can help control weight and prevent obesity, a major risk factor for many diseases.

- **Back Pain.** By increasing muscle strength and endurance and improving flexibility and posture, regular exercise helps to prevent back pain.

- **Osteoporosis.** Regular weight-bearing exercise promotes bone formation and may prevent many forms of bone loss associated with aging.

Studies on the psychological effects of exercise have found that regular physical activity can improve your mood and the way you feel about yourself. Researchers also have found that exercise is likely to reduce depression and anxiety and help you to better manage stress.

Keep these health benefits in mind when deciding whether or not to exercise. And remember, any amount of physical activity you do is better than none at all.

How Much Should I Exercise?

For the greatest overall health benefits, experts recommend that you do 20 to 30 minutes of aerobic activity three or more times a week and some type of muscle strengthening activity and stretching at least twice a week. However, if you are unable to do this level of activity, you can gain substantial health benefits by accumulating 30 minutes

371

or more of moderate-intensity physical activity a day, at least five times a week.

If you have been inactive for a while, you may want to start with less strenuous activities such as walking or swimming at a comfortable pace. Beginning at a slow pace will allow you to become physically fit without straining your body. Once you are in better shape, you can gradually do more strenuous activity.

Moderate-Intensity Activity

Moderate-intensity activities include some of the things you may already be doing during a day or week, such as gardening and housework. These activities can be done in short spurts—10 minutes here, 8 minutes there. Alone, each action does not have a great effect on your health, but regularly accumulating 30 minutes of activity over the course of the day can result in substantial health benefits.

To become more active throughout your day, take advantage of any chance to get up and move around. Here are some examples:

- Take a short walk around the block
- Rake leaves
- Play actively with the kids
- Walk up the stairs instead of taking the elevator
- Mow the lawn
- Take an activity break—get up and stretch or walk around
- Park your car a little farther away from your destination and walk the extra distance

The point is not to make physical activity an unwelcome chore, but to make the most of the opportunities you have to be active.

Aerobic Activity

Aerobic activity is an important addition to moderate-intensity exercise. Aerobic exercise is any extended activity that makes you breathe hard while using the large muscle groups at a regular, even pace. Aerobic activities help make your heart stronger and more efficient. They also use more calories than other activities. Some examples of aerobic activities include:

- Brisk walking
- Jogging

- Bicycling
- Swimming
- Aerobic dancing
- Racket sports
- Rowing
- Ice or roller skating
- Cross-country or downhill skiing
- Using aerobic equipment (i.e., treadmill, stationary bike)

To get the most health benefits from aerobic activity, you should exercise at a level strenuous enough to raise your heart rate to your target zone. Your target heart rate zone is 50 to 75 percent of your maximum heart rate (the fastest your heart can beat). To find your target zone, look for the category closest to your age in the chart shown in Table 40.2 and read across the line. For example, if you are 35 years old, your target heart rate zone is 93-138 beats per minute.

To see if you are exercising within your target heart rate zone, count the number of pulse beats at your wrist or neck for 15 seconds, then multiply by four to get the beats per minute. Your heart should be beating within your target heart rate zone. If your heart is beating faster than your target heart rate, you are exercising too hard and should slow down. If your heart is beating slower than your target heart rate, you should exercise a little harder.

When you begin your exercise program, aim for the lower part of your target zone (50 percent). As you get into better shape, slowly build up to the higher part of your target zone (75 percent). If exercising within your target zone seems too hard, exercise at a pace that is comfortable for you. You will find that, with time, you will feel more comfortable exercising and can slowly increase to your target zone.

Table 40.2. Target Heart Rates

Age	Target Heart Rate Zone 50-75%	Average maximum Heart Rate 100%
20-30 years	98-146 beats/min.	195
31-40 years	93-138 beats/min.	185
41-50 years	88-131 beats/min.	175
51-60 years	83-123 beats/min.	165
61 + years	78-116 beats/min.	155

Stretching and Muscle Strengthening Exercises

Stretching and strengthening exercises such as weight training should also be a part of your physical activity program. In addition to using calories, these exercises strengthen your muscles and bones and help prevent injury.

Tips to a Safe and Successful Physical Activity Program

- Make sure you are in good health. Answer the questions below before you begin exercising (Source: British Columbia Department of Health).

    1. Has a doctor ever said you have heart problems?
    2. Do you frequently suffer from chest pains?
    3. Do you often feel faint or have dizzy spells?
    4. Has a doctor ever said you have high blood pressure?
    5. Has a doctor ever told you that you have a bone or joint problem, such as arthritis, that has been or could be aggravated by exercise?
    6. Are you over the age of 65 and not accustomed to exercise?
    7. Are you taking prescription medications, such as those for high blood pressure?
    8. Is there a good medical reason, not mentioned here, why you should not exercise?

    If you answered "yes" to any of these questions, you should see your doctor before you begin an exercise program.

- Follow a gradual approach to exercise to get the most benefits with the fewest risks. If you have not been exercising, start at a slow pace and as you become more fit, gradually increase the amount of time and the pace of your activity.

- Choose activities that you enjoy and that fit your personality. For example, if you like team sports or group activities, choose things such as soccer or aerobics. If you prefer individual activities, choose things such as swimming or walking. Also, plan your activities for a time of day that suits your personality. If you are a morning person, exercise before you begin the rest of your day's activities. If you have more energy in the evening, plan activities that can be done at the end of the day. You will be more likely to stick to a physical activity program if it is convenient and enjoyable.

- Exercise regularly. To gain the most health benefits it is important to exercise as regularly as possible. Make sure you choose activities that will fit into your schedule.

- Exercise at a comfortable pace. For example, while jogging or walking briskly you should be able to hold a conversation. If you do not feel normal again within 10 minutes following exercise, you are exercising too hard. Also, if you have difficulty breathing or feel faint or weak during or after exercise, you are exercising too hard.

- Maximize your safety and comfort. Wear shoes that fit and clothes that move with you, and always exercise in a safe location. Many people walk in indoor shopping malls for exercise. Malls are climate controlled and offer protection from bad weather.

- Vary your activities. Choose a variety of activities so you don't get bored with any one thing.

- Encourage your family or friends to support you and join you in your activity. If you have children, it is best to build healthy habits when they are young. When parents are active, children are more likely to be active and stay active for the rest of their lives.

- Challenge yourself. Set short-term as well as long-term goals and celebrate every success, no matter how small.

Whether your goal is to control your weight or just to feel healthier, becoming physically active is a step in the right direction. Take advantage of the health benefits that regular exercise can offer and make physical activity a part of your lifestyle.

Additional Resources

The following organizations have materials on physical activity and weight control available to the public:

President's Council on Physical Fitness and Sports
701 Pennsylvania Avenue, NW Suite 250
Washington, DC 20004
(202) 272-3421

National Heart, Lung, and Blood Institute Information Center
P.O. Box 30105
Bethesda, MD 20824-0105
(301) 251-1222

American College of Sports Medicine
P.O. Box 1440
Indianapolis, IN 46206-1440
(317) 637-9200

Weight-Control Information Network
1 WIN Way
Bethesda, MD 20892-3665
(301) 570-2177
800) WIN-8098
(301) 570-2186 Fax
E-mail: WIN@ matthewsgroup.com

The Weight-Control Information Network (WIN) is a service of the National Institute of Diabetes and Digestive and Kidney Diseases, part of the National Institutes of Health. Authorized by Congress (Public Law 103-43), WIN assembles and disseminates to health professionals and the general public information on weight control, obesity, and nutritional disorders. WIN responds to requests for information; develops, reviews, and distributes publications; and develops communication strategies to encourage individuals to achieve and maintain a healthy weight. Publications produced by WIN are reviewed for scientific accuracy, content, and readability. Materials produced by other sources are also reviewed for scientific accuracy and are distributed, along with WIN publications, to answer requests.

Part Five

Dietary Supplements and Food Additives

Chapter 41

A Guide to Dietary Supplements

Set between a Chinese restaurant and a pizza and sub sandwich eatery, a Rockville health food store offers yet another brand of edible items: Bottled herbs like cat's claw, dandelion root, and blessed thistle. Vitamins and minerals in varying doses. Herbal and nutrient concoctions whose labels carry claims about relieving pain, "energizing" and "detoxifying" the body, or providing "guaranteed results."

This store sells dietary supplements, some of the hottest selling items on the market today. Surveys show that more than half of the U.S. adult population uses these products. In 1996 alone, consumers spent more than $6.5 billion on dietary supplements, according to Packaged Facts Inc., a market research firm in New York City.

But even with all the business they generate, consumers still ask questions about dietary supplements: Can their claims be trusted? Are they safe? Does the Food and Drug Administration approve them?

Many of these questions come in the wake of the 1994 Dietary Supplement Health and Education Act, or DSHEA, which set up a new framework for FDA regulation of dietary supplements. It also created an office in the National Institutes of Health to coordinate research on dietary supplements, and it called on President Clinton to set up an independent dietary supplement commission to report on the use of claims in dietary supplement labeling.

In passing DSHEA, Congress recognized first, that many people believe dietary supplements offer health benefits and second, that

"An FDA Guide to Dietary Supplements," *FDA Consumer*, September-October 1998.

consumers want a greater opportunity to determine whether supplements may help them. The law essentially gives dietary supplement manufacturers freedom to market more products as dietary supplements and provide information about their products' benefits—for example, in product labeling.

The Council for Responsible Nutrition, an organization of manufacturers of dietary supplements and their suppliers, welcomes the change. "Our philosophy has been ... to maintain consumer access to products and access to information [so that consumers can] make informed choices," says John Cordaro, the group's president and chief executive officer.

But in choosing whether to use dietary supplements, FDA answers consumers' questions by noting that under DSHEA, FDA's requirement for premarket review of dietary supplements is less than that over other products it regulates, such as drugs and many additives used in conventional foods.

This means that consumers and manufacturers have responsibility for checking the safety of dietary supplements and determining the truthfulness of label claims.

What Is a Dietary Supplement?

Traditionally, dietary supplements referred to products made of one or more of the essential nutrients, such as vitamins, minerals, and protein. But DSHEA broadens the definition to include, with some exceptions, any product intended for ingestion as a supplement to the diet. This includes vitamins; minerals; herbs, botanicals, and other plant-derived substances; and amino acids (the individual building blocks of protein) and concentrates, metabolites, constituents and extracts of these substances.

It's easy to spot a supplement because DSHEA requires manufacturers to include the words "dietary supplement" on product labels. Also, starting in March 1999, a "Supplement Facts" panel will be required on the labels of most dietary supplements.

Dietary supplements come in many forms, including tablets, capsules, powders, softgels, gelcaps, and liquids. Though commonly associated with health food stores, dietary supplements also are sold in grocery, drug and national discount chain stores, as well as through mail-order catalogs, TV programs, the Internet, and direct sales.

FDA oversees safety, manufacturing and product information, such as claims, in a product's labeling, package inserts, and accompanying literature. The Federal Trade Commission regulates the advertising of dietary supplements.

One thing dietary supplements are not is drugs. A drug, which sometimes can be derived from plants used as traditional medicines, is an article that, among other things, is intended to diagnose, cure, mitigate, treat, or prevent diseases. Before marketing, drugs must undergo clinical studies to determine their effectiveness, safety, possible interactions with other substances, and appropriate dosages, and FDA must review these data and authorize the drugs' use before they are marketed. FDA does not authorize or test dietary supplements.

A product sold as a dietary supplement and touted in its labeling as a new treatment or cure for a specific disease or condition would be considered an unauthorized—and thus illegal—drug. Labeling changes consistent with the provisions in DSHEA would be required to maintain the product's status as a dietary supplement.

Another thing dietary supplements are not are replacements for conventional diets, nutritionists say. Supplements do not provide all the known—and perhaps unknown—nutritional benefits of conventional food.

Anatomy of the New Requirements for Dietary Supplement Labels

Information that will be required on the labels of dietary supplements includes:

- Statement of identity (e.g., "ginseng")

- Net quantity of contents (e.g., "60 capsules")

- Structure-function claim and the statement "This statement has not been evaluated by the Food and Drug Administration. This pro-duct is not intended to diagnose, treat, cure, or prevent any disease."

- Directions for use (e.g., "Take one capsule daily.")

- Supplement Facts panel (lists serving size, amount, and active ingredient)

- Other ingredients in descending order of predominance and by common name or proprietary blend.

- Name and place of business of manufacturer, packer or distributor. This is the address to write for more product information.

(Effective March 1999)

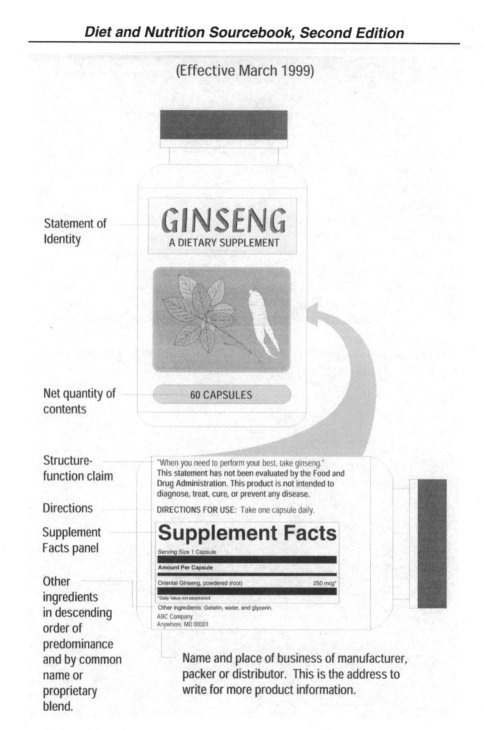

Figure 41.1. *Anatomy of the New Requirements for Dietary Supplement Labels.*

Monitoring for Safety

As with food, federal law requires manufacturers of dietary supplements to ensure that the products they put on the market are safe. But supplement manufacturers do not have to provide information to FDA to get a product on the market, unlike the food additive process often required of new food ingredients. FDA review and approval of supplement ingredients and products is not required before marketing.

Food additives not generally recognized as safe must undergo FDA's premarket approval process for new food ingredients. This requires manufacturers to conduct safety studies and submit the results to FDA for review before the ingredient can be used in marketed products. Based on its review, FDA either authorizes or rejects the food additive.

In contrast, dietary supplement manufacturers that wish to market a new ingredient (that is, an ingredient not marketed in the United States before 1994) have two options. The first involves submitting to FDA, at least 75 days before the product is expected to go on the market, information that supports their conclusion that a new ingredient can reasonably be expected to be safe. Safe means that the new ingredient does not present a significant or unreasonable risk of illness or injury under conditions of use recommended in the product's labeling.

The information the manufacturer submits becomes publicly available 90 days after FDA receives it.

Another option for manufacturers is to petition FDA, asking the agency to establish the conditions under which the new dietary ingredient would reasonably be expected to be safe. To date, FDA's Center for Food Safety and Applied Nutrition has received no such petitions.

Under DSHEA, once a dietary supplement is marketed, FDA has the responsibility for showing that a dietary supplement is unsafe before it can take action to restrict the product's use. This was the case when, in June 1997, FDA proposed, among other things, to limit the amount of ephedrine alkaloids in dietary supplements (marketed as ephedra, Ma huang, Chinese ephedra, and epitonin, for example) and provide warnings to consumers about hazards associated with use of dietary supplements containing the ingredients. The hazards ranged from nervousness, dizziness, and changes in blood pressure and heart rate to chest pain, heart attack, hepatitis, stroke, seizures, psychosis, and death. The proposal stemmed from FDA's review of adverse event reports it had received, scientific literature, and public comments. FDA has received many comments on the 1997 proposal and was reviewing them at press time.

Also in 1997, FDA identified contamination of the herbal ingredient plantain with the harmful herb Digitalis lanata after receiving a report of a complete heart block in a young woman. FDA traced all use of the contaminated ingredient and asked manufacturers and retailers to withdraw these products from the market. (For information about other potentially dangerous dietary supplements, see "Supplements Associated with Illnesses and Injuries" at the end of this chapter.)

DSHEA also gives FDA authority to establish good manufacturing practices, or GMPs, for dietary supplements. In a February 1997 advance notice of proposed rulemaking, the agency said it would establish dietary supplement GMPs if, after public comment, it determined that GMPs for conventional food are not adequate to cover dietary supplements, as well. GMPs, the agency said, would ensure that dietary supplements are made under conditions that would result in safe and properly labeled products. At press time, FDA was reviewing comments on the 1997 notice.

Some supplement makers may already voluntarily follow GMPs devised, for example, by trade groups.

Besides FDA, individual states can take steps to restrict or stop the sale of potentially harmful dietary supplements within their jurisdictions. For example, Florida has already banned all ephedra-containing products, and other states have said they are considering similar action.

Also, the industry strives to regulate itself, the Council for Responsible Nutrition's Cordaro says. He cites the GMPs that his trade group and others developed for their member companies. FDA is reviewing these GMPs as it considers whether to pursue mandatory industry-wide GMPs. Another example of self-regulation, Cordaro says, is the voluntary use of a warning about ephedra products that his organization drafted. He says that about 90 percent of U.S. manufacturers of products containing ephedra alkaloids now use this warning label.

Understanding Claims

Claims that tout a supplement's healthful benefits have always been a controversial feature of dietary supplements. Manufacturers often rely on them to sell their products. But consumers often wonder whether they can trust them.

Under DSHEA and previous food labeling laws, supplement manufacturers are allowed to use, when appropriate, three types of claims: nutrient-content claims, disease claims, and nutrition support claims, which include "structure-function claims."

Nutrient-content claims describe the level of a nutrient in a food or dietary supplement. For example, a supplement containing at least 200 milligrams of calcium per serving could carry the claim "high in calcium." A supplement with at least 12 mg per serving of vitamin C could state on its label, "Excellent source of vitamin C."

Disease claims show a link between a food or substance and a disease or health-related condition. FDA authorizes these claims based on a review of the scientific evidence. Or, after the agency is notified, the claims may be based on an authoritative statement from certain scientific bodies, such as the National Academy of Sciences, that shows or describes a well-established diet-to-health link. As of this writing, certain dietary supplements may be eligible to carry disease claims, such as claims that show a link between:

- the vitamin folic acid and a decreased risk of neural tube defect-affected pregnancy, if the supplement contains sufficient amounts of folic acid

- calcium and a lower risk of osteoporosis, if the supplement contains sufficient amounts of calcium

- psyllium seed husk (as part of a diet low in cholesterol and saturated fat) and coronary heart disease, if the supplement contains sufficient amounts of psyllium seed husk.

Nutrition support claims can describe a link between a nutrient and the deficiency disease that can result if the nutrient is lacking in the diet. For example, the label of a vitamin C supplement could state that vitamin C prevents scurvy. When these types of claims are used, the label must mention the prevalence of the nutrient-deficiency disease in the United States.

These claims also can refer to the supplement's effect on the body's structure or function, including its overall effect on a person's well-being. These are known as structure-function claims.

Examples of structure-function claims are:

- Calcium builds strong bones.
- Antioxidants maintain cell integrity.
- Fiber maintains bowel regularity.

Manufacturers can use structure-function claims without FDA authorization. They base their claims on their review and interpretation of the scientific literature. Like all label claims, structure-function claims must be true and not misleading.

Structure-function claims can be easy to spot because, on the label, they must be accompanied with the disclaimer "This statement has not been evaluated by the Food and Drug Administration. This product is not intended to diagnose, treat, cure, or prevent any disease."

Manufacturers who plan to use a structure-function claim on a particular product must inform FDA of the use of the claim no later than 30 days after the product is first marketed. While the manufacturer must be able to substantiate its claim, it does not have to share the substantiation with FDA or make it publicly available.

If the submitted claims promote the products as drugs instead of supplements, FDA can advise the manufacturer to change or delete the claim.

Because there often is a fine line between disease claims and structure-function claims, FDA in April [1998] proposed regulations that would establish criteria under which a label claim would or would not qualify as a disease claim. Among label factors FDA proposed for consideration are:

- the naming of a specific disease or class of diseases
- the use of scientific or lay terminology to describe the product's effect on one or more signs or symptoms recognized by health-care professionals and consumers as characteristic of a specific disease or a number of different specific diseases
- product name
- statements about product formulation
- citations or references that refer to disease
- use of the words "disease" or "diseased"
- art, such as symbols and pictures
- statements that the product can substitute for an approved therapy (for example, a drug).

FDA's proposal is consistent with the guidance on the distinction between structure-function and disease claims provided in the 1997 report by the President's Commission on Dietary Supplement Labels.

If shoppers find dietary supplements whose labels state or imply that the product can help diagnose, treat, cure, or prevent a disease (for example, "cures cancer" or "treats arthritis"), they should realize that the product is being marketed illegally as a drug and as such has not been evaluated for safety or effectiveness.

FTC regulates claims made in the advertising of dietary supplements, and in recent years, that agency has taken a number of enforcement actions against companies whose advertisements contained false and misleading information. The actions targeted, for example, erroneous claims that chromium picolinate was a treatment for weight loss and high blood cholesterol. An action in 1997 targeted ads for an ephedrine alkaloid supplement because they understated the degree of the product's risk and featured a man falsely described as a doctor.

Fraudulent Products

Consumers need to be on the lookout for fraudulent products. These are products that don't do what they say they can or don't contain what they say they contain. At the very least, they waste consumers' money, and they may cause physical harm.

Fraudulent products often can be identified by the types of claims made in their labeling, advertising and promotional literature. Some possible indicators of fraud, says Stephen Barrett, M.D., a board member of the National Council Against Health Fraud, are:

- Claims that the product is a secret cure and use of such terms as "breakthrough," "magical," "miracle cure," and "new discovery." If the product were a cure for a serious disease, it would be widely reported in the media and used by health-care professionals, he says.

- "Pseudomedical" jargon, such as "detoxify," "purify" and "energize" to describe a product's effects. These claims are vague and hard to measure, Barrett says. So, they make it easier for success to be claimed "even though nothing has actually been accomplished," he says.

- Claims that the product can cure a wide range of unrelated diseases. No product can do that, he says.

- Claims that a product is backed by scientific studies, but with no list of references or references that are inadequate. For instance, if a list of references is provided, the citations cannot be traced, or if they are traceable, the studies are out-of-date, irrelevant, or poorly designed.

- Claims that the supplement has only benefits—and no side effects. A product "potent enough to help people will be potent enough to cause side effects," Barrett says.

- Accusations that the medical profession, drug companies and the government are suppressing information about a particular treatment. It would be illogical, Barrett says, for large numbers of people to withhold information about potential medical therapies when they or their families and friends might one day benefit from them.

Though often more difficult to do, consumers also can protect themselves from economic fraud, a practice in which the manufacturer substitutes part or all of a product with an inferior, cheaper ingredient and then passes off the fake product as the real thing but at a lower cost. Varro Tyler, Ph.D., Sc.D., a distinguished professor emeritus of pharmacognosy (the study of medicinal products in their crude, or unprepared, form) at Purdue University in West LaFayette, Ind., advises consumers to avoid products sold for considerably less money than competing brands. "If it's too cheap, the product is probably not what it's supposed to be," he says.

Quality Products

Poor manufacturing practices are not unique to dietary supplements, but the growing market for supplements in a less restrictive regulatory environment creates the potential for supplements to be prone to quality-control problems. For example, FDA has identified several problems where some manufacturers were buying herbs, plants and other ingredients without first adequately testing them to determine whether the product they ordered was actually what they received or whether the ingredients were free from contaminants.

To help protect themselves, consumers should:

- Look for ingredients in products with the U.S.P. notation, which indicates the manufacturer followed standards established by the U.S. Pharmacopoeia.

- Realize that the label term "natural" doesn't guarantee that a product is safe. "Think of poisonous mushrooms," says Elizabeth

Yetley, Ph.D., director of FDA's Office of Special Nutritionals. "They're natural."

• Consider the name of the manufacturer or distributor. Supplements made by a nationally known food and drug manufacturer, for example, have likely been made under tight controls because these companies already have in place manufacturing standards for their other products.

• Write to the supplement manufacturer for more information. Ask the company about the conditions under which its products were made.

Reading and Reporting

Consumers who use dietary supplements should always read product labels, follow directions, and heed all warnings.

Supplement users who suffer a serious harmful effect or illness that they think is related to supplement use should call a doctor or other health-care provider. He or she in turn can report it to FDA MedWatch by calling 1-800-FDA-1088 or going to www.fda.gov/medwatch/report/ hcp.htm on the MedWatch Website. Patients' names are kept confidential.

Consumers also may call the toll-free MedWatch number or go to www.fda.gov/medwatch/report/consumer/consumer.htm on the MedWatch Website to report an adverse reaction. To file a report, consumers will be asked to provide:

• name, address and telephone number of the person who became ill

• name and address of the doctor or hospital providing medical treatment

• description of the problem

• name of the product and store where it was bought.

Consumers also should report the problem to the manufacturer or distributor listed on the product's label and to the store where the product was bought.

Today's Dietary Supplements

The report of the President's Commission on Dietary Supplement Labels, released in November 1997, provides a look at the future of dietary supplements. It encourages researchers to find out whether consumers want and can use the information allowed in dietary supplement labeling under DSHEA. It encourages studies to identify more clearly the relationships between dietary supplements and health maintenance and disease prevention. It urges FDA to take enforcement action when questions about a product's safety arise. And it suggests that FDA and the industry work together to develop guidelines on the use of warning statements on dietary supplement labels.

FDA generally concurred with the commission's recommendations in the agency's 1998 proposed rule on dietary supplement claims.

While much remains unknown about many dietary supplements—their health benefits and potential risks, for example—there's one thing consumers can count on: the availability of a wide range of such products. But consumers who decide to take advantage of the expanding market should do so with care, making sure they have the necessary information and consulting with their doctors and other health professionals as needed.

"The majority of supplement manufacturers are responsible and careful," FDA's Yetley says. "But, as with all products on the market, consumers need to be discriminating. FDA and industry have important roles to play, but consumers must take responsibility, too."

Expert Advice

Before starting a dietary supplement, it's always wise to check with a medical doctor. It is especially important for people who are:

- pregnant or breastfeeding
- chronically ill
- elderly
- under 18
- taking prescription or over-the-counter medicines. Certain supplements can boost blood levels of certain drugs to dangerous levels.

Varro Tyler, Ph.D., Sc.D., distinguished professor emeritus of pharmacognosy at Purdue University, cites as examples garlic and the supplement ginkgo biloba. Both can thin the blood, which can be hazardous, he says, for people taking prescription medicines that also thin the blood.

In addition to medical doctors, other health-care professionals, such as registered pharmacists, registered dietitians and nutritionists, also can be sources of information about dietary supplements.

Supplements Associated with Illnesses and Injuries

The following information is from an FDA statement before the Senate Committee on Labor and Human Resources, October 21, 1993.

Herbal Ingredients

Chaparral (a traditional American Indian medicine)
Possible Health Hazards: liver disease, possibly irreversible

Comfrey
Possible Health Hazards: obstruction of blood flow to liver, possibly leading to death

Slimming / dieter's teas
Possible Health Hazards: nausea, diarrhea, vomiting, stomach cramps, chronic constipation, fainting, possibly death

Ephedra (also known as Ma huang, Chinese Ephedra, and epitonin)
Possible Health Hazards: ranges from high blood pressure, irregular heartbeat, nerve damage, injury, insomnia, tremors, and headaches to seizures, heart attack, stroke, and death

Germander
Possible Health Hazards: liver disease, possibly leading to death

Lobelia (also known as Indian tobacco)
Possible Health Hazards: range from breathing problems at low doses to sweating, rapid heartbeat, low blood pressure, and possibly coma and death at higher doses

Magnolia-Stephania preparation
Possible Health Hazards: kidney disease, possibly leading to permanent kidney failure

Willow bark
Possible Health Hazards: Reye syndrome, a potentially fatal disease associated with aspirin intake in children with chickenpox or flu symptoms; allergic reaction in adults. (Willow bark is marketed as an aspirin-free product, although it actually contains an ingredient that converts to the same active ingredient in aspirin.)

Wormwood
Possible Health Hazards: neurological symptoms, characterized by numbness of legs and arms, loss of intellect, delirium, and paralysis

Vitamins and Essential Minerals

Vitamin A (in doses of 25,000 or more International Units a day)
    Possible Health Hazards: birth defects, bone abnormalities, and severe liver disease

Vitamin B$_6$ (in doses above 100 milligrams a day)
    Possible Health Hazards: balance difficulties, nerve injury causing changes in touch sensation

Niacin (in slow-released doses of 500 mg or more a day or immediate-release doses of 750 mg or more a day)
    Possible Health Hazards: range from stomach pain, vomiting, bloating, nausea, cramping, and diarrhea to liver disease, muscle disease, eye damage, and heart injury

Selenium (in doses of about 800 micrograms to 1,000 mcg a day)
    Possible Health Hazards: tissue damage

Other Supplements

Germanium (a nonessential mineral)
    Possible Health Hazards: kidney damage, possibly death

L-tryptophan (an amino acid)
    Possible Health Hazards: eosinophilia myalgia syndrome, a potentially fatal blood disorder that can cause high fever, muscle and joint pain, weakness, skin rash, and swelling of the arms and legs

Supplement Your Knowledge

    Some sources for additional information on dietary supplements are:

Federal Agencies

Food and Drug Administration
Office of Consumer Affairs
HFE-88
Rockville, MD 20857
1-800-FDA-4010 (Food Information Line)
(202) 205-4314 (in the Washington, D.C., area)
Website: www.cfsan.fda.gov/~dms/supplmnt.html

Federal Trade Commission
Public Reference Branch
Room 130
Washington, DC 20580
Website: www.ftc.gov

National Institute on Aging
NIA Information Center
P.O. Box 8057
Gaithersburg, MD 20898-8057
1-800-222-2225
1-800-222-4225 TTY
Website: http://128.231.160.11/nia/health/pubpub/hormrev.htm

Health Professional Organization

American Dietetic Association
216 W. Jackson Blvd.
Chicago, IL 60606-6995
1-800-366-1655 (recorded messages)
1-900-225-5267 (to talk to a registered dietitian)
Website: www.eatright.org

—by Paula Kurtzweil

Paula Kurtzweil is a member of FDA's public affairs staff.

Chapter 42

Vitamin and Mineral Supplements

Dietary supplements can have therapeutic effects. In large doses, though, they can also cause serious problems.

Once upon a time, nutrition therapy meant making sure that a patient got enough food from each of four important groups. If a patient had a disorder that robbed him of some essential vitamin or mineral, it also meant supplementing the diet to correct the deficiency.

We have come a long way since then. Researchers are now discovering that certain nutrients, when given in amounts that sometimes greatly exceed the Recommended Dietary Allowance (RDA), can do significantly more than correct deficiencies.

Perhaps vitamin E best illustrates this major change in direction. The adult RDA for the vitamin is 8–12 IU [international units]. That's enough to prevent muscle weakness, hemolytic anemia, poor reflexes, and decreased sensation in the hands and feet. But the results of several major studies strongly suggest that much higher doses also protect patients from coronary artery disease (CAD) and a host of other serious disorders.

Similarly, research on folic acid, selenium, vitamin C, and chromium has turned these nutrients into nutritional drugs—one expert calls them nutriceuticals—that may very well have a wide array of therapeutic effects. Here we bring you up to date on how these "drugs" are being used and how to monitor patients for adverse effects.

Published in *RN*, November 1997, Vol. 60, No. 11. Copyright © 1997, Medical Economics, Montvale, NJ. Reprinted by permission.

Vitamin E and Heart Disease

One of the most convincing trials involving vitamin E found that oral intake of 800 IU a day for about a year reduced the number of non-fatal MIs [myocardial infarctions][1]. In addition, a recent review of the literature concluded that taking 100–200 IU a day for more than six years can reduce the risk of CAD [coronary artery disease][2]. It's likely the vitamin protects the heart and arteries by acting as an antioxidant, which blocks the damaging effects of a group of harmful chemicals called free radicals.

Among the possible adverse effects to watch for among adults taking large doses of vitamin E are nausea, GI [gastrointestinal] upset, headache, fatigue, and breast soreness.[3] One researcher has reported seeing several cases of thrombophlebitis in his practice, but controlled trials have not been able to confirm his observations.[4]

There are also reports that suggest that patients on warfarin (Coumadin) should avoid taking 100 IU or more of vitamin E a day. The vitamin may prolong prothrombin time in this patient population, increasing the risk of bleeding. It may also be contraindicated in patients with a vitamin K deficiency because it further increases the body's need for vitamin K.

It's important that you advise patients not to take iron and vitamin E supplements together. Iron apparently interferes with the body's ability to absorb or use the vitamin.

Folic Acid and the Threat of CAD

We have known for decades that folic acid helps prevent a form of megaloblastic anemia. Research over the last couple of years has clearly demonstrated that it can also protect the unborn against neural tube defects (NTDs).[5] Women who have already given birth to a child with an NTD should take 4 mg a day, starting at least one month before trying to conceive again. Others planning to get pregnant should get 0.4–0.8 mg of the vitamin on a daily basis. (The RDA for the general population is 0.4 mg.)

There has also been some evidence to suggest that 0.4–1 mg of folic acid a day may reduce the threat of CAD by decreasing the amount of homocysteine in the bloodstream. How the amino acid contributes to heart disease remains unclear, but a number of studies indicate elevated serum levels may be as strong a risk factor as smoking.[6]

If the physician orders folic acid supplements, or your patient is self-medicating, there are a few precautions to keep in mind. On occasion, the vitamin may mask some of the signs of vitamin B_{12} deficiency. That's more of a risk among the elderly, who are prone to the disorder. A simple way around the problem is to have the patient take supplemental B_{12} as well.

Patients on phenytoin (Dilantin) have to be careful about taking folic acid. Case studies suggest that 1 mg or more of the vitamin can lower serum phenytoin levels, increasing the risk of seizures. However, since phenytoin itself can cause folic acid deficiency, it's a catch-22 situation. Starting patients on both phenytoin and folic acid immediately after a diagnosis of epilepsy may help resolve the conflict.

Vitamin C May Play Many Roles

Large doses of ascorbic acid have been recommended for a wide variety of ailments; some of these claims are well-founded, some are not. Among the diverse reasons some physicians prescribe it: to treat upper respiratory infections, cancer, and hypercholesterolemia, and to combat some of the damaging effects of cigarette smoking. While the RDA for the vitamin is only 50–95 mg, therapeutic dosages can range from 500 to 10,000 mg a day.

If your patient is taking supplemental vitamin C, watch for diarrhea and GI upset. Hemolytic anemia, another adverse effect, has been reported in at least one premature infant; it has also been known to occur in African-American patients with a genetic disorder called glucose-6-phosphate dehydrogenase deficiency.

Patients who suddenly stop taking large doses of the vitamin may develop rebound scurvy, so advise patients to cut back slowly. There is also a risk of renal stones, though that claim remains somewhat controversial.[7]

Of more concern, however, are possible drug interactions. Vitamin C supplements may decrease the therapeutic effects of tricyclic antidepressants, for instance. We still do not know for sure if that interaction is clinically significant but at the very least, you should monitor patients to see if the symptoms of depression begin to re-emerge.

Five to 10 gm of the vitamin have also been reported to reduce the anticoagulant effects of warfarin. If a patient is taking both agents, inform the physician of the potential interaction and monitor prothrombin time closely. Advise patients not to take cholestyramine (Questran) and vitamin C at the same time because they bind to one another in the GI tract.

Can Zinc Tame the Common Cold?

In the last few years, researchers have tried to determine if zinc lozenges can help relieve the common cold. The latest Cleveland Clinic trial concluded that it can, although not all studies have confirmed this. Nevertheless, the sale of zinc tablets has skyrocketed.

Typically, patients take about 13 mg of zinc every two hours until their symptoms clear up.[8] That's about 200 mg a day, which far exceeds the adult RDA of 12–19 mg. Over the short-term, patients can expect some nausea and a bad aftertaste. Some experts warn that chronic use can cause copper deficiency, a drop in HDL cholesterol—the good cholesterol—and a weakened immune response. One study, for instance, found that 150 mg a day caused copper deficiency-induced neutropenia.[9]

There's also a zinc/drug interaction to be aware of. Zinc may inhibit tetracycline absorption. So tell patients who take the supplements not to do so for at least two hours after taking the antibiotic.

Chromium Holds Promise for Diabetics

Evidence has been building to suggest that chromium may help control non-insulin dependent diabetes. Some experts suspect this trace mineral helps normalize blood glucose by increasing the effects of insulin on the cell, in effect making cells more insulin-sensitive.

There's no RDA for chromium, but experts estimate that adults and children over age 7 need 50–200 mcg a day. One clinical trial in China has found, however, that as much as 1,000 mcg of chromium picolinate helps to normalize glycosylated hemoglobin, blood glucose, and serum cholesterol levels.[10] Although there's no consensus yet among nutritionists, several U.S. studies suggest that patients with impaired glucose tolerance what is sometimes called pre-diabetes—may also benefit from the mineral.[11]

If your patient is taking chromium tablets and a hypoglycemic drug, monitor him closely. Chromium supplements can reduce the need for insulin, sulfonylureas, and metformin (Glucophage); so, if a patient's drug dosage isn't adjusted, he can develop hypoglycemia.

Selenium and Beta Carotene

Two nutrients have entered into the search for a way to prevent cancer: selenium and beta carotene. In places where the soil contains low levels of the trace element selenium (Se), the incidence of cancer is usually quite high; in Se-rich areas, the incidence is low. The latest double blind trial couldn't confirm that selenium protects against skin cancer but did reveal that 200 mcg a day reduced the risk of colorectal, prostate, and lung cancer.[12] (The RDA is only 40–75 mcg.)

While 200 mcg is considered a safe daily dose, even over the long-term, amounts that far exceed 200 mcg can produce hair loss, nausea, abdominal pain, and diarrhea. They can also cause the skin to give off a garlic-like odor.

The evidence for beta carotene supplements is less convincing. While there's good reason to believe that a diet rich in carotene—containing fruits and vegetables—helps thwart cancer and CAD, clinical trials have failed to show that carotene supplements will accomplish the same goals. While there's no RDA for the nutrient, at least one study suggests that 30 mg a day may actually increase the risk of lung cancer in smokers.[13]

Summary

As more research dollars are invested in nutritional pharmacology, it's likely the list of therapeutic supplements will continue to grow. Keeping up to date with these new developments will allow you to offer a safe, effective complement to conventional drug therapy.

References

1. Stephens, N. G., Parsons, A., *et al*. (1996). Randomized controlled trial of vitamin E in patients with coronary disease: Cambridge Heart Antioxidant Study (CHAOS). *Lancet*, 347(9004), 781.

2. Jha, P., Flather, M., *et al*. (1995). The antioxidant vitamins and cardiovascular disease. *Ann. Intern. Med.*, 123(11), 860.

3. Meyers, D. G., Maloley, P. A., & Weeks, D. (1996). Safety of antioxidant vitamins. *Arch. Intern. Med.*, 156(9), 925.

4. Kappus, H., & Diplock, A. T. (1992). Tolerance and safety of vitamin E: A toxicological position report. *Radical Biology and Medicine*, 13, 55.

5. Frame, P. S., Berg, A. O., & Woolf, S. (1997). U.S. Preventive Services Task Force: Highlights of the 1996 report. *Am. Fam. Phys.*, 55(2), 567.

6. Graham. I. A., Daly, L. E., *et al*. (1997). Plasma homocysteine as a risk factor for vascular disease. *JAMA*, 277(22), 1775.

7. Mahan, L. K., & Escott-Stump, S. (1996). *Krause's food, nutrition, & diet therapy (9th ed.).* Philadelphia: W. B. Saunders.

8. Mossad, S. B., Mackinin, M. L., *et al.* (1996). Zinc gluconate lozenges for treating the common cold: A randomized double-blind, placebo-controlled study. *Ann. Intern. Med.*, 125(2), 81.

9. Prasad, A. S., Brewer, G. J., *et al.* (1978). Hypocupremia induced by zinc therapy in adults. *JAMA*, 240(20), 2166.

10. Anderson, R., Cheng, N., *et al.* (1996). Beneficial effects of chromium for people with Type II diabetes. *Diabetes*, 45(Suppl. 2), 124A.

11. Food and Nutrition Board. (1989). *Recommended dietary allowances (10th ed.).* Washington, DC: National Academy Press.

12. Clark, L. C., Combs, G. F., *et al.* (1996). Effects of selenium supplementation for cancer prevention in patients with carcinoma of the skin. *JAMA*, 276(24), 1957.

13. Omenn, G. S., Goodman, G. E., *et al.* (1996). Effects of a combination of beta carotene and vitamin A on lung cancer and cardiovascular disease. *N. Engl. J. Med.*, 334(18), 1150.

—by Paul Cerrato

Paul Cerrato, series editor and a senior editor, has taught nutrition at Vermont College, City University of New York, and at nursing homes in the New York metropolitan area. Series co-editor, Sandra Chase, PharmD, is a clinical pharmacist at Thomas Jefferson University Hospital in Philadelphia, a clinical associate professor at the Philadelphia College of Pharmacy and Science, and a member of the *RN* editorial board.

Chapter 43

Fluoride: The Wonder Nutrient

Despite hopes to the contrary, magic bullets are few in the world of medical science. The exception may be fluoride. It is credited with being the primary factor in a dramatic reduction in dental caries in the last twenty years.

Fluoride is a natural component of minerals in rocks and soils. All water contains fluoride, but it is sometimes necessary to add it to some public supplies to attain the optimal amount for dental health.

The story of how fluoride came to have an essential role in the effort to achieve a cavity-free generation is not one of laboratory science. Rather it is one of careful scientific observation of a naturally occurring phenomenon, followed by wide experimentation.

First noticed in the early part of this century when researchers observed that persons with "mottled teeth" experienced fewer dental caries than those without the discoloration. The phenomenon was traced to high amounts of naturally occurring fluoride in their drinking water. "Mottled teeth" is also known as fluorosis, a cosmetic defect characterized by white flecks, or in some severe cases, stained teeth.

Fluoride was first introduced into the drinking water of Grand Rapids, Michigan as part of a two-city community trial in 1945. The Grand Rapids undertaking was so successful that the control city of Muskegon soon insisted on fluoridating its water.

Since then, literally thousands of studies on fluorides and fluoridation have been completed, and more than 3,700 studies have been

"Fluoride: The Wonder Nutrient," *Food Insight*, September/October 1997; reprinted with permission.

conducted since 1970 alone. The most recent national study on children conducted from 1986–1987 by the National Institute of Dental Research found "a clear and continuing benefit of community water fluoridation in preventing tooth decay."

The fluoridation of drinking water has expanded steadily, as has the use of fluorides in other ways. "Originally viewed as beneficial primarily for children, fluoride agents are now recognized as effective for all ages and of increasing importance in an aging population," according to Irwin Mandel, D.D.S., professor emeritus, Columbia University School of Dental and Oral Surgery. Virtually all toothpaste used in the United States contains fluoride. Fluoride mouthwashes and tablets are used in schools and homes, and topical fluorides are applied in dental offices. Around the world, where fluoridation of water supplies may not be realistic, fluoride-containing toothpaste is used. Unfortunately, those who consume high amounts of bottled water in place of fluoridated tap water may not be receiving its oral health benefits.

Fluoride has not achieved its fame nor results without its share of critics. It has been accused of being illegal, a communist plot, immoral, and unconstitutional. It has been blamed for everything from cancer and birth defects to premature aging and, more recently, Alzheimer's disease and AIDS.

However, according to the American Dental Association, "The simple fact remains that there has never been a single valid, peer-reviewed laboratory, clinical, or epidemiological study that showed that drinking water with fluoride at optimal levels caused cancer, heart disease, or any other multitude of diseases of which it has been accused."

Based on the findings from hundreds of studies, both the National Institute of Dental Research and the U.S. Public Health Service support fluoridation as a safe, effective, equitable means of controlling dental caries.

Chapter 44

Olestra and Other Fat Substitutes

Americans' growing preference for reduced-fat diets has food manufacturers cooking up new substances to replace most, if not all, of the fat in a food.

Some of these fat substitutes, with trade names such as Simplesse and Avicel, already are on the market and being used in a variety of foods, including cheese, chips, frozen desserts, and candy. Others remain in development. At least one—olestra—is under FDA review. [For an update on the status of Olestra see "Olestra—Approved with Special Labeling" at the end of this chapter.]

The idea behind all these substitutes is to reduce a food's fat and calories while maintaining the texture provided by fat. They often fall short, however. While most contain fewer calories than fat, they don't withstand the cooking temperatures that natural fats do.

Olestra appears to be an exception. Because olestra is formed by chemical combination of sucrose (sugar) with fatty acids, it has properties similar to those of a naturally occurring fat. But, unlike the natural products, this synthetic substitute provides no calories or saturated fat because it is undigestible: It passes through the digestive tract but is not absorbed into the body.

As promising as that sounds, olestra and similar fat substitutes that may come along in the future raise new concerns: What effect can they have on the gastrointestinal system if they are not absorbed?

This chapter includes text from "Olestra and Other Fat Substitutes," *FDA Backgrounder*, November 28, 1995; and "Olestra—Approved with Special Labeling," *FDA Consumer*, March 1996.

403

Can they affect absorption of fat-soluble vitamins? Can they interfere with absorption of other nutrients or with drugs? What particular effects might they have in people with conditions that affect nutrition, such as intestinal disease?

Unlike other food additives, which make up only a minute amount of the diet, fat substitutes, such as olestra, have the potential to make up a substantial portion of the diet because they replace fat, a major dietary component. This raises another concern: how best to determine if there are possible toxic effects from such fat substitutes. The usual method for studying toxicity of food additives—giving upwards of 100 times the likely human intake of the substance to laboratory animals—is impractical for fat substitutes like olestra. It is not possible to feed laboratory animals the large amount of fat substitutes that would be required to conduct a traditional toxicology test as is done with other food additives to determine safety.

FDA's Center for Food Safety and Applied Nutrition (CFSAN) is exploring these concerns in its review of a food additive petition for olestra. The manufacturer, Procter and Gamble of Cincinnati, is seeking approval to use olestra in salty or sharp-tasting snacks, such as potato chips, cheese puffs, and crackers. This is the first and only filed petition for a fat-based fat substitute now before the agency. P&G filed the petition in 1987.

Fat in the Diet

Replacing fat in the diet is not as easy as it may sound. Contrary to public perception, natural fats actually have many useful roles in the diet. They are one of the nutrient categories essential for proper growth and development and maintenance of good health. They carry the fat-soluble vitamins A, D, E, and K and aid in their absorption in the intestine. They are the only source of linoleic acid, an essential fatty acid. And they are an especially important source of calories for people who are underweight and for infants and toddlers, who have the highest energy needs per kilogram of body weight of any age group.

Fat also plays important roles in food preparation and consumption. It gives taste, consistency, stability, and palatability to foods.

On the other hand, too much fat in the diet can be harmful. Fat is calorie-dense: It contains 9 calories per gram, compared to 4 calories per gram for protein and carbohydrates. So eating a lot of fat can result in excess calorie intake, which in turn can perhaps lead to undesirable weight gain.

Fat intake also is linked to several chronic diseases. There is some evidence of a link between high intakes of fat and a possible increased risk of certain cancers, such as breast, colon and prostate cancers. There also is a link between high intakes of saturated fat and cholesterol and an increased risk of coronary heart disease.

The Dietary Guidelines for Americans recommend that fat intake be limited to 30 percent or less of calories and saturated fat to less than 10 percent.

Many Americans are trying to reduce their fat intake. According to a survey by the Calorie Control Council—an association of low-calorie and diet food manufacturers—nearly two-thirds of the adult U.S. population consume low- or reduced-fat or reduced-calorie foods and beverages, and two-thirds also believe there is a need for food ingredients that replace fat.

Manufacturers are responding by adding more and more reduced-fat foods to their product lines. These products often contain fat substitutes already approved by FDA.

Fat Substitutes

Fat substitutes can be carbohydrate-, protein- or fat-based.

The first type to reach the market contained carbohydrate as the main ingredient. Avicel, for example, is a cellulose gel introduced in the mid-1960s by FMC Corp., and N-Oil is a tapioca dextrin introduced in the early 1980s by National Starch and Chemical Co. These types of fat substitutes are used in a variety of foods today, including lunch meats, salad dressings, frozen desserts, table spreads, dips, baked goods, and candy.

Protein-based fat substitutes entered the market in the early 1990s. There are two that have been affirmed as "generally recognized as safe" (GRAS): microparticulated proteins from egg white or dairy protein and whey protein concentrate. Microparticulation is a process in which the protein is shaped into microscopic round particles that roll easily over one another. These fat substitutes give a better sensation in the mouth—"mouth feel" in industry parlance—than the carbohydrate-based ones and can be used in some cooked foods. However, they're not suitable for frying.

Olestra

Olestra is a fat-based fat substitute. Unlike the other fat substitutes, it provides zero calories. This is due to its unique configuration.

Most fat substitutes mimic the molecular shape of fat—one molecule of glycerol attached to three molecules of fatty acids. With olestra, the glycerol molecule is replaced with sucrose and has six, seven or eight fatty acids attached. The fatty acids can come from a variety of vegetable oils, such as soybean, corn, palm, coconut, and cottonseed oils. The idea is that with this many fatty acids, digestive enzymes can't get to the sucrose center in the time it takes for the substance to move through the digestive tract. The sucrose center is where breakdown of the substance for absorption into the body would take place.

P&G first sought FDA approval for olestra—as a drug—in 1975. The company filed an investigational new drug application after early human studies showed that olestra lowered blood cholesterol. But additional studies showed that it did not sufficiently reduce cholesterol to warrant its use as a drug. In 1988, P&G withdrew the application.

In 1987, the company filed a food additive petition for the approval of the use of olestra as a calorie-free replacement for fat in shortening and cooking oil. In 1990, it amended the petition to limit olestra's use to 100 percent replacement for conventional fats in the preparation of savory snacks, such as potato chips, cheese puffs, and crackers.

P&G also is seeking approval for olestra in Canada and the United Kingdom.

Olestra Studies

Since 1987, P&G has submitted to FDA more than 150 studies on olestra's safety. These include:

- animal and human studies to determine whether olestra breaks down in the digestive tract

- animal studies to determine how much, if any, olestra is absorbed into the body

- animal studies to determine whether olestra can cause birth defects

- animal studies to determine whether a diet containing olestra is associated with a higher incidence of cancer

- animal and human studies to determine olestra's effects on absorption of the fat-soluble vitamins and five key water-soluble nutrients that are hard to absorb or are limited in the U.S. diet—folate, vitamin B_{12}, calcium, zinc, and iron

- animal and human studies to determine whether adding fat-soluble vitamins to diets containing olestra can offset the losses of those vitamins that may occur with olestra consumption

- human studies to determine olestra's potential to cause cramping, bloating, loose stools, diarrhea, and other gastrointestinal symptoms in healthy adults, healthy children, and adults with inflammatory bowel disease

- human studies to determine olestra's effects on normal intestinal microflora functions

- animal and human studies to determine olestra's effect on the absorption of drugs, especially those that attach to fat in the body, such as oral contraceptives.

Additional Review

To help CFSAN resolve some of the issues raised by the olestra petition, the center, in spring 1995, established a team made up of senior managers from CFSAN and FDA's Center for Veterinary Medicine, which was included because of its expertise in reviewing animal studies. The group was charged with reviewing safety data and recommending a decision to the center director on the olestra petition. In addition, CFSAN arranged for the members to discuss the data with its expert consultants from academia and with experts from other government agencies.

CFSAN sought additional input from FDA's Food Advisory Committee, which met November 17, 1995, to discuss the olestra petition. A committee working group met November 14 through 16 to review the safety data on olestra and to consider whether all safety issues had been adequately addressed.

The working group considered four areas: olestra's chemistry and consumption, toxicology and potential interference with drug absorption, gastrointestinal effects and labeling, and nutritional effects. For each area, the working group was asked to decide whether all relevant issues had been identified, whether there were sufficient data to address these issues, and whether there was a "reasonable certainty of no harm" from the proposed use of olestra. The working group unanimously concluded that, in all four areas, the relevant issues had been identified and the data were sufficient to address the relevant issues. Most of the working group also agreed that the data provided a reasonable certainty of no harm from olestra.

However, the group recommended that products containing olestra bear a label statement about the food's potential to cause intestinal discomfort or a laxative effect, without suggesting that the product is intended for use as a laxative.

Also, the committee agreed that while olestra has no effect on water-soluble nutrients, it should be formulated to contain vitamins A, D, E, and K to avoid their depletion in people who eat olestra-containing foods. Although the working group considered carotenoid depletion by olestra, most members said they were reasonably certain that no harm will result from the effect of olestra on carotenoids.

During the November 17 meeting, the full Food Advisory Committee discussed the working group's conclusions. Most committee members concurred with the working group's findings and agreed that there is a reasonable certainty of no harm from olestra's proposed uses. The committee's comments, as well as those of the working group, will be passed on to FDA for its consideration in making a decision on the olestra petition.

Olestra—Approved with Special Labeling

Products containing olestra, a fat-based substitute for conventional fats, are expected to start appearing on store shelves soon. FDA approved olestra last January 24 [1996] for use in certain snack foods. The agency is requiring all products containing olestra to be labeled with specific health information.

Procter & Gamble Co. developed olestra, which it is marketing under the trade name Olean.

Because of its unique chemical composition, olestra adds no fat or calories to food. Potato chips, crackers, tortilla chips, or other snacks made with olestra will be lower in fat and calories than snacks made with traditional fats.

Olestra may cause abdominal cramping and loose stools in some individuals, and it inhibits the body's absorption of certain fat-soluble vitamins and nutrients. FDA is requiring Procter & Gamble and other manufacturers who use olestra to label all foods made with olestra and to add essential vitamins- vitamins A, D, E, and K-to olestra.

As a condition of approval, Procter & Gamble will conduct studies to monitor consumption as well as studies on olestra's long-term effects. FDA will formally review these studies in a public meeting of the Foods Advisory Committee within 30 months from the date of olestra's approval.

The following labeling statement will be on all products made with olestra: "This Product Contains Olestra. Olestra may cause abdominal cramping and loose stools. Olestra inhibits the absorption of some vitamins and other nutrients. Vitamins A, D, E, and K have been added."

Like all food additives, olestra's safety was the primary focus of FDA evaluation. For olestra, the safety evaluation focused not only on its toxicity, but also on the product's effects on the absorption of nutrients and on the gastrointestinal system.

Studies of olestra indicated it may cause intestinal cramps, more frequent bowel movements, and loose stools in some individuals. These gastrointestinal effects do not have medical consequences. The required labeling will give consumers needed information to discontinue the product if appropriate.

Clinical testing also indicated that olestra absorbs fat-soluble vitamins (vitamins A, D, E and K) from foods eaten at the same time as olestra-containing products. Studies also demonstrated that replacing these essential nutrients in olestra-containing snacks compensates for this effect. This information will also be included in the product labeling.

In addition to inhibiting the absorption of essential vitamins, olestra reduces the absorption of carotenoids nutrients found in carrots, sweet potatoes, green leaf vegetables, and some animal tissue. The company's postmarketing monitoring of olestra consumption levels and additional studies will provide FDA with further information about olestra's effects on the absorption of carotenoids. The role of carotenoids in human health is not fully understood, and FDA is continuing to monitor all available scientific research on it.

In addressing these questions, FDA evaluated more than 150,000 pages of data on olestra, drawn from more than 150 studies. Procter & Gamble submitted these data in its original 1987 food additive petition and in several subsequent amendments.

In addition, FDA sought advice from outside experts through its Food Advisory Committee. A special working group of the committee met in public in November 1995 to review and discuss the safety questions about olestra. The working group evaluated data presented by FDA, the company, and organizations and individuals both opposing and supporting olestra's approval. A clear majority of the working group agreed that all major safety issues had been identified and addressed by the FDA review, and that the data provided reasonable certainty that the proposed use of olestra would be safe. A majority of the full Food Advisory Committee reaffirmed that judgment.

Chapter 45

Low-Calorie Sweeteners

More Than Just a Sweet Taste

Low-calorie sweeteners taste very similar to sucrose (table sugar) but are much sweeter. Most do not contain any calories. Even though some sweeteners, such as aspartame, contain calories, they are used in such small amounts that they add essentially no calories to foods and beverages. As a result, these sweeteners practically eliminate or substantially reduce calories in some foods and beverages such as carbonated soft drinks, light yogurt and sugar-free pudding.

Low-Calorie Sweeteners in the United States

The Food and Drug Administration (FDA) has to date approved three low-calorie sweeteners for use in the United States: aspartame, acesulfame-K and saccharin.

Aspartame

Aspartame tastes very similar to sucrose but is 200-times sweeter. It is broken down to compounds normally found in the foods we eat everyday: aspartic acid, phenylalanine and a small amount of methanol.

This chapter includes text from "Low-Calorie Sweeteners: Adding Reduced-Calorie Delights to a Healthful Diet," *Food Insight*, January/February 1998 and updated information from "Everything You Need to Know About Sucralose," International Food Information Council (IFIC), May 1998; both reprinted with permission from IFIC.

411

Aspartic acid and phenylalanine are essential amino acids (the building blocks of protein) and methanol is found naturally in many foods, such as fruit and vegetable juices. In fact, a glass of tomato juice provides six times as much methanol as a similar amount of diet soda. Many prepared foods contain aspartame which is also available as a tabletop sweetener.

Aspartame underwent extensive safety testing for more than a decade before the FDA concluded in 1981 that aspartame is safe for use by consumers and thus approved its use. Products made with aspartame, however, must carry a statement on the label that they contain phenylalanine. The statement is important for people with phenylketonuria, a rare hereditary disease, because they cannot properly metabolize phenylalanine.

Acesulfame-K

Acesulfame-K, or acesulfame potassium, is produced by using derivatives of acetoncetic acid (a derivative of acetic acid or vinegar). It also is 200-times sweeter than sucrose. Over 90 studies were conducted to test its safety before the FDA approved its use in 1988.

Available as a tabletop sweetener, acesulfame-K also is used in many prepared foods. When eaten alone in high concentrations, acesulfame-K may produce a slight aftertaste. However, blending acesulfame-K with other low-calorie sweeteners helps improve the taste of low-calorie products as well as their sweetness, shelf-life and stability. Also, with blended sweeteners, a synergy often occurs that makes it possible to produce the desired sweetness using a lower total amount of sweeteners.

Saccharin

Saccharin is the oldest of low-calorie sweeteners and has been used to sweeten foods and beverages since the turn of the century. It has a taste 300-times sweeter than sucrose. Saccharin is highly stable, but has a slightly bitter aftertaste.

The FDA proposed a ban on saccharin in 1977 based on animal research that suggested it was a weak bladder carcinogen. However, a congressional moratorium was placed on the ban to allow for more research on saccharin's safety. The moratorium on the ban has been extended seven times based on the need for further scientific study and continued consumer demand. The FDA withdrew the ban in 1991, but the moratorium is still in effect until the year 2002. While numerous studies since 1977 have clearly shown that saccharin does not cause cancer in humans, labels on products with saccharin must continue to have a statement that it has caused cancer in laboratory animals.

No final decision has been made regarding delisting saccharin from Health and Human Services' Public Health Services' National Toxicology Program's (NTP) Report on Carcinogens. Three separate committees have reviewed saccharin: Two internal NTP committees voted to delist saccharin, and a third, external advisory group in a close vote recommended keeping it on the list. A final decision will be made at a later date.

Waiting in the Wings

The FDA is currently considering petitions to approve other low-calorie sweeteners, including sucralose, alitame and cyclamate, all of which are already approved for use in numerous other countries.

Sucralose

Sucralose is the only low-calorie sweetener that is made from sugar. It is approximately 600-times sweeter and does not contain calories. Sucralose is highly stable under a wide variety of processing conditions. Thus, it can be used virtually anywhere sugar can, including cooking and baking, without losing any of its sugar-like sweetness.

Types of Products that Contain Sucralose

Sucralose makes low-calorie versions of a wide variety of products possible, including soft drinks, ice cream, dairy products and baked goods. One of the unique attributes of sucralose is that it can be used virtually like sugar without losing any of its sugar-like sweetness, even in applications that require prolonged exposure to high temperatures. Thus, products made with sucralose maintain their sweetness during cooking and baking, and in storage for long periods. In the United States, the FDA has granted approval for the use of sucralose in 15 food and beverage categories:

- Baked goods and baking mixes
- Beverages and beverage bases
- Chewing gum
- Coffee and tea
- Confections and frostings
- Dairy products analogs

- Fats and oils (salad dressings)
- Frozen dairy desserts and mixes
- Fruit and water ices
- Gelatins, puddings and fillings
- Jams and jellies
- Milk products
- Processed fruits and fruit juices
- Sugar substitutes
- Sweet sauces, toppings and syrups

Alitame

Alitame is formed from amino acids (L-aspartic acid, L-alanine, and a novel amide). It offers a taste that is 2,000-times sweeter than sucrose, and can be used in cooking and baking. If approved, alitame would be suitable for use in a wide variety of products, including beverages, tabletop sweeteners, frozen desserts and baked goods.

Cyclamate

Cyclamate is approved for use in Canada and more than 50 countries in Europe, Asia, South America and Africa. Cyclamate is 30-times sweeter than sucrose and is heat-stable. Since 1970, however, its use has been banned in the United States, based on a study suggesting cyclamates may be related to development of bladder tumors in rats. While 75 subsequent studies have failed to show cyclamate is carcinogenic, the sweetener has yet to be reapproved for use in this country.

Low-Calorie Delights

Low-calorie sweeteners help satisfy desires for a sweet taste, and allow people to follow a healthful eating plan that includes their favorite foods. According to Adam Drewnowski, Ph.D., professor at the University of Michigan, "Low-calorie sweeteners offer the best method to date of reducing calories while maintaining the palatability of the diet."

Low-calorie sweeteners are an option for reducing the number of calories in our diet. Although calorie reduction goes hand-in-hand with weight loss, it must be recognized that low-calorie sweeteners in and of themselves will not magically solve our struggles with weight. Successful weight management requires habits that include a balanced diet and regular physical activity.

Chapter 46

Glutamate and Monosodium Glutamate

Eating is one of life's pleasures. Taste and flavor are important to enjoying food. Think about a bowl of hot pasta with tomato sauce and parmesan cheese, a freshly grilled steak with a rich mushroom sauce, or stir-fried seafood and chicken with crisp vegetables in a savory sauce. These subtle, delicate flavors result from centuries of culinary tradition, including careful attention to ingredients and preparation. In all of these dishes, glutamate is one of the major food components that provides flavor.

What Is Glutamate?

Glutamate is an amino acid, found in all protein-containing foods. Amino acids are the building blocks of proteins. This amino acid is one of the most abundant and important components of proteins. Glutamate occurs naturally in protein-containing foods such as cheese, milk, mushrooms, meat, fish, and many vegetables. Glutamate is also produced by the human body and is vital for metabolism and brain function.

What Is Monosodium Glutamate?

Monosodium glutamate, or MSG, is the sodium salt of glutamate. When MSG is added to foods, it provides a similar flavoring function

"Everything You Need to Know about ... Glutamate and Monosodium Glutamate," International Food Information Council, January 1997.

as the glutamate that occurs naturally in food. MSG is comprised of nothing more than water, sodium, and glutamate.

Why Is MSG Used?

MSG is a flavor enhancer that has been used effectively to bring out the best taste in foods, emphasizing natural flavors. Many researchers also believe that MSG imparts a fifth taste, independent of the four basic tastes of sweet, sour, salty, and bitter. This taste, called "umami" in Japan, is described by Americans as savory. Examples of each of these tastes are:

- Sweet—Sugar
- Bitter—Coffee
- Savory—Tomato
- Sour—Lemon
- Salt—Anchovy

How Is MSG Made?

In the early 1900s, MSG was extracted from natural protein-rich foods such as seaweed. Today, MSG is made from starch, corn sugar, or molasses from sugar cane or sugar beets. MSG is produced by a natural fermentation process that has been used for centuries to make such common foods as beer, vinegar, and yogurt.

How Are Glutamate and MSG Handled by the Body?

The human body treats glutamate that is added to foods in the form of MSG the same as the natural glutamate found in food. For instance, the body does not distinguish between free glutamate from tomatoes, cheese or mushrooms and the glutamate from MSG added to foods. Glutamate is glutamate, whether naturally present or from MSG.

Does Glutamate or MSG Improve Flavors in All Foods?

The natural flavor-enhancing levels of glutamate in food varies greatly, but is high in foods such as tomatoes, mushrooms, and parmesan cheese. MSG enhances many but not all food flavors through the interaction between glutamate and other flavors. It works well with a variety of foods including meats, poultry, seafood and many vegetables. It is used to enhance the flavor of some soups, stews, meat-based sauces, and snack foods. MSG harmonizes well with salty and

Table 46.1. Glutamate Content of Foods

Food	Serving Size	Glutamate (mg/serving)
Tomato juice	1 cup	0.827
Tomato	3 slices	0.339
Meat loaf dinner	9 oz.	0.189
Human breast milk	1 cup	0.176
Mushrooms	¼ cup	0.094
Parmesan cheese	2 Tbsp	0.047
Corn	½ cup	0.031
Peas	½ cup	0.024
Cow's milk	1 cup	0.016
Canned tuna (in water)	½ can	0.008

Source: U.S. Food and Drug Administration

sour tastes, but does little for sweet foods such as cakes, pastries, or candies.

MSG can not improve bad-tasting food or make up for bad cooking. It does not allow a cook to substitute low-quality for high-quality ingredients in a recipe, and does not tenderize meat. It just makes good food taste better.

How Is MSG Used in the Home?

When you buy MSG in the grocery store, you will find suggested uses on the container label. MSG is generally added to foods before or during cooking. As a general guideline, about half a teaspoon of MSG per pound of meat or four to six servings of vegetables should be sufficient. Once the proper amount is used, adding more contributes little to food flavors.

How Much Glutamate Do People Consume?

The average American consumes about 11 grams of glutamate per day from natural protein sources and less than 1 gram of glutamate per day from MSG. This amount of added MSG is the same as adding 1 to 1.5 ounces of parmesan cheese. In contrast, the human body creates about 50 grams of glutamate daily for use as a vital component of metabolism.

Is MSG High in Sodium?

No. MSG contains only one-third the amount of sodium as table salt (13 percent vs. 40 percent) and is used in much smaller amounts. When used in combination with a small amount of table salt, MSG can help reduce the total amount of sodium in a recipe by 20 to 40 percent, while maintaining an enhanced flavor.

Are People Sensitive to MSG?

MSG is not an allergen, according to the American College of Allergy, Asthma and Immunology. The U.S. Food and Drug Administration has found no evidence to suggest any long-term, serious health consequences from consuming MSG. It is possible that some people might be sensitive to MSG, just as to many other foods and food ingredients. There are some reports that mild, temporary reactions to MSG may occur in a small portion of the population, based on tests with a large dose of MSG in the absence of food.

If you have questions about food sensitivities or allergies, contact a board-certified allergist or your personal physician.

Is MSG Safe?

Yes. MSG is one of the most extensively researched substances in the food supply. Numerous international scientific evaluations have been undertaken over many years, involving hundreds of studies. The United States and other governments worldwide support the safety of MSG as used in foods.

MSG Safety

- U.S. Food and Drug Administration (FDA): Designates MSG as safe (Generally Recognized as Safe/GRAS), with common ingredients such as salt and baking powder. (1958)

- National Academy of Sciences: Confirms the safety of MSG as a food ingredient. (1979)

- Joint Expert Committee on Food Additives of the United Nations World Health and Food and Agricultural Organizations: Designates MSG as safe and places it in its safest category for food additives. (1988)

- European Community's Scientific Committee for Food: Confirms MSG safety. (1991)

- American Medical Association: Concludes that MSG is safe, at normal consumption levels in the diet. (1992)

- FDA: Reaffirms MSG safety based upon a report from the Federation of American Societies for Experimental Biology. (1995)

Is MSG Safe for Children?

Yes. Infants, including premature babies, metabolize glutamate the same as adults. Research has shown that newborn infants are able to detect and prefer the taste of glutamate. Glutamate is actually 10 times more abundant in human breast milk than in cow's milk.

How Can I tell If Glutamate or MSG Is Added to Foods?

The U.S. Food and Drug Administration requires labeling of all ingredients on processed and packaged foods. When MSG is added to a food, it must be included on the ingredient list, as "monosodium glutamate." Glutamate-containing food ingredients, such as hydrolyzed protein and autolyzed yeast extract, also must be listed on food labels. When glutamate is a component of natural protein foods, like tomatoes, it is not listed separately on the label.

Chapter 47

Food Color Facts

The color of food is an integral part of our culture and enjoyment of life. Who would deny the mouth-watering appeal of a deep-pink strawberry ice on a hot summer day or a golden Thanksgiving turkey garnished with fresh green parsley?

Even early civilizations such as the Romans recognized that people "eat with their eyes" as well as their palates. Saffron and other spices were often used to provide a rich yellow color to various foods. Butter has been colored yellow as far back as the 1300s.

Today all food color additives are carefully regulated by federal authorities to ensure that foods are safe to eat and accurately labeled. This chapter provides helpful background information about color additives, why they are used in foods, and regulations governing their safe use in the food supply.

What Is a Color Additive?

Technically, a color additive is any dye, pigment or substance that can impart color when added or applied to a food, drug, cosmetic or to the human body.

The Food and Drug Administration (FDA) is responsible for regulating all color additives used in the United States. All color additives

Food and Drug Administration (FDA), 5600 Fishers Lane, Rockville, MD 20857 in cooperation with International Food Information Council Foundation, 1100 Connecticut Ave. NW, Suite 430, Washington, D.C. 20036, January 1993, updated March 1998; reprinted with permission.

permitted for use in foods are classified as "certifiable" or "exempt from certification" (see Table 47.1).

Certifiable color additives are manmade, with each batch being tested by the manufacturer and FDA. This "approval" process, known as color additive certification, assures the safety, quality, consistency, and strength of the color additive prior to its use in foods.

There are nine certified colors approved for use in food in the United States. One example is FD&C Yellow No.6, which is used in cereals, bakery goods, snack foods, and other foods.

Color additives that are exempt from certification include pigments derived from natural sources such as vegetables, minerals or animals, and man-made counterparts of natural derivatives. For example,

Table 47.1. Color Additives Permitted for Direct Addition to Human Food in the United States

Certifiable Colors	Colors Exempt from Certification
FD&C Blue No.1 (Dye and Lake)	Annatto extract
FD&C Blue No.2 (Dye and Lake)	B-Apo-8'-carotenal*
FD&C Green No.3 (Dye and Lake)	Beta-carotene
FD&C Red No.3 (Dye)	Beet powder
FD&C Red No.40 (Dye and Lake)	Canthaxanthin
FD&C Yellow No.5 (Dye and Lake)	Caramel color
FD&C Yellow No.6 (Dye and Lake)	Carrot oil
Orange B*	Cochineal extract (carmine)
Citrus Red No.2*	Cottonseed flour, toasted partially defatted, cooked
	Ferrous gluconate*
	Fruit juice
	Grape color extract*
	Grape skin extract* (enocianina)
	Paprika
	Paprika oleoresin
	Riboflavin
	Saffron
	Titanium dioxide*
	Turmeric
	Turmeric oleoresin
	Vegetable juice

*These food color additives are restricted to specific uses.

caramel color is produced commercially by heating sugar and other carbohydrates under strictly controlled conditions for use in sauces, gravies, soft drinks, baked goods, and other foods.

Whether a color additive is certifiable or exempt from certification has no bearing on its overall safety. Both types of color additives are subject to rigorous standards of safety prior to their approval for use in foods.

Certifiable color additives are used widely because their coloring ability is more intense than most colors derived from natural products; thus, they are often added to foods in smaller quantities. In addition, certifiable color additives are more stable, provide better color

Table 47.2. Color Additives Certifiable for Food Use

Name/Common Name	Hue	Common Food Uses
FD&C Blue No.1 Brilliant Blue FCF	Bright blue	Beverages, dairy products powders, jellies, confections, condiments, icings, syrups, extracts
FD&C Blue No.2 Indigotine	Royal Blue	Baked goods, cereals, snack foods, ice cream, confections, cherries
FD&C Green No.3 Fast Green FCF	Sea Green	Beverages, puddings, ice cream, sherbet, cherries, confections, baked goods, dairy products
FD&C Red No.40 Allura Red AC	Orange-red	Gelatins, puddings, dairy products, confections, beverages, condiments
FD&C Red No.3 Erythrosine	Cherry-red	Cherries in fruit cocktail and in canned fruits for salads, confections, baked goods, dairy products, snack foods
FD&C Yellow No.5 Tartrazine	Lemon Yellow	Custards, beverages, ice cream, confections, preserves, cereals
FD&C Yellow No.6 Sunset Yellow	Orange	Cereals, baked goods, snack foods, ice cream, beverages, dessert powders, confections

uniformity and blend together easily to provide a wide range of hues. Certifiable color additives generally do not impart undesirable flavors to foods, while color derived from foods such as beets and cranberries can produce such unintended effects.

Of nine certifiable colors approved for use in the United States, seven color additives are used in food manufacturing (see Table 47.2). Regulations known as Good Manufacturing Practices limit the amount of color added to foods. Too much color would make foods unattractive to consumers, in addition to increasing costs.

What Are Dyes and Lakes?

Certifiable color additives are available for use in food as either "dyes" or "lakes." Dyes dissolve in water and are manufactured as powders, granules, liquids, or other special purpose forms. They can be used in beverages, dry mixes, baked goods, confections, dairy products, pet foods and a variety of other products.

Lakes are the water insoluble form of the dye. Lakes are more stable than dyes and are ideal for coloring products containing fats and oils or items lacking sufficient moisture to dissolve dyes. Typical uses include coated tablets, cake and donut mixes, hard candies, and chewing gums.

Why Are Color Additives Used in Foods?

Color is an important property of foods that adds to our enjoyment of eating. Nature teaches us early to expect certain colors in certain foods, and our future acceptance of foods is highly dependent on meeting these expectations.

Color variation in foods throughout the seasons and the effects of food processing and storage often require that manufacturers add color to certain foods to meet consumer expectations. The primary reasons of adding colors to foods include:

- To offset color loss due to exposure to light, air, extremes of temperature, moisture, and storage conditions.

- To correct natural variations in color. Off-colored foods are often incorrectly associated with inferior quality. For example, some tree-ripened oranges are often sprayed with Citrus Red No.2 to correct the natural orangy-brown or mottled green color of their peels (Masking inferior quality, however, is an unacceptable use of colors.)

- To enhance colors that occur naturally but at levels weaker than those usually associated with a given food.

- To provide a colorful identity to foods that would otherwise be virtually colorless. Red colors provide a pleasant identity to strawberry ice while lime sherbet is known by its bright green color.

- To provide a colorful appearance to certain "fun foods." Many candies and holiday treats are colored to create a festive appearance.

- To protect flavors and vitamins that may be affected by sunlight during storage.

- To provide an appealing variety of wholesome and nutritious foods that meet consumers' demands.

How Are Color Additives Regulated?

In 1900, there were about 80 man-made color additives available for use in foods. At that time there were no regulations regarding the purity and uses of these dyes. Legislation enacted since the turn of the century, however, has greatly improved food color additive safety and stimulated improvements in food color technology.

The Food and Drug Act of 1906 permitted or "listed" seven man-made color additives for use in foods. The Act also established a voluntary certification program, which was administered by the U.S. Department of Agriculture (USDA); hence man-made color additives became known as "certifiable color additives".

The Federal Food, Drug & Cosmetic (FD&C) Act of 1938 made food color additive certification mandatory and transferred the authority for its testing from USDA to FDA. To avoid confusing color additives used in food with those manufactured for other uses, three categories of certifiable color additives were created:

- Food, Drug and Cosmetic (FD&C)—Color additives with application in foods, drugs, or cosmetics;

- Drug and Cosmetic (D&C)—Color additives with applications in drugs or cosmetics;

- External Drug and Cosmetic (External D&C)—Color additives with applications in externally applied drugs (e.g. ointments) and in externally applied cosmetics.

In 1960, the Color Additive Amendments to the FD&C Act placed color additives on a "provisional" list and required further testing using up-to-date procedures. One section of the amendment known as the Delaney Clause, prohibits adding to any food substance that has been shown to cause cancer in animals or man regardless of the dose. Under the amendments, color additives exempt from certification also are required to meet rigorous safety standards prior to being permitted for use in foods.

According to the Nutrition Labeling and Education Act of 1990, a certifiable color additive used in food must be listed in the ingredient statement by its common or usual name. All labels printed after July 1, 1991 must comply with this requirement.

How Are Color Additives Approved for Use in Foods?

To market a new color additive, a manufacturer must first petition FDA for its approval. The petition must provide convincing evidence that the proposed color additive performs as it is intended. Animal studies using large doses of the color additive for long periods are often necessary to show that the substance would not cause harmful effects at expected levels of human consumption. Studies of the color additive in humans also may be submitted to FDA.

In deciding whether a color additive should be approved, the agency considers the composition and properties of the substance, the amount likely to be consumed, its probable long-term effects and various safety factors. Absolute safety of any substance can never be proven. Therefore, FDA must determine if there is a reasonable certainty of no harm from the color additive under its proposed conditions of use.

If the color additive is approved, FDA issues regulations that may include the types of foods in which it can be used, the maximum amounts to be used and how it should be identified on food labels. Color additives proposed for use in meat and poultry products also must receive specific authorization by USDA.

Federal officials then carefully monitor the extent of Americans' consumption of the new color additive and results of any new research on its safety.

In addition, FDA operates an Adverse Reaction Monitoring System (ARMS) to help serve as an ongoing safety check of all activities. The system monitors and investigates all complaints by individuals or their physicians that are believed to be related to food and color additives; specific foods; or vitamin and mineral supplements. The

ARMS computerized database helps officials decide whether reported adverse reactions represent a real public health hazard, so that appropriate action can be taken.

Additional Information About Color Additives

Are certain people sensitive to FD&C Yellow No.5 in foods?

FDA's Advisory Committee on Hypersensitivity to Food Constituents concluded in 1986 that FD&C Yellow No.5 may cause hives in fewer that one out of 10,000 people. The committee found that there was no evidence the color additive in foods provokes asthma attacks nor that aspirin-intolerant individuals may have a cross-sensitivity to the color. As with other color additives certifiable for food use, whenever FD&C Yellow No.5 is added to foods, it is listed on the product label. This allows the small portion of people who may be sensitive to the color to avoid it.

What is the status of FD&C Red No.3?

In 1990, FDA discontinued the provisional listing of all lake forms of FD&C Red No.3 and its dye form used in external drugs and cosmetics. The uses were terminated because one study of the color additive in male rats showed an association with thyroid tumors. In announcing the decision, FDA [stated] that any human risk posed by FD&C Red No.3 was extremely small and was based less on safety concerns than the legal mandate of the Delaney Clause. FD&C Red No.3 remains permanently listed for use in food and ingested drugs, although FDA has announced its intent to propose rescinding those listings.

Why are decisions sometimes changed about the safety of food color additives?

Since absolute safety of any substance can never be proven, decisions about the safety of color additives or other food ingredients are made on the best scientific evidence available. Because scientific knowledge is constantly evolving, federal officials often review earlier decisions to assure that the safety assessment of a food substance remains up-to-date. Any change made in previous clearances should be recognized as an assurance that the latest and best scientific knowledge is being applied to enhance the safety of the food supply.

Do food color additives cause hyperactivity?

Although this theory was popularized in the 1970s, well-controlled studies conducted since then have produced no evidence that food color additives cause hyperactivity or learning disabilities in children. A Consensus Development Panel of the National Institutes of Health concluded in 1982 that there was no scientific evidence to support the claim that colorings or other food additives cause hyperactivity. The panel said that elimination diets should not be used universally to treat childhood hyperactivity, since there is no scientific evidence to predict which children may benefit.

Chapter 48

Fresh Look at Food Preservatives

Unless you grow all your food in your own garden and prepare all your meals from scratch, it's almost impossible to eat food without preservatives added by manufacturers during processing. Without such preservatives, food safety problems would get out of hand, to say nothing of the grocery bills. Bread would get moldy, and salad oil would go rancid before it's used up.

Food law says preservatives must be listed by their common or usual names on ingredient labels of all foods that contain them—which is most processed food. You'll see calcium propionate on most bread labels, disodium EDTA on canned kidney beans, and BHA on shortening, just to name a few. Even snack foods—dried fruit, potato chips, and trail mix—contain sulfur-based preservatives.

Manufacturers add preservatives mostly to prevent spoilage during the time it takes to transport foods over long distances to stores and then our kitchens. It's not unusual for sourdough bread manufactured in California to be eaten in Maine, or for olive oil manufactured in Spain to be used on a California salad. Rapid transport systems and ideal storage conditions help keep foods fresh and nutritionally stable. But breads, cooking oils, and other foods, including the complex, high-quality convenience products consumers and food services have come to expect, usually need more help.

Preservatives serve as either antimicrobials or antioxidants— or both. As antimicrobials, they prevent the growth of molds, yeasts, and bacteria. As antioxidants, they keep foods from becoming rancid,

FDA Consumer, October 1993.

browning, or developing black spots. Rancid foods may not make you sick, but they smell and taste bad. Antioxidants suppress the reaction that occurs when foods combine with oxygen in the presence of light, heat, and some metals. Antioxidants also minimize the damage to some essential amino acids—the building blocks of proteins—and the loss of some vitamins.

Safety Questions

Consumers often ask the Food and Drug Administration about the safety of preservatives, and if there's a system in place to make sure preservatives are safe.

Many preservatives are regulated under the food additives amendment, added to the Federal Food, Drug, and Cosmetic Act in 1958. The amendment strengthened the law to ensure the safety of all new ingredients that manufacturers add to foods. Under these rules, a food manufacturer must get FDA approval before using a new preservative, or before using a previously approved preservative in a new way or in a different amount. In its petition for approval, the manufacturer must demonstrate to FDA that the preservative is safe for consumers, considering:

- the probable amount of the preservative that will be consumed with the food product, or the amount of any substance formed in or on the food resulting from use of the preservative

- the cumulative effect of the preservative in the diet

- the potential toxicity (including cancer-causing) of the preservative when ingested by humans or animals.

Also, a preservative may not be used to deceive a consumer by changing the food to make it appear other than it is. For example, preservatives that contain sulfites are prohibited on meats because they restore the red color, giving meat a false appearance of freshness. (The U.S. Department of Agriculture regulates meats, but depends on the FDA regulation to prohibit sulfites in meats.)

The food additive regulations require the preservative to be of food grade and be prepared and handled as a food ingredient. Also, the quantity added to food must not exceed the amount needed to achieve the manufacturer's intended effect.

Regulations about the use of nitrites demonstrate the scrutiny given to the use of additives. Nitrites, used in combination with salt, serve as antimicrobials in meat to inhibit the growth of bacterial spores that cause botulism, a deadly food-borne illness. Nitrites are also used as preservatives and for flavoring and fixing color in a number of red meat, poultry, and fish products.

Since the original approvals were granted for specific uses of sodium nitrite, safety concerns have arisen. Nitrite salts can react with certain amines (derivatives of ammonia) in food to produce nitrosamines, many of which are known to cause cancer. A food manufacturer wanting to use sodium nitrites must show that nitrosamines will not form in hazardous amounts in the product under the additive's intended conditions of use. For example, regulations specify that sodium nitrite, used as an antimicrobial against the formation of botulinum toxin in smoked fish, must be present in 100 to 200 parts per million. In addition, other antioxidants, such as sodium ascorbate or sodium erythorbate, may be added to inhibit the formation of nitrosamines.

As scientists learn more about the action of certain chemicals in our bodies, FDA uses the new data to reevaluate the permitted uses of preservatives. Two examples are the commonly used preservatives butylated hydroxyanisole (BHA) and sulfites.

BHA

BHA and the related compound butylated hydroxytoluene (BHT) have been used for years, mostly in foods that are high in fats and oils. They slow the development of off-flavors, odors, and color changes caused by oxidation. When the food additives amendment was enacted, BHA and BHT were listed as common preservatives considered generally recognized as safe (GRAS). GRAS regulations limit BHA and BHT to 0.02 percent or 200 parts per million (ppm) of the fat or oil content of the food product.

Lawrence Lin, Ph.D., of FDA's Center for Food Safety and Applied Nutrition, explains, "The 0.02 percent allowed relates only to the product's fat content. For example, if a product weighs 100 grams and one of those grams is fat, the quantity of BHA in the product cannot exceed 0.02 percent of that one gram of fat."

BHA is also used as a preservative for dry foods, such as cereals. But because such foods contain so little fat, the amount of BHA allowed cannot be measured against the percentage of fat, explains Lin. Therefore, as manufacturers petitioned FDA for approvals for this use, the agency set limits for each type of food. On cereals, for example, FDA limited BHA to 50 ppm of the total product.

In 1978, under contract with FDA, the Life Sciences Research Office of the Federation of American Societies for Experimental Biology

(FASEB) examined the health aspects of BHA as part of FDA's comprehensive review of GRAS safety assessments. FASEB concluded that although BHA was safe at permitted levels, additional studies were needed.

Since that evaluation, other studies suggested that at very high levels in the diets of laboratory animals, BHA could cause tumors in the forestomach of rats, mice and hamsters, and liver tumors in fish. Many experts examined the data and concluded the tests did not establish that such problems could exist in humans, mostly because humans do not have forestomachs. Other studies showed that BHA was protective, inhibiting the effect of some chemical carcinogens, depending on the conditions of the tests.

Studies on BHA were reviewed by scientists from the United Kingdom, Canada, Japan, and the United States. Their findings were published in 1983 in the *Report of the Working Group on the Toxicology and Metabolism of Antioxidants* and reviewed in the 1990 *Annual Review of Pharmacology and Toxicology*. The 1983 report stated that data from a Japanese study showed a high incidence of cancerous tumors and papillomas (benign tumors of the skin or mucous membranes) of the forestomach of treated rats and that the effect was dose-related. The report also mentioned the possible existence of a no-effect level, based on dose response, and noted that the level which produced cancer in this study was many thousands of times higher than the level to which humans are exposed.

Sulfites

Sulfites are used primarily as antioxidants to prevent or reduce discoloration of light-colored fruits and vegetables, such as dried apples and dehydrated potatoes. They are also used in wine-making because they inhibit bacterial growth but do not interfere with the desired development of yeast.

Sulfites are also used in other ways, such as for bleaching food starches and as preventives against rust and scale in boiler water used in making steam that will come in contact with food. Some sulfites are used in the production of cellophane for food packaging.

FDA prohibits the use of sulfites in foods that are important sources of thiamin (vitamin B_1), such as enriched flour, because sulfites destroy the nutrient.

Though most people don't have a problem with sulfites, some do. FDA's sulfite specialist, consumer safety officer Joann Ziyad, Ph.D., points to a bookcase full of binders and says, "Those are the case histories of adverse reactions to sulfites that have been reported to FDA. Since 1985, when the agency started reporting on sulfites through the Adverse Reaction Monitoring System, over 1,000 adverse reactions have been recorded."

As reports of adverse reactions mounted, FDA asked FASEB to reexamine the use of sulfites. FASEB's report, released in 1985, concluded that sulfites posed no hazard to most Americans, but that they were a hazard of unpredictable severity to people who were sensitive to the substance. Based on the FASEB study, FDA estimated that more than 1 million asthmatics are sensitive or allergic to the substance.

In 1986, FDA ruled that sulfites used specifically as preservatives must be listed on the label, regardless of the amount in the finished product. Sulfites used in food processing but not serving as preservatives in the final food must be listed on the label if present at levels of 10 parts per million or higher. Regulations issued in 1990 extended these required listings to standardized foods.

Also in 1986, FDA banned the use of sulfites on fruits and vegetables intended to be eaten raw, such as in salad bars and grocery store produce sections. Grocers and restaurateurs were using them to maintain the color and crispness of fresh produce. (Even before the FDA ban, industry trade groups had persuaded many of their members to stop using sulfites on fresh produce.)

In addition, sulfite-sensitive consumers are learning how to avoid sulfites. Consumer awareness combined with FDA actions have slowed the number of adverse reaction reports. Ziyad says that from 1990 to 1992, fewer than 40 were reported, and at press time, there had been only three reports in 1993.

Ziyad says the only way FDA can know about sulfite-sensitivity problems is through consumer and physician reports. Adverse reaction reporting is totally voluntary, and FDA encourages physicians to report patients' reactions to sulfites. But there are times when such reactions are not medically treated because the individual doesn't go to the doctor with the condition or the symptoms are not recognized. Such information would help FDA evaluate the current status of problems with foods among sulfite-sensitive individuals.

The agency's Adverse Reaction Monitoring System collects and acts on complaints concerning all food ingredients including preservatives. If you experience an adverse reaction from eating a food that contains sulfites, describe the circumstances and your reaction to the FDA district office in your area (see local phone directory) and send your report in writing to: Adverse Reaction Monitoring System (HFS-636) 200 C St., S.W. Washington, DC 20204.

A Sulfite by Any Other Name ...

People who are sulfite-sensitive should know which foods may possibly contain sulfites. But it's not always obvious by the chemical names on the label which ingredients are sulfites. Currently, there are six sulfiting agents allowed in packaged foods. The names by which they are listed on food labels are:

- sulfur dioxide
- sodium sulfite
- sodium and potassium bisulfite
- sodium and potassium metabisulfite

They are used in the following food categories at these typical maximum residual sulfur dioxide equivalent levels:

- baked goods: 30 ppm
- beer: 25 ppm
- wine: 275ppm
- tea: 90 ppm
- condiments and relishes: 30 ppm
- vinegar: 75 ppm
- dairy products: 200 ppm
- processed seafood products, other than dried or frozen: 25 ppm
- shrimp, fresh & frozen: 100 ppm
- lobster, frozen: 100 ppm
- gelatin: 40 ppm
- grain products: 200 ppm
- gravies and sauces: 75 ppm
- jam and jellies: 30 ppm
- nut products: 25 ppm
- plant protein isolates: 110 ppm
- dried fruit: 2,000 ppm
- fruit juices: 1,000 ppm in concentrates; 300 ppm in regular-strength juice
- glace fruit: 150 ppm
- maraschino cherries: 150 ppm
- dehydrated vegetables: 200 ppm
- dehydrated potatoes: 500 ppm
- canned vegetables: 30 ppm
- frozen potatoes: 50 ppm
- vegetable juice: 100 ppm

- filled crackers: 75 ppm
- soup mixes: 20 ppm in dry mix
- sugar: 20 ppm
- sweet sauces and syrups: 60 ppm
- molasses: 300 ppm

The symptom most reported by sulfite-sensitive people is difficulty breathing. Other problems range from stomach ache and hives to anaphylactic shock. In addition to knowing which food preservatives are sulfites and which foods are likely to contain them, sulfite-sensitive consumers can help themselves avoid health problems by following these suggestions:

- Read food labels and choose foods that don't contain sulfites.

- Be aware that foods served in restaurants, especially potato products and some canned foods, could contain sulfites. Ask the waiter if sulfites are used in what you plan to order.

For example, lemon juice in your tea or splashed on your salad could be a source of sulfites. Fresh-squeezed lemon is OK, but bottled lemon juice often contains sodium bisulfite.

Puzzling It Out

Preservatives are a puzzle for many consumers that can sometimes raise safety concerns. Even though these concerns are usually unfounded, some industry publications are reporting attempts to find naturally occurring substitutes for synthetic antioxidants. In a 1990 article, one such publication, *Inform*, says alternatives to synthetics are commercially available in the United States, although most are generally more costly or have other drawbacks. For example, tocopherol (vitamin E), generally is not as effective in vegetable fats and oils as it is in animal fats. Also, some herbs and herb extracts, such as rosemary and sage, can do the work of antioxidants, but they impart strong color or flavors. And just because these are plant-derived doesn't necessarily mean they are always safe. *Inform* points to the FDA rule that newly identified natural antioxidants, like other new food additives, must undergo rigorous toxicological tests before they can be approved.

As an additional alternative to synthetic antioxidants, the edible oil industry is increasingly using ultraviolet-barrier packaging and filling under nitrogen to protect the product's stability.

FDA scientists will continue to carefully evaluate all research presented to the agency on new preservatives to ensure that substances added to food to preserve quality and safety are themselves safe.

—by Judith E. Foulke

Judith E. Foulke is a staff writer for *FDA Consumer*.

Chapter 49

Dietary Supplements and Alternative Diets

Preventing and Treating Chronic Disease

Throughout evolution, human beings adapted to a wide range of naturally occurring foods, but the types of food and the mix of nutrients (in terms of carbohydrates, fats, and proteins) remained relatively constant. Food supplies were often precarious, and the threat of death from starvation was a constant preoccupation for most early humans.

However, about 10,000 years ago the agricultural revolution began making profound dietary changes in many human populations. The ability to produce and store large quantities of dried foods led to preferential cultivation of some foods, such as grains, which constituted new challenges to the human digestive system. Then about 200 years ago, the Industrial Revolution introduced advances in food production, processing, storage, and distribution. Recent technological innovations, along with increased material well-being and lifestyles that have allowed people more freedom in deciding what and when they wish to eat, have led to even further major dietary changes in

Office of Alternative Medicine (OAM), National Institutes of Health, Adapted from *Alternative Medicine: Expanding Medical Horizons*, a report prepared under the auspices of the Workshop on Alternative Medicine, held in Chantilly, VA, on September 14-16, 1992. The NIH cautions users not to seek the therapies described on these pages without the consultation of a licensed health care provider. Inclusion of a treatment or resource does not imply endorsement by the OAM, the NIH, or the Department of Health and Human Services (DHHS).

developed countries. Because changes in the dietary patterns of the more technologically developed countries, such as the United States, have been so dramatic and rapid, the people consuming these affluent diets have had little time to adapt biologically to the types and quantities of food that are available to them today. The longer term adverse health effects of the diet prevailing in these countries—characterized by an excess of energy-dense foods rich in animal fat, partially hydrogenated vegetable oils, and refined carbohydrates but lacking in whole grains, fruits, and vegetables—have become apparent only in recent decades.

Because of the recent, rapid rise in chronic illness related directly or indirectly to diet, the focus nutrition research has shifted away from eliminating nutritional deficiency to dealing with chronic diseases caused by nutritional excess. Another concern among nutrition researchers is the accumulation of evidence indicating that less-than-adequate intake of some micronutrients over a long period may increase the risks of developing coronary heart disease, cancers, cataracts, and birth defects. In recent decades the data on the relationship between certain dietary habits and nutritional intake have been growing exponentially. Designing interventions based on this wealth of research has become increasingly more difficult and complex.

Dietary Supplements

The Federal Government's approach to dietary intervention, formulated by boards composed of nutrition scientists, generally does not recommend supplementing the typical American diet with vitamins or nutrients beyond the recommended daily allowances (RDAs), nor does it suggest that some foods never be eaten. In contrast, many alternative dietary approaches contend that no amount of manipulation of the typical American diet is enough to promote optimum health or prevent eventual chronic illness. These alternative approaches represent a continuum of philosophies ranging from the concept that supplementing the typical American diet somewhat beyond the RDAs is necessary to promote optimum health, to the idea that supplementation well beyond the RDAs is often required to reverse the effects of long-term deficiencies. Other approaches advocate drastic dietary modification, either eliminating or adding certain types of foods or macronutrients, to treat specific types of conditions such as cancer and cardiovascular disease. Finally, there is the view that certain major staples of typical American diet, such as meat and dairy products, are basically unhealthy and should be generally avoided.

There is a growing body of data supporting the notion that the RDAs for minerals, such as calcium and magnesium, may be too low and that supplementation may be necessary to prevent the onset of chronic diseases. In addition, the RDAs for a number of vitamins and micronutrients, such as vitamin C, vitamin D, vitamin E, folate, and beta-carotene, may not be adequate to prevent chronic illness. For example, recent studies have found that the RDA for folate may need to be doubled for women as well as men.

Orthomolecular Medicine

Orthomolecular medicine—the therapeutic use of high-dose vitamins to treat chronic disease—promotes improving health and treating disease by using the optimum concentration of substances normally present in the body. Increasing the intake of such nutrients to levels well above those usually associated with preventing overt deficiency disease may have health benefits for some people. There is at least preliminary evidence that orthomolecular remedies may be effective in treating AIDS; bronchial asthma; cancer; cardiovascular disease, heart attacks, and stroke; lymphedema; and mental and neurological disorders.

Alternative Diets

A variety of alternative diets are offered for treating cancer, cardiovascular disease, and food allergies. Virtually all these interventions focus on eating more fresh and freshly prepared vegetables, fruits, whole grains, and legumes. Allergy to food has become a major area of research. Food intolerance is being studied as a causal or contributing factor in rheumatoid arthritis, and there is evidence that food-elimination diets may help many hyperactive children.

Some alternate dietary lifestyles are believed to offer a greater resistance to illness. These include several variations of the vegetarian diet, such as those consumed by Seventh-Day Adventists and proponents of the macrobiotic diet. Studies have found a significant lowering of risk factors for heart disease and certain forms of cancer in these two groups. Recent studies have also reported that certain cultural eating styles, such as the Asian and Mediterranean diets, appear to lower risk factors for heart disease and certain forms of cancer as well. Although there have been few controlled studies of the benefits of many traditional diets, such as those originally consumed by Native American Indians, diseases such as diabetes and cancer were not a problem for these populations until their diets became more Western, or affluent.

Because dietary and nutritional therapy interventions affect an array of biochemical and physiological processes in the body, evaluating their effectiveness may require equally complex methods. Furthermore, developing a comprehensive health care policy that incorporates diet and nutritional interventions may require taking into account Federal feeding programs and dissemination strategies that might present barriers to the effective propagation of adequate nutritional knowledge.

Chapter 50

Nutrition in a Can?

Manufacturers of liquid nutritional supplements such as Ensure, Sustical, Boost, and ReSource would have consumers believe that all middle-aged and older adults can benefit from using these products. According to them, liquid supplements (which are also available as puddings and powders) can help nearly everyone in this age group lose weight, gain weight, maintain weight, build muscle, or boost energy.

Such claims are unfounded. Virtually all nutritionists agree that liquid supplements are a poor choice for the average person when used as a substitute for meals on a regular basis. According to the American Pharmaceutical Association (APA), "although dietary supplements can be obtained without a prescription, they are complex agents with specific indications, and medical assessment should precede their use." In other words, supplements should be reserved for situations in which they're medically necessary (see "When Supplements Make Sense," below).

Once distributed primarily through hospitals, supplements can now be purchased at pharmacies, supermarkets, and convenience stores. Many manufacturers have gone so far as to promote them as meal substitutes, both for the well and the ill. And they're spending millions of dollars to drum up business just as the first wave of baby boomers turns 50. According to *The Wall Street Journal*, the advertising budget for Ensure, the market leader, rose from $3.6 million in 1991 to $44 million last year. In each of the past two years, sales have risen almost 50% for an estimated total of $500 million in 1995.

The ingredients found in supplements are almost certainly not harmful, but they do not provide the "balanced nutrition" manufacturers promise. Many products contain skim milk, water, sugars, vegetable oil, thickeners, and flavoring agents. One 8-ounce serving has about two-dozen vitamins and minerals, 10 to 16 grams of protein, 200 to 360 calories, 35 grams of carbohydrates, and 10 grams of fat. While this usually provides 15 to 50% of the recommended daily allowances for minerals and vitamins, it leaves out carotenoids, isoflavones, fiber, and many other important nutrients found in fruits, vegetables, and other wholesome foods.

Regularly substituting one of these drinks for a meal is a bad idea because you won't get the complete array of nutrients you need. And if you simply add a supplement to your regular diet without exercising more, you'll gain weight. Some people find the taste of supplements to be oily or medicinal, and a few experience side effects (primarily diarrhea). Furthermore, at $1 to $2 a serving, their expensive.

If you're looking for a nutritious snack or drink, it makes far more sense to reach for a piece of fruit, a container of non-fat yogurt, a glass of juice or skim milk, some nuts, or a slice of whole-grain bread spread with peanut butter. Such foods are much more nutritious—and often less expensive—than any liquid supplement the industry has yet to offer.

If you still think you need a supplement, consider taking a multivitamin instead and see your doctor, especially if you retain water, have diabetes or kidney problems, take blood-thinning medications such as warfarin or aspirin, or have a medical condition that requires regular monitoring.

When Supplements Make Sense

Liquid supplements were developed for those who are undernourished, not for people in good health with sound diets. Those most likely to benefit are the frail elderly (many of whom live alone and are thus more likely to eat poorly than those who are less isolated) and patients who are severely underweight. Others who may benefit include those with:

- chronic illness, such as colitis, diabetes, or congestive heart failure, accompanied by weight loss, weakness, and fatigue;

- mobility problems caused by illnesses such as arthritis, which may make food preparation difficult;

- swallowing and chewing problems, which may be caused by Parkinson's disease, stroke, or other illness;

- weight loss, caused by chemotherapy, cancer, or illnesses such as AIDS.

Chapter 51

Nutrition Quackery

Enzymes, botanicals, immune boosters and super green algae are a few of the products being promoted today as cures for every thing from fatigue to cancer.

But are consumers just being manipulated? While some people believe these products work, consumers need to be aware of the potential dangers these products pose and what they can do if they suspect a product or service is worthless—or even harmful.

The Harm in the Hype

Just because a product is an herb or "natural" does not mean it is necessarily safe.

For example, in February 1995, the American Medical Association reported a case of a woman who needed a liver transplant after the herbal preparation chaparral apparently caused severe hepatitis. Chaparral's active ingredient is a potent antioxidant, nordihydroguaiaretic acid, or NDGA. Advocates maintain that chaparral, made of the ground leaves of an evergreen desert shrub known as the creosote bush or greasewood, acts as a "free-radical scavenger" to slow aging and to improve other disorders. These claims remain unsupported by scientific studies. The AMA has urged physicians to question patients about their use of nontraditional medications.

"Nutrition Quackery: 'Miracle Cures' Come with Strings Attached," *Food Insight*, March/April 1995; reprinted with permission.

The Quest for Miracle Cures

Yet despite reported dangers, health and nutrition quackery thrives.

Quacks, defined in Webster's as those "...who, with little or no foundation, pretend to have skill or knowledge in a particular field," take advantage of the natural human tendency to want sure and quick answers to health conditions.

"With increased public awareness about health and fitness, consumers seem more willing than ever to spend hard-earned dollars to maintain or improve their health," said the U.S. Office of Consumer Affairs. "Quacks are keenly aware of this: they know too that media exposure has made many scientific terms at least vaguely familiar to consumers and frequent announcements of scientific breakthroughs have blunted skepticism about inflated claims for medications and treatments ... Chronic conditions are cash cows and terminal illnesses are golden opportunities to swindle people who are so desperate they'll try anything."

Indeed, of the $800 billion spent annually on health care, the federal government estimates that fraud and abuse account for $50 billion to $80 billion.

In addition to products, consumers should be wary of "specialists" who use unproven methods to detect dietary deficiencies. For example, hair analysis, although useful to detect heavy metal poisoning, is not a reputable way to test for general dietary deficiencies. Those deficiencies are usually diagnosed through blood, urine, tissue saturation or metabolic tests.

Other dubious practices include blaming food allergies as the culprit for symptoms ranging from headache and general malaise to depression. A true food allergy involves the immune system and sometimes can be life-threatening.

According to S. Allan Bock, M.D., "Adverse food reactions have multiple causes and mechanisms. These reactions need to be properly evaluated like other medical conditions. Consumers can start first with their family physician or practitioner to see if a referral to a specialist is necessary."

Consumers should also be wary of practitioners who rule out entire food groups and categories of food without undertaking medical diagnostic procedures.

Good Riddance to Bad Advice

What can consumers do to avoid being misled or defrauded? The best advice is still "let the buyer beware."

The first line of defense is to contact a qualified health professional with questions about a specific health condition and products that purport to help alleviate or cure that condition.

Sarah Short, Ph.D., EdD., R.D., writing on the role of the professional in health quackery in the June 1994 issue of the *Journal of the American Dietetic Association* said, "Know your subject area... be able to explain what is in the news. It is impossible to do too much homework."

"We need a Herculean educational program ... so that so-called magic products do not look so attractive," Short said.

What basic advice do experts give?

Be Skeptical. Regardless of the product, treatment or claim, if it sounds too good to be true, it probably is. Consumers should be skeptical and check out all dubious offers.

"Me rise of the 'alternative' slogan has given quacks a propaganda advantage. The media consider alternative medicine newsworthy and have therefore given these practitioners a lot of publicity," Barrett said. But "alternative" doesn't mean better, he warns.

Verify the Credentials of Information Sources. A survey by Ira Milner, R.D., coordinator of the Task Force for Nutrition Diploma Mills for the National Council Against Health Fraud, found that over half the "nutritionists" who advertised in the phone book only had a degree from a correspondence school. Check to see whether advanced degrees, such as Ph.D.s, are from accredited institutions.

Seek Qualified Professionals. Don't act on health or nutrition advice except from a qualified professional. In the 1990s, quacks are using the new communications technologies, including on-line services and CD-ROMs, to deliver bad advice and sell worthless products. However, its unlikely that anyone could make a proper diagnosis via computer.

Instead, look for a registered dietitian who has a minimum of four years of college study in the field of human nutrition, health, and food; has completed an internship; must maintain his or her practice credential through continuing education; and has an up-to-date state license (in states that require one).

Registered dietitians are skilled in developing a workable plan based on your food preferences and health needs for a lifetime of good eating. Ask your doctor, local hospital, health maintenance organization, clinic or health department for a referral.

Or you may call the National Center for Nutrition and Dietetics of the American Dietetic Association weekdays 10 a.m.–5 p.m. EST at 1-800-366-1655.

Build Your Diet on Whole Foods. Foods are more than the sum of their nutrients pulled apart and isolated into pills, powders and potions. Science continually discovers the marvels of little-known components in whole foods that work together to provide health benefits.

Enjoy a Variety of Foods. Choose foods in servings and portion sizes recommended in the Food Guide Pyramid.

Don't Exclude Foods or Food Groups. What you don't eat can affect your health, too. Be wary of products promoting one specific food or food component. Restricting food intake to only a certain combination of foods, or foods from certain food groups, may indeed rob you of the balance of nutrients needed for optimal well-being.

New Era, Old Claims

Although specific products, claims, and practices may have changed over the years, nutrition quackery still succeeds because people believe in the offer of a better, healthier life. The U.S. Office of Consumer Affairs urges consumers to be wary of products that:

- Claim to be quick, painless, and effortless.
- Claim to have special, secret, foreign, ancient, or natural ingredients.
- Claim to be effective for a wide variety of conditions.
- Rely on personal stories of success rather than on scientific data for documentation.
- Claim that the medical community or government agencies refuse to acknowledge the effectiveness of the cure, product, or treatment.

If It Happens to You

If you believe you've been victimized by a product or practitioner, contact:

- **Your Physician.** If you have a medical problem that is aggravated by or an adverse reaction to a product, contact your doctor first. You or your physician can then contact FDA's MedWatch at 1-800-322-1088, to file a formal complaint about the product and begin an FDA investigation of the incident. You can also begin with your local FDA Office.

- **Your Local or State Consumer Affairs Office of the State Attorney General** for action against an unlicensed practitioner.

- **The Federal Trade Commission (National Advertising Division) and the Council of Better Business Bureaus** for complaints about false or misleading advertising.

- **The Local Postal Inspector**, for products ordered through the mail.

Part Six

Nutrition Research

Chapter 52

Nutrients and Micronutrients: Progress in Understanding

Dietary Excess, Deficiency, and/or Imbalance

Diseases associated with dietary excess, deficiency and/or imbalance rank among the leading causes of illness and death in the United States. Major diseases in which diet plays a critical role include coronary heart disease, many types of cancer, cerebrovascular stroke, hypertension, obesity, dental caries, gingivitis and periodontal diseases, and noninsulin-dependent diabetes mellitus. For example, heart disease is the leading cause of death in the United States, with coronary heart disease accounting for 1.5 million myocardial infarctions and nearly 500,000 deaths each year. Cancer of the colon, breast, and prostate, closely associated epidemiologically with nutritional risk factors, causes more than 140,000 deaths every year.

Nutritional factors are also linked or associated with osteoporosis, iron deficiency anemia, neural tube defects, cleft lip and palate, and a host of other oral diseases. An estimated 40 percent of women in the United States will suffer from osteoporosis-related fractures by the time they reach 70 years of age. In all too many American inner cities and rural communities, school children living in poverty continue to develop rampant dental caries and other diseases associated with malnutrition. Disorders of overeating and undereating are common in older adults, with up to 40 percent having inadequate dietary intake of three or more nutrients. Many older adults suffer from

Excerpted from *Insights on Human Health*, National Institute of Dental Research (NIDR), September 1997 (subheads added).

protein-calorie malnutrition; up to 50 percent of nursing home residents in the United States may be malnourished.

In 1894, the first government official to offer Americans dietary advice, W.O. Atwater of the U.S. Department of Agriculture, sounded a warning on fatty and sugar-containing foods. Atwater advocated a diet low in fat, moderate in protein and high in complex carbohydrates. A century later, his sage advice and a number of improved public health and education measures appear to have made a significant difference in the morbidity and mortality of the American people; life expectancy has almost doubled in these 100 years. Today, it is common to stroll through the aisles of grocery stores and experience shoppers reading and evaluating their food item selection based on the nutritional facts label located on many packaged items. The public has a desire for improved quality of life and also possesses an increased awareness of nutrients and micronutrients and their role in reproduction, development, maintaining health and preventing disease throughout the life span.

Oral Tissues Can Provide Clues about Nutritional Status

Oral tissues and fluids exquisitely mirror subtle changes in nutritional status and are often the first sites of the body to exhibit clinical signs of malnutrition and micronutrient excesses, deficiencies or imbalances. The relatively high rates of epithelial stem cell division in the oral mucosal tissues, the production of saliva and its constituents, the rates of alveolar bone growth and resorption, and the inability of enamel to remodel all provide readily available opportunities to monitor the physiological status of humans throughout the life span. Virtually every classical nutritional deficiency disease, such as scurvy and pellagra, as well as a host of immune deficiencies, have signs and symptoms in the oral cavity. The lips, tongue, oral mucosa, gingiva, periodontal ligament and alveolar bone can all reflect nutritional status. Nutrients interact with physiological systems in the oral cavity such as cell division, deoxyribonucleic acid, or DNA, repair, protein synthesis and secretion, and immune-response mechanisms in such a manner as to increase or decrease the risk of disease.

Regulations and Nutrition

As early as 1906, public concern about unsafe foods, unregulated elixirs and misbranded products reached a level that led to the first attempts at federal legislative controls, resulting in the Pure Food and

Drug Act of 1906. In the ensuing years, rules in regard to the nutritional composition of some foods and supplements of vitamins and minerals acquired a legislative and regulatory history. A category of foods was established for special dietary use. The labeling of such foods was required to provide information about their vitamin, mineral and other dietary properties. By 1941, the Food and Drug Administration, or FDA, established regulations governing the labeling of vitamin and mineral substances and establishing minimal daily requirements, or MDR, to express the daily need for a vitamin and mineral. This need to promote health and prevent disease was assumed to be usually satisfied by a so-called good or balanced diet. At this time in history, the regulations had not considered the quantity or varieties of nutrients and/or micronutrients that could be included in a supplement or a fortified food. The Nutrition Labeling and Education Act (passed by Congress in 1990) required the FDA to develop an entirely new system of food labeling for packaged food. Succinctly, the FDA was requested to provide enforceable definitions for terms such as low fat, light and high fiber; to standardize portions; to strictly limit health claims; and to develop a standardized and mandatory chart of nutrients for all packaged foods.

Dietary Supplement Health and Education Act (DSHEA)

Ironically, despite attempts to regulate dietary supplements and food content of nutrients, which were often stayed pending judicial review and withdrawn, there were no formal labeling regulations for dietary supplements from 1973 to 1994. This changed with the Dietary Supplement Health and Education Act, or DSHEA, which was enacted by Congress in 1994. This act defined dietary supplements, placed the responsibility for ensuring their safety on manufacturers, established the manner in which literature may be used in connection with their sale, specified types of statements of nutritional support that may be made on labels, specified certain labeling requirements and provided for the establishment of regulations for good manufacturing practices. The legislation also created an Office of Dietary Supplements, which has since been established at the National Institutes of Health, or NIH. This office has a mandate to coordinate scientific research relating to dietary supplements within all of the NIH, and the office serves to advise other federal agencies on issues relating to dietary supplements.

In enacting DSHEA, Congress estimated that almost 50 percent of Americans regularly consume dietary supplements of vitamins, minerals or herbs as a means of improving nutrition. Congress appreciated that increasingly more Americans were assuming a responsibility to promote their own health. These emerging trends were also evident in the economy; sales of vitamins and minerals were $4.8 billion in 1995, followed by sales of botanical products at $2.5 billion and sports nutrition supplements at $0.8 billion. Within the vitamin/mineral category, multivitamin preparations constitute 31 percent of retail sales followed in amount of sales by vitamin E, vitamin C, iron, calcium and B vitamins. Some 1,500 to 1,800 botanicals are sold in the United States as dietary or ethnic traditional medicines. The top 10 purchased from selected health stores in 1995 were echinacea, garlic, goldenseal, ginseng, saw palmetto, aloe, ma huang, Siberian ginseng and cranberry. It would seem that the public is increasingly turning to complementary or alternative health promotion and disease prevention sources as we approach the end of this millennium.

In signing the DSHEA into law in 1994, President Clinton stated, " ... in an era of greater consciousness among people about the impact of what they eat, on how they live, indeed, how long they live, it is appropriate that we have finally reformed the way the government treats consumers and these supplements in a way that encourages good health." The president appointed a commission on Dietary Supplement Labels one year later. After public and executive hearings, the commission issued its draft report in June 1997. Included within this draft report are health claims that the FDA has approved over the past 5 years using the advice of scientific experts and based on publicly available scientific studies. Additional claims are considered when the manufacturer can demonstrate that the product is safe at levels used to support the claim.

The status of the health claims, as they apply to labeling, is divided into three groups:

- the approved health claims that can be used on dietary supplement and conventional food labeling;

- the approved health claims that could be used on conventional food labeling only;

- the health claims not authorized for labeling on supplements or conventional food based on lack of sufficient evidence to support the claim

In the first group, approval to label supplements and conventional food was given to the diet claim that calcium and its use, especially in teens and young adult women, [can help] avoid osteoporosis later in life. No upper limits were given; in its original proposal, the FDA felt that intakes above 2,000 milligrams daily were not likely to provide any additional benefits. A second example is soluble fiber from whole oats, which can be labeled in both supplements and in foods to reduce the risk of coronary heart disease. A third is the FDA approval of labeling supplements and foods containing sugar alcohols for their ability to reduce the extent of dental caries. The sugar alcohols considered in this group include xylitol, sorbitol, mannitol, malitol, isomalt, lacitol, hydrogenated starch hydrolysates and glucose syrups or combinations. The criteria for inclusion in this group included that the substance must be safe and lawful and not lower the plaque pH below 5.7. These requirements differ from the body's response to sucrose. Metabolism of this sugar creates an acid pH and a cariogenic environment. On April 4, 1997, the FDA was requested to add another naturally occurring four-carbon monosaccharide sugar alcohol, erythritol, to the list of sweeteners that do not promote the disease (dental caries) for which the U.S. population is at risk. Dental caries, though declining, particularly in children, represents a large portion of dental disease and remains widespread throughout the population.

Health Claims for Folate

A fourth FDA approved health claim that can be used to label dietary supplements and conventional foods is a public health preventive measure for the use of folate to prevent neural tube defects. The scientific research on the determination of a nutritional component that resulted in widespread benefits is one of the most important nutritional advances in recent years. The term neural tube defect, or NTD, applies to any malformation of the embryonic brain and/or spinal cord. Thirty years ago, it was suggested that maternal intake of certain vitamins during pregnancy affected the incidence of serious fetal malformation. Over the past few years, scientific inquiry has learned that folate (folic acid, a B vitamin) plays a crucial part in the development of neural tube closure during the embryonic period of human embryogenesis. The embryonic neural tube forms between the third and fourth week after fertilization, usually before a pregnancy is confirmed. During this time, the flattened neuroectoderm sheet folds inward, creating a u-shaped groove; thereafter, the lateral surfaces of the neural groove fuse posteriorly to form a tube. Failure of fusion during this crucial period, which occurs with inadequate amounts of the nutrient folate, jeopardizes further embryonic development of

Table 52.1. Approval of Health Claims for Dietary Supplement Labels

Approved Health Claims for Supplements and Conventional Foods

- Calcium supplementation for prevention of osteoporosis
- Soluble fibers from whole oats can reduce coronary heart disease
- Use of sugar alcohols for prevention of dental caries
- Folate supplements for prevention of neural tube defects

Approved Health Claims for Conventional Foods Only

- Dietary lipids and cancer
- Dietary saturated fat and cholesterol and coronary heart disease
- Fiber-containing grain products, fruits and vegetables and cancer
- Fruits and vegetables and cancer (for foods that are naturally a good source of vitamin A, vitamin C or dietary fiber)
- Fruits, vegetables and grain products that contain fiber, particularly soluble fiber, and coronary heart disease
- Sodium and hypertension

Health Claims Not Authorized

- Antioxidant vitamin and cancer
- Calcium-rich foods and hypertension
- Dietary fiber and cancer
- Dietary fiber and cardiovascular disease
- Omega-3 fatty acids and coronary heart disease
- Zinc and immune function in the elderly

Source: Commission on Dietary Supplement Labels. Draft report. Washington, D.C.: Office of Disease Prevention and Health Promotion, Public Health Service, U.S. Dept. of Health and Human Services, June 1997.

the central nervous system and the structures dependent on it. The defects may range in severity from anencephaly, or the absence of the cerebrum, to incomplete formation of the spinal cord (spina bifida), cranial bones, vertebral arches, meninges and overlying skin. NTD is among the most common of severe birth defects. The rate of occurrence with the first pregnancy is about 1 to 2 in 1,000 births. The incidence among African-Americans is less than 1 in 3,000. Couples who have produced a baby with an NTD have a 2 to 5 percent risk of such a defect recurring in a subsequent pregnancy. The same increased risk applies to the children of an affected parent. Second-degree relatives of an affected individual (nieces, nephews) have about a 1 in 100 risk; for first cousins, there is a risk of about 1 in 200. A number of congenital anomalies and diseases that are clearly familial do not fit the expectation for mendelian inheritance. More likely, these conditions, such as NTD, result from multifactorial inheritance of a continuously distributed variable, with a threshold (predisposition) separating the affected individual from the healthy individual. The predisposition may represent the sum of genetic and environmental influences. Maternal serum alpha-fetoprotein is elevated in about 99 percent of the amniotic fluids of fetuses with open NTDs and this test can be used to screen pregnancies at high risk. Although the Public Health Service in 1992 recommended that women during their entire childbearing years take 0.4 milligrams of folic acid per day to avoid neural tube birth defects, only 15 percent of women appear to take micronutrients, such as folic acid, in this recommended amount. A British medical council supported clinical research trials, which were randomized, controlled, double-blinded and multicentered; the results showed a 72 percent decrease in the recurrence of NTDs when women ingested 4 mg per day of folic acid from the date of randomization (before conception) to 12 weeks thereafter. Comprehensive K-12 education of the general public that results in science, mathematics and health literacy is essential to promote health, prevent disease, understand risk factors and provide a science-based foundation for considerations of diagnostics and therapeutics.

Although not yet considered by the FDA, the preventive effects of micronutrients such as folic acid or multivitamins in congenital craniofacial malformations, such as cleft lip and/or cleft palate, would appear to have many characteristics in common with NTD. A clinical study carried out in the Czech Republic demonstrated the prevention of facial cleft anomalies with a regimen of multivitamin and folic acid supplementation before conception and during pregnancy. The supplementation is associated with a 65.4 percent decrease in cleft lip/palate recurrence in families at risk: families that had one occurrence of cleft lip/palate among the first-degree relatives of the awaited child. Further studies are needed to establish whether the presumed preventive agent was folic acid or multivitamin supplement or both.

Problems Associated with Some Excessive Nutrient Intakes

These examples suggest that nutrients, when present or used as a supplement to the diet, especially in pregnant women, can exert a beneficial effect in the prevention of developmental anomalies in the human baby. Of course, we also anticipate a dose response in most issues in biology, so that we anticipate upper limits to the beneficial effects. For example, excessive amounts of nutrients can produce a teratogenic or developmental defect; this is well-exemplified by the teratogenic effects of excessive amounts of retinoic acid or vitamin A. Vitamin A is an unsaturated aliphatic alcohol and includes compounds that have the biological activity of retinol. It is essential for embryogenesis, growth and epithelial differentiation and is required for the production and regeneration of the visual purple for night vision. In the diet, it is found in dairy products, liver, fortified food and vitamin supplements. Beta carotene and other carotenoids are plant-synthesized precursors of vitamin partially converted to retinol during or after absorption. In the United States about 25 percent of adults ingest supplements containing vitamin A and about 5 percent take supplements of vitamin A alone. In animals, retinoids (but not carotenoids) have been found to be teratogenic. In the mid-1980s, it was discovered that use of isotretinoin, a synthetic retinoid used to treat cystic acne in adolescents, if consumed by a female during the first trimester increased the risk of malformation in a fetus 25-fold. The retinoic acid embryopathy included defects in craniofacial, skeletal, cardiac, thymic and central nervous system structures. This evidence is consistent with a common teratogenic mechanism by which natural and synthetic retinoids affect the development of cephalic neural crest cells, presumably by inducing programmed cell death or apoptosis, and thereby interfere with a number of developmental processes by reducing the number of cells required for normal morphogenesis of the head, face and jaws, skeleton and digits, heart, thymus gland and even the closure of the neural tube. In terms of molecular mechanisms, we are beginning to appreciate how retinoic acid binds to cognate receptors that, in turn, bind to unique regions within the promoter region of regulatory and/or structural genes. Recent evidence suggests that the expression of the homeo- box gene Hoxb-1, which regulates axial patterning in the embryo, is highly responsive to vitamin A and that excess vitamin A may induce altered pattern formation with apoptosis. A study from the Boston University School of Medicine found that infants born to women who took more than 10,000 international units of preformed vitamin A per day in the form of supplements had a one in 57 chance of having a malformation attributable to the supplement. The increased frequency of defects was concentrated among the infants born to women who had consumed high levels of vitamin A before the seventh week of gestation. The recommended daily allowance for women as published by the National Research Council is 800 retinol equivalents or approximately 2,700 IU of vitamin A per day. However, the daily ingestion of vitamin A in food plus the supplement brings the total amount of vitamin A close to 10,000 IU (approximately threefold more than the recommended amount). On the basis of this emerging scientific literature on the teratogenic effects of vitamin A, some manufacturers have reduced the level of vitamin A in multivitamin supplements or substituted beta carotene.

Establishing Standards for Nutritional Health Promotion

The need to provide national standards to serve the goals of health promotion through nutrition, to maintain good health and to serve as a science-based foundation for evaluating the adequacy of diets of groups of people has evolved in our astonishing 20th century. Despite the availability of only limited data to make these important public health decisions, national nutritional standards were published in 1943 as the Recommended Dietary Allowances, or RDAs, by the Food and Nutrition Board, a committee of the National Research Council under the auspices of the National Academy of Science. Since 1974, the RDAs have been defined as the gold standard levels of intake of essential nutrients, which on the basis of scientific knowledge are judged by the Food and Nutrition Board to be adequate to meet the known nutrient needs of practically all healthy people. RDAs are generally established based upon the following evidence:

- studies of subjects maintained on diets containing low or deficient levels of a nutrient, followed by correction of the deficit with measured amounts of the nutrient;

- nutrient balance studies that measure nutrient status in relation to intake;

- biochemical measurements of tissue saturation or adequacy of molecular function in relation to nutrient intake;

- nutrient intake of fully breast-fed infants and of apparently healthy people from their food supply;

- epidemiological observations of nutrient status in populations in relation to intake;

- in some cases, extrapolation of data from animal experiments. The RDAs are not based on dietary supplements or on special diets. The last edition of the RDAs was published in 1989.

Scientific knowledge regarding the role of nutrients has continued to expand since the inception of the RDAs. Contemporary studies address topics ranging from the prevention of classical nutritional deficiency diseases, such as rickets, to the reduction of risk of chronic diseases such as osteoporosis, cancer, diabetes and cardiovascular disease. In partnership with Health Canada, the Food and Nutrition Board has recently changed its approach to setting nutrient reference values. The new title is Dietary Reference Intakes, or DRIs. DRIs refers to at least three types of reference values:

- Estimated Average Requirement, or EAR, the intake value that is estimated to meet the requirement defined by a specific indicator of adequacy in 50 percent of an age- and gender-specific group;

- RDA, the dietary intake level that is sufficient to meet the dietary requirements of nearly all people in the group;

- Tolerable Upper Intake Limit, or UL, the maximum level of daily nutrient that is unlikely to pose risks of adverse health effects in almost all of the people in the group for whom it is designed.

The DRI project has been divided into seven nutrient groups and two subcommittees, each of which reports to the Standing Committee on the Scientific Evaluation of Dietary Reference Intakes. The seven nutrient groups are

- calcium, vitamin D, phosphorus, magnesium, fluoride;
- folate and other B vitamins;
- antioxidants (for example, vitamins C and E, selenium);
- macronutrients (for example, protein, fat, carbohydrates);

- trace elements (for example, iron, zinc);
- electrolytes and water;
- other food components (for example, fiber, phytoestrogens).

The panel for the first group hopes to release its report in 1997. The second group began its work in March 1997 with an expected report release date of April 1998. The Upper Reference Levels, or URL, subcommittees are working with the first group to establish UL levels. It is hoped that the entire group of nutrients will be reviewed and the DRIs released by the year 2000. [Information about the first two reports, one regarding calcium and related nutrients and the second on B vitamins and choline, can be found in Chapters 3 and 4 of this book.]

Conducting clinical research to assess the validity of statements on nutritional support is a complex endeavor. A claim that a product providing a feeling of well-being may be confounded with the placebo effect requires double-blinded studies using placebo to assess such statements. A statement that a product enhances immune function requires an appropriate challenge with acceptable immunological methodology that is sensitive and specific enough to accurately determine whether the product significantly improves resistance to very common diseases and disorders such as colds or flu. Such research is resource-intensive. The costs are such that pursuit of clinical testing may be of little interest to commercial manufacturing firms. Determination of disease prevention in the general population or even in a population at risk of developing a specific disease is even more expensive than determining an effect in a population with the disease. Consequently, the scientific information currently available on the specific effect of nutrition or supplements as applicable to health promotion and disease prevention or reduction remains fragmentary and incomplete. Randomized and prospective clinical trials are very important.

Nutrition and The Immune System

The immune system is critical toward understanding many infectious diseases and disorders. The effect of nutrients and micronutrients, or their absence, on the immune system is often studied in individuals or populations suffering from malnutrition either because of economic circumstances or in the context of a devastating disease such as AIDS. Many books on nutrition and immunology are available, and the *Journal of Nutritional Immunology* is now in its fourth year.

Malnutrition often presents devastating effects upon the antigen-specific arms of the immune system and on generalized host-defensive mechanisms. Protein-calorie malnutrition and/or deficiencies of single nutrients that assist in nucleic acid metabolism generally lead to atrophy of lymphoid tissue and dysfunctions of cell-mediated immunity. Deficiencies of specific nutrients that act as co-factors in enzymatic reactions can lead to impaired production of key enzymes and proteins. Iron deficiency is known to have effects on the internal structure and function of lymphocytes and reduce the ability of phagocytic cells to kill microorganisms. Zinc is the fundamental component of thymic hormones, the metal that allows these protein hormones to function in their roles in stimulating the activities of thymus-derived lymphocytes, or T-lymphocytes. Selenium serves as an antioxidant, contributing to antibody responses as well as to the cytotoxicity of natural killer cells. Humoral immunity continues to be maintained in malnutrition, although new primary responses to T-cell-dependent antigens are less than normal.

The nutrition and immunology of AIDS are complex and entwined. The immunologic dysfunctions associated with malnutrition have been termed nutritionally acquired immune deficiency syndromes, or NAIDS. Infants and small children are at great risk because they possess only immature, inexperienced immune systems and small protein reserves. Additional basic, translational, patient-oriented and community-based research is needed to understand the complex interacting effects of nutrients on immune functions.

Conclusion

The human condition in part reflects the balance between human behavior, the environment and biology. Each of us is dependent upon nutrients and micronutrients from our conception through senescence, and these dependencies change with stages of development, chronological age, gender, physical activity and health status. We require carbohydrates, proteins, lipids, vitamins, minerals and water. The specific requirement for each nutrient and micronutrient varies with age, stage in the life cycle, gender, physical activity, style of living, and psychological and sociocultural factors. The role of nutrition in health promotion, maintaining well-being, prevention of disease and disorders, and recovery from disease (for example, soft- and hard-tissue repair and regeneration) should not be underestimated. Important discoveries in molecular biology, physiology, intermediary metabolism, genetics and immunology continue to provide new opportunities for the improvement of health. The modern techniques for addressing the fundamental questions about the nature of living organisms that have evolved from these discoveries are just now being applied to nutritional research. Further application should advance biomedical nutritional discoveries at an unprecedented pace, permit the refinement and individualization of dietary guidance and nutritional interventions, and ultimately have a major impact on health.

For Additional Information

Organizations

American Institute of Nutrition
9650 Rockville Pike
Bethesda, Md. 20814
(301) 530-7050

National Institute of Dental Research Information Office
National Institutes of Health
Bethesda, Md. 20892
(301) 496-4261

National Institute of Diabetes and Digestive and Kidney Diseases
Nutritional Sciences Branch
National Institutes of Health
Bethesda, Md. 20892
(301) 594-8883

Publications

Butterworth CE Jr, Bendich A. Folic acid and the prevention of birth defects. *Ann Rev Nutr* 1996;16:73-97.

Commission on Dietary Supplement Labels, *Draft report*. Washington, D.C.: Office of Disease & Prevention and Health Promotion, 1997 (PHS) (DHHS).

Healthy People 2000: National Health Promotion and Disease Prevention Objectives. Washington, D.C.: U.S. Government Printing Office; 1-202-783-3238.

Tolarova M, Harris J. Reduced recurrence of orofacial clefts after periconceptional supplementation with high-dose folic acid and multivitamins. *Teratology* 1995;51:71-8.

Pfahl M, Chytil F. Regulation of metabolism by retinoic acid and its nuclear receptors. *Annu Rev Nutr* 16:257-83.

Chapter 53

Nutrition and the Immune System

Immune function protects healthy tissue from disease-promoting factors. Nutrient availability has the potential to affect almost all aspects of the immune system. Nutritional immunomodulation of patients in clinical settings has received a great deal of attention during the past few years.[1] As concern grows about acquired immunodeficiency syndrome[2] and the alarming increase in cases of tuberculosis in the United States,[3] the influence of nutrition and diet in enhancing or suppressing the immune response of healthy persons to promote optimal health is an important issue.

Several excellent reviews of research delineate the relationship of single nutrients to immune function.[4] In human beings, nutrient deficiencies often occur together, as do excess intakes. Research on the effects of multiple nutrient imbalances has been limited, yet nutrient interactions may be a key to explaining seemingly contradictory results of studies. In the Alpha-Tocopherol, Beta-Carotene Cancer Prevention Study in Finland,[5] the reported apparent adverse effect of supplemental beta carotene on prevalence of lung cancer might have been attributable to the interaction of a supplemental level of the antioxidant with low levels of other nutrients, (eg, selenium) altering immune cells and carcinogenesis.[6]

This article focuses on reports that examine imbalance of more than one nutrient and interactive effects on immunocompetence.

Nutrient-Nutrient Interactions and the Effect on Immunity

Vitamin-Nutrient Interactions

Vitamin E and selenium. Among the first reports of the role of selenium in mammalian metabolism was one of an interaction between selenium and vitamin E. Schwarz and Foltz[13] found that selenium in small amounts could prevent the liver necrosis observed in rats deficient in vitamin E. So began the saga of a relationship between these two nutrients. In an early report of the relationship and immune function, Spallholz *et al.*[14] noted that the effect of dietary selenium and vitamin E on antibody titer was additive.

During the past 20 years, studies have been conducted to assess the influence of vitamin E and selenium on immune function in several species of animals. Both nutrients function in the maintenance of biological membranes, selenium as a component of glutathione peroxidase, which reduces hydrogen peroxide and other hydroperoxides in the cytosol to prevent formation of free radicals[15], and vitamin E as an antioxidant that prevents lipid hydroperoxide formation by quenching free radicals.[16] Together they protect unsaturated membrane phospholipids and protein sulfhydryl groups from oxidants that may impair cellular function.[17]

Other reports also provide evidence of an interaction between the two nutrients.[18,19] Deficiency studies of a nutrient allow identification of the function of that nutrient. For example, Eskew *et al.*[20] induced a double deficiency in rats. In comparison with animals low in either selenium or vitamin E, a decrease in magnitude of splenic cytolytic T-lymphocyte activity and splenocyte response to mitogen stimulation was noted in the doubly deficient group. Conversely, the same animals demonstrated an increase in ADCC [antibody-dependent cellular cytotoxicity] activity, which was not surprising to Eskew *et al.* because they expected reactive oxygen metabolites that are involved in mediating cytotoxic reactions to be present in higher amounts when less antioxidant was present. Findings that some components of the immune system are not impaired but actually may be enhanced with low levels of these antioxidant nutrients were reported in other studies as well.[21,22]

Marsh *et al.*[23] described a mechanism by which immune function might be impaired by combined vitamin E and selenium deficiency, that is, reduced thymic growth. Combined deficiency was associated with a gradual degeneration of the epithelium and depletion of lymphocytes within lymphoid tissue. These researchers concluded that the major targets of deficiency of these two nutrients were the primary lymphoid organs.

In studies with dogs and pigs, a combined deficient diet suppressed lymphocyte response to mitogens more than diets deficient in either vitamin E or selenium alone.[24] Perhaps a substance such as a lipid oxidation product was present in the blood of the deficient animals and suppressed immune function. It has been suggested that in addition to the increased lipid and protein oxidation that accompanies lack of vitamin E and selenium, membrane function may be destroyed and membrane enzymes and receptors inactivated.[24,25] Perhaps lack of antioxidants, particularly vitamin E, results in abnormally high levels of prostaglandins, which impairs immune function. Vitamin E has been reported to control prostaglandin E_2 synthesis.[26]

Humoral immunity (eg, levels of immunoglobulins) was improved in rats given selenium and vitamin E compared with rats deficient in both nutrients.[27] A pronounced effect occurred on immunoglobulin M, and vitamin E seemed to compensate for the effects of selenium deficiency on immunoglobulin G.

Two studies in pigs revealed interactions between dietary vitamin E and selenium with respect to resistance to infectious disease. Sows were given oral supplements containing vitamin E alone, selenium alone, or both vitamin E and selenium. Vitamin E and selenium deficiencies resulted in reduced phagocytic activity by PMNs [polymorphonuclear neutrophil leukocytes] from peripheral blood. The combined deficiency exerted a more severe effect on PMN function, with impairment of intracellular killing in addition to reduced phagocytic uptake, and extension of the detrimental effects to colostral as well as blood leukocytes.[28] In a similar study in cattle, however, animals given both nutrients had higher percentages of B cells than animals supplemented with either vitamin E or selenium.[29] In another study, weanling pigs were made deficient in vitamin E and selenium over a 25-day period. They were infected with *Salmonella typhisuis* during the last 4 days of the dietary treatment. The proliferative response to three different mitogens (concanavalin A, phytohemagglutinin, and pokeweed mitogen) was not affected when cultures of peripheral blood lymphocytes were grown in medium containing fetal bovine serum. However, the addition of autologous serum suppressed proliferation in cells from pigs deficient in selenium and vitamin E.[22] These results suggest that adequate levels of selenium and/or vitamin E must be present *in vitro* to support lymphocyte mitogenesis.

In an investigation of lymphocytes conducted with T cells from chickens deficient in selenium and vitamin E, Chang *et al.*[30] suggested that impaired immune capability was associated primarily with problems in maturation of T lymphocytes within the thymus and functional and proliferative capabilities of lymphocytes in the periphery.

A conclusion can be drawn from these studies: Although selenium can spare vitamin E and vice versa, at least to a certain degree,[31,32] when selenium and vitamin E are not present in adequate levels, immune function is impaired more severely than when only one is inadequate. Both nutrients are needed for optimal response.

Average intakes of selenium measured in the Total Diet Study for 1982 to 1986[33] for the United States exceeded the Recommended Dietary Allowances (RDAs).[34] Dietary content of selenium varies with soil content, however, so deficient intakes are likely in some countries.[35] Vitamin E intakes seem to be highly variable but are probably adequate for most healthy people, which is why the RDA is based on usual intakes.[34] In vitamin E deficiency, impaired immunocompetence occurs earlier than more classical symptoms of vitamin E deficiency.[36] This suggests that immune status might be a logical parameter to evaluate in the development of dietary recommendations.

Even though deficiency of vitamin E and selenium is unlikely among healthy persons in the United States, supplementation with vitamin E and selenium is quite common, especially among subpopulations such as the elderly.[37] Limited evidence exists about the relationship between supplementation of vitamin E and selenium and the effect on immune response. Several studies have been conducted in human subjects in which supplementation with vitamin E only or multiple vitamins and minerals yielded positive results on immune function.[38-40] Nevertheless, only one study with chicks was identified in which supplementation of vitamin E and selenium to diets already adequate in these nutrients was assessed.[41] Compared with unsupplemented groups, groups fed the vitamin E and selenium supplement had enhanced immune function, including higher geometric mean titers of the tube agglutination test against a microbial antigen and higher numbers of rosette-forming cells in the peripheral blood. Information is certainly incomplete about the potential benefit on immunocompetence associated with supplementation of vitamin E and selenium. Of course, the adverse effect of excessive intakes of selenium on immune function has been documented.[14]

Vitamin E and Vitamin C. Another example of an interaction with vitamin E involves vitamin C. A synergistic effect of supplemental vitamins E and C on inhibition of release of arachidonic acid was observed in an *in vitro* study.[42] Because inhibition of arachidonic acid has been reported to result in stimulation of immune cell responses and suppression of tumor growth in animals and human beings,[43,44] ElAttar and Lin[42] suggested that supplemental vitamins C and E might be effective in minimizing the chemotherapy and radio-therapy required for treatment of patients with cancer. More research is needed in this area.

Vitamin E and Vitamin A. An antagonistic effect between vitamins E and A has been noted in several studies. Although supplements of both vitamin E and A were observed to increase antibody production and phagocytosis, when either one was increased immune function was less.[45,46] This effect may occur because of the suppression of gastrointestinal absorption and of tissue reserves of vitamin E by high levels of vitamin A.[47] The possibility exists that supplements of only beta carotene, a precursor of vitamin A, could have interfered with vitamin E availability in the clinical trial in Finland referred to earlier. This could have resulted in the higher incidence of lung cancer compared with groups supplemented with both beta carotene and vitamin E or not supplemented with beta carotene.[5] Another study, however, reported that supplemental vitamin E apparently interfered with vitamin A.[48] Bactericidal activity of neutrophils was suppressed by supplementation of either nutrient, whereas supplements of both enhanced neutrophil activity.

Vitamin A and Vitamin D. Vitamin A nutriture is clearly linked to optimal immune responses. Dietary deficiencies of vitamin A or retinol have been shown to produce impairment of mitogen-induced proliferation in rats,[49] reduced antibody responses to pneumococcal polysaccharide,[50] and decreased NK cell and IFN-γ [interferon-γ] activity in rats.[51] Resistance to infectious disease was observed to be impaired in vitamin A-deficient rodents and chickens.[52]

Experiments to examine the interaction between vitamin A and vitamin D have been carried out in human macrophagelike cell lines *in vitro*. Both vitamins are known to have hormonelike effects on the maturation and differentiation of monocytes. One set of studies has demonstrated apparent antagonism between vitamins A and D. Cell lines U937 and THP-1 were treated with either vitamin alone or both simultaneously. Vitamin A alone upregulated expression of the surface marker CD11b and increased the production of eicosanoids and prostanoids. The addition of both vitamin D and vitamin A did not induce additional products of the arachidonic acid cascade.[53] On the other hand, vitamin D alone upregulated the lipopolysaccharide receptor (CD14) on the surface of U937 cells and suppressed the vitamin

471

A-induced expression of the Fc receptor for immunoglobulin E (CD23).[54] These results were interpreted as evidence of functional antagonism between the two compounds. Sellmayer *et al.*[53] suggest that each vitamin induces the differentiation of a distinct monocytic subtype.

In contrast, another research team has reported that retinoic acid and vitamin D act synergistically to induce macrophagelike properties in U937 cells. Doubly treated cells were more phagocytic and exhibited an enhanced oxidative burst.[55] More recently, the effects of these two vitamins on cytokine production by lipopolysaccharide-stimulated U937 cells were examined. Retinoic acid alone failed to induce IL[interleukin]1ß, TNF-α [tumor necrosis factor-α], or IL6 even in the presence of lipopolysaccharide. Vitamin D alone induced cytokine mRNA but not cytokine secretion. When both retinoic acid and vitamin D were incubated together with U937 cells, both cytokine mRNA and secretion were enhanced. Tiami *et al.*[56] reported that this synergism was not seen in two other human macrophagelike cell lines, THP-1 and HL-60.

Mineral-Nutrient Interactions

Magnesium. Evidence reviewed by Kubena[57] indicates that magnesium functions in the development, distribution, and function of immune cells and soluble factors that are critical for humoral and cell-mediated immunity. Magnesium depletion occurs in disorders ranging from alcoholism to cardiovascular disease and is associated with the use of a variety of medications. Because it is essential for the activity of more than 300 enzymes, it is not surprising that magnesium influences the metabolism of many other nutrients. For example, alterations of potassium, calcium, phosphorus, and sodium metabolism are associated with magnesium deficiency.[58] Similarly, magnesium homeostasis may be affected by other nutrients.

In vitro (cell culture) studies illustrate that certain functions of the immune system are affected when the availability of minerals changes. In one such study, Jackson *et al.*[59] found that calcium, magnesium, and manganese were needed for normal function of leukocytes (cell adhesion), but excess calcium ions displaced magnesium, thus reducing adhesion.[59] Other interactions between magnesium and vitamin E,[60] iron, copper, zinc,[61] manganese, calcium,[62,63] and other nutrients[62] that influence the function of immune cells have been reported. Although intake of magnesium below recommended levels is usual among some population groups in developed countries,[64] supplementation with single or multiple micronutrients is common.[37]

Whether the interactive effects of mineral imbalance on immune function that have been found to occur *in vitro* also occur *in vivo* is not known but needs to be investigated.

Magnesium is but one example of a mineral that is interrelated with other nutrients and thus might enhance or impair immune function differently in the presence of low or high amounts of the other nutrients.

Copper. Other mineral nutrients have been examined for their effects on immune function and resistance to infectious disease. Single nutrient deficiencies of copper and iron, for example, are known to affect several aspects of the immune response adversely.[65,66] Mineral nutrients serve as important cofactors for enzymes that are vital for lymphocyte and macrophage function. In addition, the ability of the host to sequester mineral nutrients (eg, iron) and to compete successfully with microbes for limiting supplies is thought to be an important aspect of resistance to some infections.[66] Compared with the extensive literature on the effect of single mineral nutrient deficiencies on immunity, relatively few studies have examined interactive effects. Some investigators have examined combinations during a dietary depletion phase, and others have studied combinations during supplementations.

Several studies in cattle have demonstrated interesting combined effects of dietary copper and other nutrients on PMN phagocyte function, lymphocyte proliferation, and antibody production. Investigators have documented functional copper deficiency in cattle fed diets high in iron[67] or molybdenum.[67,68] Secondary copper deficiency resulted in significant reductions in phagocytosis of latex beads by PMNs, which could be reversed by deleting iron or adding copper to the diet.[67] The suppression of PMN function was more severe in secondary, rather than in primary, copper deficiency. Antibody production, on the other hand, was unaffected in copper-deficient cattle immunized with chicken γ-globulin.[67]

Detrimental effects of combined dietary deficiencies of copper and selenium on phagocyte functions have also been documented in cattle. Cattle deficient in copper and selenium had PMNs that phagocytized the yeast *Candida albicans* as efficiently as cells from normal cattle, but were significantly impaired with regard to nitroblue tetrazolium reduction and, most importantly, intracellular killing of *C. albicans*. The effect of combined copper and selenium deficiencies in this model was found to be additive, so that each metal nutrient affected PMN function by an independent pathway.[69]

An alternative approach in cattle has been to investigate the effects of combined dietary supplementation of copper with or without molybdenum and sulfur. The addition of molybdenum and sulfur to the diet resulted in reduced phytohemagglutinin-stimulated lymphoproliferation and reduced baseline proliferation in peripheral blood cells. No effect was seen on antibody production after immunization with ovalbumin. The suppression of lymphocyte proliferation may have been a result of secondary copper deficiency, because cattle fed the molybdenum and sulfur supplement had reduced plasma copper levels.[70]

The detrimental effect of high sulfur diets on PMN function in sheep was examined by supplementing the diets with thiamin, copper, or molybdenum. The addition of thiamin was observed to enhance killing of *C. albicans* by PMNs, whereas copper supplementation improved the phagocytic uptake of these yeast cells by PMNs.[71]

Thus, selected immune responses in ruminants appear to be quite susceptible to reduced copper availability, which, in turn, can result from excess iron or molybdenum in the diet. High sulfur intake appears to be suppressive for PMN functions and lymphocyte proliferation, and this effect can be spared by copper and thiamin supplements. These results underscore the importance of appropriate nutrient balance and the highly interactive nature of mineral nutrients in maintaining immune cell functions in domestic animals. The relevance of these observations for human health has yet to be investigated.

Zinc. Zinc is undoubtedly the most intensely studied nutrient with regard to its effects on immune responses. In both human beings and in animals used experimentally, dietary zinc deficiency has a profound suppressive effect on thymic function, T-lymphocyte development, lymphoproliferation, T-cell-dependent B-cell functions, and resistance to infections.[72] Conversely, zinc supplementation has been shown to enhance certain immune responses in people.[38,39]

Several laboratories have reported interactions between zinc and other nutrients with respect to immune functions and resistance to infectious disease. For example, interactions between zinc and copper have been examined *in vivo* in mice and *in vitro* in human peripheral blood leukocytes. Mice receiving excess copper (100 or 200 ppm) in their drinking water for 8 weeks demonstrated suppressed mitogen-induced lymphoproliferative responses and reduced numbers of splenic plaque-forming cells in the classic Jerne plaque assay after immunization with sheep erythrocytes. The latter is a T-cell-dependent B-cell response. This immunosuppression by dietary copper was reversed in mice that received injections of zinc (1.14 mg/kg), which implies that the T-cell defects were the result of secondary zinc deficiency produced by excess copper.[73] In cultures of human peripheral blood leukocytes, the addition of copper salts suppressed the production of the proinflammatory cytokines IL1 and IL6, whereas zinc salts stimulated IL1 production and had no effect on IL6. When added together, copper and zinc stimulated the production of TNF-α, but not IL1, in a synergistic fashion upon the addition of lipopolysaccharide.[74] These results suggest that interactive effects of zinc and copper on the immune response may involve differential cytokine stimulation.

A study of persons in Thailand examined the effects of supplementing children's diets with either zinc alone (25 mg/day), vitamin A alone (1,500 RE/day), or the combination of zinc and vitamin A. The combined supplement normalized conjunctival epithelium in a synergistic manner and significantly increased the proliferative response of peripheral blood lymphocytes to tuberculin purified protein derivative but not to concanavalin A or tetanus toxoid. Interestingly, the immunoenhancing effects of zinc and vitamin A were observed in girls but not in boys.[75,76]

The relationship between zinc and protein has been examined in two models of experimental infectious disease. McMurray and Yetley[77] studied moderate protein deficiency (10% ovalbumin) and zinc deficiency (<5 ppm), separately and combined, in guinea pigs vaccinated with the tuberculosis vaccine, Mycobacterium bovis BCG. Protein deficiency, with or without concomitant zinc deficiency, resulted in reduced splenic cellularity and reduced delayed hypersensitivity reactions to purified protein derivative in the skin. All three deficient groups failed to control the early replication of BCG in the tissues. Suppression of phytohemagglutinin-induced proliferation of peripheral blood lymphocytes at high mitogen doses was observed only in the group with combined protein and zinc deficiency.[77]

Similar results were obtained in mice rendered protein deficient, zinc deficient, or protein and zinc deficient and infected with a lethal dose of *Salmonella typhimurium* by injection intraperitoneally. Protein deficiency alone increased weight loss and mortality, but zinc deficiency alone did not. The combined deficiency, however, shortened the survival of infected mice even more than protein deficiency alone.[78]

Zinc has been shown to antagonize the detrimental effects of toxic dietary metals, such as nickel, on the immune response. Mice fed nickel alone and immunized with keyhole-limpet hemocyanin (KLH) exhibited suppressed antigen-specific immune responses *in vivo* (serum anti-KLH antibodies) and *in vitro* (KLH-induced lymphoproliferation). Zinc supplementation reversed the effects and produced immune responses that were not different from those of control animals.[79]

Fat-Nutrient Interactions

Fatty acids may influence the immune system in a number of ways. Alteration in membrane composition is known to result in changes in fluidity and transmembrane receptor function in immune cells.[80] Arachadonic acid metabolism may be altered by dietary fat quantity and quality; results are changes in highly immunomodulatory prostaglandin production.[17]

Fatty Acids and Vitamin E. Immunosuppression associated with fatty acids, particularly polyunsaturated fatty acids, might be beneficial in conditions involving an overactive immune response, such as rheumatoid arthritis or psoriasis,[81] but it is not desirable under other circumstances, for example, injury.[82] Interaction with other nutrients could moderate such an effect. For instance, alterations in macrophages from rats fed a diet rich in polyunsaturated fatty acids were reversed by adding vitamin E.[83] Similarly, inhibition of proliferation of lymphocytes *in vitro* by several fatty acids, especially the polyunsaturated, was observed, but the condition improved when vitamin E was present in cell cultures.[80] This suggested that suppression might be attributable to oxidative products from fatty acids, as a similar benefit was noted when vitamin C, another antioxidant, was introduced. Calder and Newsholme[80] concluded that fatty acids might affect lymphocyte proliferation primarily by changing the composition of the cell membrane and, thus, fluidity and function.

Studies investigating the relationship between dietary fat fed to mothers and immune function of offspring include one in which the effect of sunflower oil, which is highly polyunsaturated, did not differ from that of animal fat, although immune function in young pigs benefited from supplemental vitamin E.[84] On the other hand, in a study monitoring development of cell-mediated immunity in newborn pigs, those born to mothers fed fish oil tended to acquire the ability to respond to mitogens (phytohemagglutinin and concanavalin A) more slowly than those born to mothers fed beef tallow or no added fat.[85] Vitamin E fed to mothers did not allow more rapid acquisition of cell-mediated immunity except when fed at high levels, that is, up to four times the recommended intake.

An explanation for the benefit of high levels of vitamin E on immune function when n-3 fatty acids are fed comes from work by

Fritsche *et al.*,[86] who demonstrated that feeding fish oil severely reduced tocopherol content of immune cells, which was followed by lowered immune response. Rats were fed diets with one of two types of dietary fat (corn oil or fish oil) and three levels of supplemented vitamin E (30, 300, and 900 mg/kg). Animals were immunized with sheep erythrocytes and the number of Jerne plaque-forming spleen cells was determined. The most robust antibody response was observed in the rats fed fish oil with high levels of vitamin E. The data suggested that the α-tocopherol levels in splenocytes were actually increased in the fish oil-fed, but not in the corn oil-fed, animals supplemented with vitamin E. Further, levels of immunosuppressive prostaglandin E_2 were reduced in rats fed fish oil; this effect was independent of vitamin E supplementation.[86]

Support for this mechanism was provided by a human study. The suppressed response of T lymphocytes to mitogens that occurred when n-3 fatty acids were fed to human beings was normalized by increased intakes of vitamin E (22 mg/day).[87] Because of the importance of vitamin E to lymphocyte proliferation and other aspects of immune function, its interaction with fatty acids merits further study.

Fat and Selenium. The interactions between dietary fat and other nutrients, and between different fatty acids themselves, have been examined with respect to effects on immunity. A study in rats demonstrated interesting interactions between dietary fat and selenium. Neonatal rats were fed diets that contained high or low levels of corn oil combined with either high or low levels of selenium. The rats were immunized with a heterologous protein (bovine serum albumin), and the serum antibody titers were determined. Rats consuming the combined diet with excess fat and excess selenium experienced a significant suppression in circulating antibody levels 1 to 2 weeks after immunization.[88]

Fat and Vitamin A. Fatty acid and vitamin A deficiencies, alone and combined, were studied for their effects on the induction of carcinogen-induced lung tumors in rats.[89] Groups of animals were fed either 6% peanut oil or no added oil, combined with either 2,000 IU vitamin A per 100 g of diet or no added vitamin A. Vitamin A deficiency alone enhanced tumor burden, whereas fatty acid deficiency alone protected against tumor formation both in terms of the percentage of animals with tumors and the mean number of tumors per animal. In rats consuming the diet deficient in both vitamin A and fat, the fatty acid deficiency apparently protected the rats against the enhanced tumor burden expected to be induced by vitamin A deficiency. The authors proposed alterations in carcinogen metabolism or glutathione-mediated detoxification mechanisms to explain their results.[89]

It is clear from the studies just reviewed that dietary fat and other nutrients can interact and affect the immune response notably. There is also evidence, however, that the individual fatty acids can interact with each other to alter immunologic reactivity. Various doses of palmitic, stearic, oleic, and linoleic acids, alone or combined together in a "physiologic" mixture (ie, at the same relative concentrations found in certain natural fats), were added to cultures of human peripheral blood leukocytes. The cultures were stimulated with the polyclonal T-cell mitogen phytohemagglutinin, and proliferation and cytokine production were measured. All fatty acids stimulated IL1ß production, and all but linoleic acid stimulated proliferation. IL2 production was stimulated by palmitic acid and suppressed by stearic and oleic acids. IFN-γ was stimulated only by palmitic acid and the mixture, whereas TNF-α was suppressed only by palmitic and stearic acids. The mixture tended to attenuate the positive or negative effects of individual fatty acids in this system.[90]

Applications

Research reviewed here suggests that nutrient supplementation may enhance but may also suppress immune function mediated by effects of the supplement on other nutrients. Because of the influence of the immune system on overall health, as well as on infectious disease and tumor resistance, enhancing or sometimes suppressing immune function is of great interest. Consumers may attempt to achieve these goals through the use of supplements, frequently of single nutrients at high levels. Research clearly indicates that nutrients playing vital roles in immune function may often affect or be affected by other nutrients. Dietitians should thus encourage the intake of a variety of nutrient-dense foods to promote proper balance among all nutrients. For consumers who are not deficient in one or more nutrients but nevertheless are intent on using supplements, products that provide multiple nutrients (ie, multivitamin and multimineral) without supplying excess amounts should be encouraged. Far more research into nutrient-nutrient interactions and immune function, particularly in human subjects, is needed. At this time, the best dietary advice to enhance immune function in healthy people seems to be variety, balance, and moderation.

References

1. McClave SA, Lowen CC, Snider HL. Immunonutrition and enteral hyperalimentation of critically ill patients. *Dig Dis Sci.* 1993; 37:1153-1161.

2. Watson RR. Nutrition, immunomodulation and AIDS: an overview. *J Nutr.* 1992;112:715.

3. McMurray DN, Bartow RA. Immunosuppression and alteration of resistance to pulmonary tuberculosis in guinea pigs by protein undernutrition. *J Nutr.* 1992;122:738-743.

4. Chandra RK, Sarchielli P. Nutritional status and immune responses. *Clin Lab Med.* 1993;13:455-461.

5. The Alpha-Tocopherol, Beta Carotene Cancer Prevention Study Group. The effect of vitamin E and beta carotene on the incidence of lung cancer and other cancers in male smokers. *N Engl J Med.* 1994; 330:1029-1035.

6. Blumberg A. The Alpha-Tocopherol, Beta-Carotene Cancer Prevention Study in Finland. *Nutr Rev.* 1994; 52:242-250.

7. Reichlin S. Neuroendocrine-immune interactions. *N Engl J Med.* 1993; 329:1246-1253.

8. Scott P. Selective differentiation of CD4+ T helper cell subsets. *Curr Opinion Immunol.* 1993; 5:391-397.

9. Murphy DB. T cell-mediated immunosuppression. *Curr Opinion Immunol.* 1993; 5:411-417.

10. Lotzova E. Definition and functions of natural killer cells. *Nat Immun.* 1993; 12:169-176.

11. Coligan JE, Kraisbeek AM, Margulies DH, Shevach EM, Strober W, eds. *Current Protocols in Immunology.* New York, NY: John Wiley & Sons; 1994.

12. Rose N, Friedman H, eds. *Manual of Clinical Immunology.* 3rd ed. Washington, DC: American Society for Microbiology; 1986.

13. Schwarz K, Foltz CM. Selenium as an integral part of factor 3 against dietary necrotic liver degeneration. *J Am Chem Soc.* 1957; 79:3292-3293.

14. Spallholz JE, Martin JL, Gerlach MS, Heinzerling RH. Immunologic responses of mice fed diets supplemented with selenite selenium. *Proc Soc Exp Biol Med.* 1973; 143:685-689.

15. Burk RF. Biological activity of selenium. *Ann Rev Nutr.* 1983; 3:53-70.

16. Urano S, Matsuo M. A radical scavenging reaction of alpha-to-copherol with methyl radicals. *Lipids.* 1976; 11:380-386.

17. Chow CK. Nutritional influences on cellular antioxidant defense systems. *Am J Clin Nutr.* 1979; 32:1066-1081.

18. Finch JM, Turner RJ. Enhancement of ovine lymphocyte responses: a comparison of selenium and vitamin E supplementation. *Vet Immunol Immunopathol.* 1989; 23:245-256.

19. Pollock JM, McNair J, Kennedy S, Kennedy DG, Walsh DM, Goodall EA, Mackie DP, Crockard AD. Effects of dietary vitamin E and selenium on in vitro cellular immune responses in cattle. *Res Vet Sci.* 1994; 56:100-107.

20. Eskew ML, Scholz RW, Reddy CC, Todhunter DA, Zarkower A. Effects of vitamin E and selenium deficiencies on rat immune function. *Immunology.* 1985; 54:173-180.

21. Turner RJ, Finch JM. Immunological malfunctions associated with low selenium-vitamin E diets in lambs. *J Comp Pathol.* 1990; 109:99-109.

22. Lessard M, Yang WC, Elliott GC, Rebar AH, Van Vleet JF, Deslauriers N, Brission GJ, Schultz RD. Cellular immune responses in pigs fed a vitamin E- and selenium deficient diet. *J Anim Sci.* 1991; 69:1575-1582.

23. Marsh JA, Combs GF, Whitacre ME, Dietert RR. Effect of selenium and vitamin E dietary deficiencies on chick lymphoid organ development. *Proc Soc Exp Biol Med.* 1986; 182:425-436.

24. Lessard M, Yang WC, Elliot GS, Deslauriers N, Brisson GJ, Van Vleet JF, Schultz RD. Suppressive effect of serum from pigs and dogs fed a diet deficient in vitamin E and selenium on lymphocyte proliferation. *Vet Res.* 1993; 24:291-303.

25. Parker L. Interactions among antioxidants in health and disease: vitamin E and its redox cycle. *Proc Soc Exp Biol Med.* 1992; 200:271-276.

26. Meydani SN, Meydani M, Verdon CP, Shapiro AA, Blumberg JB, Hayes KC. Vitamin E supplementation suppresses prostaglandin E2 synthesis and enhances the immune response of aged mice. *Mech Ageing Dev.* 1986; 34:191-201.

27. Bauersachs S, Kirchgessner M, Paulicks BR. Effects of different levels of dietary selenium and vitamin E on the humoral immunity of rats. *J Trace Elem Electrolytes Health Dis.* 1993; 7:145-152.

28. Wuryastuti H, Stowe HD, Bull RW, Miller ER. Effects of vitamin E and selenium on immune responses of peripheral blood, colostrum and milk leukocytes of sows. *J Anim Sci.* 1993; 71:2464-2472.

29. Pollock JM, McNair J, Kennedy S, Kennedy DG, Walsh DM, Goodall EA, Mackie DP, Crockard AD. Effects of dietary vitamin E and selenium on in vitro cellular immune responses in cattle. *Res Vet Sci.* 1994; 56:100-107.

30. Chang W, Hom JSH, Dietert RR, Combs GF, Marsh JA. Effect of dietary vitamin and selenium deficiency on chicken splenocyte proliferation and cell surface marker expression. *Immunopharmacol Immunotoxicol.* 1994; 16:208-223.

31. Hogan JS, Smith KL, Weiss WP, Todhunter DA, Schockey WL. Relationships among vitamin E, selenium, and bovine blood neutrophils. *J Dairy Sci.* 1990; 73:2372-2378.

32. Makimura S, Kodama A, Kishita M, Takagi H, Adachi K. Secondary antibody response to Haemophilus somnus antigen in breeding Japanese black cattle fed selenium-deficient and α-tocopherol-fortified diets. *J Vet Med Sci.* 1993; 55:872-873.

33. Pennington JAT, Young BE, Wilson DB. Nutritional elements in U.S. diets: results from the Total Diet Study, 1982-86. *J Am Diet Assoc.* 1989; 89:659-664.

34. Food and Nutrition Board. *Recommended Dietary Allowances. 10th ed.* Washington, DC: National Academy Press; 1989.

35. Levander OA, Buck RF. Selenium. In: Shils ME, Olson JA, Shike M, eds. *Modern Nutrition in Health and Disease. 8th ed.* Philadelphia, Pa: Lea & Febiger; 1994:242-251.

36. Bendich A, Gabriel E, Machlin LJ. Dietary vitamin E requirement for optimum immune responses in the rat. *J Nutr.* 1986; 116:675-681.

37. McIntosh WA, Kubena KS, Walker J, Smith D, Landmann WA. The relationship between beliefs about nutrition and dietary practices of the elderly. *J Am Diet Assoc.* 1990; 90:671-676.

38. Chandra RK. Effect of vitamin and trace-element supplementation on immune responses and infection in elderly subjects. *Lancet*. 1992; 340:1124-1127.

39. Bogden JD, Oleske JM, Lavenhar MA, Munves EM, Kemp FW, Bruening KS, Holding KJ, Denny TN, Guarino MA, Holland BK. Effects of one year of supplementation with zinc and other micronutrients on cellular immunity in the elderly. *J Nutr*. 1990; 3:214-225.

40. Haberal M, Hamaloglu E, Bora S, Oner G, Bilgin N. The effects of vitamin E on immune regulation after thermal injury. *Burns Incl Therm Inj*. 1988; 14:388-393.

41. Panda SK, Rao AT. Effect of a vitamin E-selenium combination on chickens infected with infectious bursal disease virus. *Vet Rec*. 1994; 134:242-243.

42. ElAttar TMA, Lin HS. Effect of vitamin C and vitamin E on prostaglandin synthesis by fibroblasts and squamous carcinoma cells. *Prostaglandins Leukot Med*. 1992; 47:253-257.

43. Lynch NR, Salmon JC. Tumor growth inhibition and potentiation of immunotherapy by indomethacin. *J Natl Cancer Inst*. 1979; 62:117-121.

44. Gelin J, Anderson C, Lundholm K. Effect of indomethacin, cytokines, and cyclosporin A on tumor growth and subsequent development of cancer cachexia. *Cancer Res*. 1991; 51:660-663.

45. Tengerdy RP, Nockels CF. Vitamin E or vitamin A protects chickens against *E. coli* infection. *Poultry Sci*. 1975; 54:1292-1296.

46. Tengerdy RP, Brown JC. Effect of vitamin E and A on humoral immunity and phagocytosis in *E. coli* infected chicken. *Poultry Sci*. 1977; 56:957-963.

47. Pudelkiewicz WJ, Webster L, Matterson LD. Effects of high levels of dietary vitamin A acetate on tissue tocopherol and some related observations. *J Nutr*. 1964; 84:113-117.

48. Eicher SD, Morrill JL, Blecha F. Vitamin concentration and function of leukocytes from dairy calves supplemented with vitamin A, vitamin E, and ß-carotene *in vitro*. *J Dairy Sci*. 1994; 77:560-565.

49. Krantha SS, Taylor CE, Ross AC. The impact of vitamin A deficiency and repletion with retinol and ß-carotene on concanavalin A-induced lymphocyte proliferation. *Nutr Res*. 1992; 12:1527-1539.

50. Pasatiempo AMG, Taylor CE, Ross AC. Vitamin A status and the immune response to pneumococcal polysaccharide: effects of age and early stages of retinol deficiency in rats. *J Nutr*. 1991; 121:556-562.

51. Bowman TA, Goonewardene IM, Pasatiempo AMG, Ross AC, Taylor CE. Vitamin A deficiency decreases natural killer cell activity and interferon production in rats. *J Nutr*. 1990; 120:1264-1273.

52. Ross AC. Vitamin A status: relationship to immunity and the antibody response. *Proc Soc Exp Biol Med*. 1992; 200:303-320.

53. Sellmayer A, Goeschl C, Obermeier H, Volk R, Reder E, Weber C, Weber PC. Differential induction of eicosanoid synthesis in monocytic cells treated with retinoic acid and 1,25 dihydroxy-vitamin D3. *Prostaglandins*. 1994; 47:203-220.

54. Oberg F, Botling J, Nilsson K. Functional antagonism between vitamin D_3, and retinoic acid in the regulation of CD14 and CD23 expression during monocytic differentiation of U937 cells. *J Immunol*. 1993; 150:3487-3495.

55. Tiami H, Chatau MT, Cabanne S, Marti J. Synergistic effect of retinoic acid and 1,25 dihydroxyvitamin D3 on the differentiation of the human monocytic cell line U937. *Leuk Res*. 1991; 15:1145-1152.

56. Tiami M, Defacque H, Commes T, Favero J, Caron E, Marti J, Dornand J. Effect of retinoic acid and vitamin D on the expression of interleukin-1ß, tumor necrosis factor-α and interleukin-6 in the human monocytic cell line U937. *Immunology*. 1993; 79:229-235.

57. Kubena KS. The role of magnesium in immunity. *J Nutr Immunol*. 1993; 2:107-126.

58. Durlach J. *Magnesium in Clinical Practice*. London, England: John Libbey; 1988.

59. Jackson AM, Alexandroff AB, Lappin MB, Esuvaranathan K, James K, Chisholm GD. Control of leucocyte function-associated antigen-1-dependent cellular conjugation by divalent cations. *Immunology*. 1994; 81:120-126.

60. Wegliki WB, Stafford RE, Freeman AM, Cassidy MM, Philips TM. Modulation of cytokines and myocardial lesions by vitamin E and chloroquine in a Mg-deficient rat model. *Am J Physiol*. 1993; 264:C723-C726.

61. Carpentieri U, Myers J, Daeschner CW III, Haggard ME. Effects of iron, copper, zinc, calcium and magnesium on human lymphocytes in culture. *Biol Trace Elem Res.* 1988; 16:165-176.

62. Martz E. Immune T lymphocyte to tumor cell adhesion: magnesium sufficient, calcium insufficient. *J Cell Biol.* 1980; 84:584-598.

63. Dransfield I, Cabanas C, Craig A, Hogg N. Divalent cation regulation of the function of the leukocyte integrin LFA-1. *J Cell Biol.* 1992; 116:219-226.

64. Kubena KS, Durlach J. Historical review of the effects of marginal intake of magnesium in chronic experimental magnesium deficiency. *Magnesium Res.* 1990; 3:219-226.

65. Prohaska JR, Failla ML. Copper and immunity. In: Klurfeld DM, ed. *Human Nutrition—A Comprehensive Treatise. vol 8: Nutrition and Immunology.* New York, NY: Plenum Press; 1993:309-332.

66. Sherman AR, Spear AT. Iron and immunity. In: Klurfeld DM, ed. *Human Nutrition—A Comprehensive Treatise. vol 8: Nutrition and Immunology.* New York, NY: Plenum Press; 1993:285-307.

67. Niederman CN, Blodgett D, Eversole D, Schurig GG, Thatcher CD. Effect of copper and iron on neutrophil function and humoral immunity of gestating beef cattle. *J Am Vet Med Assoc.* 1994; 204:1796-1800.

68. Boyne R, Arthur JR. Effects of molybdenum or iron induced copper deficiency on the viability and function of neutrophils from cattle. *Res Vet Sci.* 1986; 41:417-419.

69. Boyne R, Arthur JR. Effects of selenium and copper deficiency on neutrophil function in cattle. *J Comp Pathol.* 1981; 91:271-276.

70. Ward JD, Spears JW, Kegley EB. Effect of copper level and source (copper lysine vs copper sulfate) on copper status, performance and immune responses in growing steers fed diets with or without supplemental molybdenum and sulfur. *J Anim Sci.* 1993; 71:2748-2755.

71. Olkowski AA, Gooneratne SR, Christensen DA. Effects of diets of high sulfur content and varied concentrations of copper, molybdenum and thiamine on in vitro phagocytic and candidacidal activity of neutrophils in sheep. *Res Vet Sci.* 1990; 48:82-86.

72. Fraker PJ, King LE Garry BA, Medina CA. The immunopathology of zinc deficiency in humans and rodents. In: Klurfeld

DM, ed. *Human Nutrition — A Comprehensive Treatise, vol 8: Nutrition and Immunology*. New York, NY: Plenum Press; 1993:267-283.

73. Pocino M, Malave I, Baute L. Zinc administration restores the impaired immune response observed in mice receiving excess copper by the oral route. *Immunopharmacol Immunotoxicol*. 1990; 12:697-713.

74. Scuderi P. Differential effects of copper and zinc on human peripheral blood monocyte cytokine secretion. *Cell Immunol*. 1990; 126:391-405.

75. Udomkesmalee E, Dhanamitta S, Sirisinha S, Charoenkiatkul S, Tantipopipat S, Banjong O, Rojroongwasinkul N, Kramer TR, Smith JC Jr. Effect of vitamin A and zinc supplementation on the nutriture of children in Northeast Thailand. *Am J Clin Nutr*. 1992; 56:50-57.

76. Kramer TR, Udomkesmalee E, Dhanamitta S, Sirisinha S, Charoenkiatkul S, Tuntipopipat S, Banjong O, Rojroongwasinkul N, Smith JC Jr. Lymphocyte responsiveness of children supplemented with vitamin A and zinc. *Am J Clin Nutr*. 1993; 58:566-570.

77. McMurray DN, Yetley EA. Response to Mycobacterium bovis BCG vaccination in protein- and zinc-deficient guinea pigs. *Infect Immun*. 1983; 39:755-761.

78. Peck MD, Alexander JW. Interaction of protein and zinc malnutrition with the murine response to infection. *JPEN*. 1992; 16:232-235.

79. Schiffer RB, Sunderman FW Jr, Baggs RB, Moynihan JA. The effects of exposure to dietary nickel and zinc upon humoral and cellular immunity in SJL mice. *J Neuroimmunol*. 1991; 34:229-239.

80. Calder PC, Newsholme EA. Influence of antioxidant vitamins on fatty acid inhibition of lymphocyte proliferation. *Biochem Mol Biol Int*. 1993; 29:175-183.

81. Gallin JL, Goldstein IM, Snyderman R, eds. *Inflammation: Basic Principles and Clinical Correlates*. New York, NY: Raven Press; 1988. 359-383.

82. Sobrado J, Moldawer LL, Pomposelli JJ, Mascioli EA, Babyan VK, Bistrian BR, Blackburn GL. Lipid emulsions and reticuloendothelial system function in healthy and burned guinea pigs. *Am J Clin Nutr*. 1985; 42:855-863.

83. Rosa LF, Guimaraes AR, Sitnik RH, Curi R. Effect of dietary vitamin E supplementation on macrophage metabolism during aging: study in rats fed fat-rich diets during aging. *Biochem Mol Biol Int*. 1994; 34:147-158.

84. Babinsky L, Langhout DJ, Verstegen MWA, den Hartog LA, Joling P, Nieuwland M. Effect of vitamin E and fat source in sows' diets on immune response of suckling and weaned piglets. *J Anim Sci*. 1991; 69:1833-1842.

85. Nemec M, Butler G, Hidiroglou M, Farnworth ER, Nielsen K. Effect of supplementing gilts' diets with different levels of vitamin E and different fats on the humoral and cellular immunity of gilts and their progency. *J Anim Sci*. 1994; 72:665-676.

86. Fritsche KL, Cassity NA, Huang S. Dietary (n-3) fatty acid and vitamin E interactions in rats: effects on vitamin E status, immune cell prostaglandin E production and primary antibody response. *J Nutr*. 1992; 122:1009-1018.

87. Kramer TR, Schoene N, Douglass LW, Judd JT, Ballard-Barbash R, Taylor PR, Bhagavan HN, Nair PP. Increased vitamin E intake restores fish-oil-induced suppressed blastogenesis of mitogen-stimulated T lymphocytes. *Am J Clin Nutr*: 1991; 54:896-902.

88. Harik-Khan R, Shamsa F, Johnson PV, Picciano MF, Segre M. Effect of time on neonatal immune responses to dietary selenium and fat. *J Trace Elem Electrolytes Health Dis*. 1993; 7:87-93.

89. Khanduja KL, Koul IB, Sehgal S. Influence of combined deficiency of fat and vitamin A on benzo(a)pyrene-induced lung carcinogenesis in rats. *Indian J Exp Biol*. 1994; 32:124-127.

90. Karsten S, Schafer G, Schauder P. Cytokine production and DNA synthesis by human peripheral lymphocytes in response to palmitic, stearic, oleic, and linoleic acid. *J Cell Physiol*. 1994; 161:15-22.

K. S. Kubena (corresponding author) is a professor in the Human Nutrition Section, Department of Animal Science and Faculty of Nutrition and D. N. McMurray is a professor in the Department of Medical Microbiology and Immunology and Faculty of Nutrition, Texas A&M University, College Station, TX 77843.

Chapter 54

Nutrition and Asthma

Asthma is a chronic lung disease characterized by obstruction, inflammation, and hyperresponsiveness of the airway to a variety of nonspecific stimuli. The obstruction is recurrent, is at least partially reversible, and manifests clinically as dyspnea, wheezing, and/or coughing. For children aged 6 to 11 years, the reported prevalence of asthma obtained from the first National Health and Nutrition Examination Survey conducted from 1971 to 1975 was 4.8%.[1] In the second study conducted from 1976 to 1980, the prevalence of asthma in the same age group increased to 7.6%.[1] For adults, the prevalence of active asthma was estimated to be 2.6%. The follow-up incidence of new cases was estimated at 2.1 cases per 1000 population per year.[2]

Acute episodes of asthma can be triggered by a variety of stimuli, including exercise, cold air, viral infection, emotional factors, and allergens. The allergens are usually inhalant, but can include food and food additives. Approximately 80% of children with asthma and 40% of adults with asthma are allergic[3] and may have an allergic component to their asthma, although some researchers would argue that almost all asthma has an allergic basis.[4]

The role of nutrition in asthma may be 2-fold. First, a food allergy can be a provoking stimulus for acute episodes of asthma. In these cases, avoidance of an allergenic food may lead to amelioration of asthmatic symptoms. In addition, the suboptimal status of specific nutrients may play a role in the cause of asthma in some patients. Supplementation of these nutrients, such as vitamin C and magnesium, may be of use in the treatment of some cases of asthma. This is an active area of research, particularly with the current widespread interest in nonmedicinal, nutritional, or "natural" cures and treatments for diseases. This review summarizes and analyzes the available data on the role of nutrition in the provocation and treatment of asthma.

Food Allergy

When an allergen, such as a food protein, enters the gastrointestinal tract, it encounters a unique mucosal immune system involving lymphocytes, mast cells, and IgA.[5] The allergen is first taken up by specialized M cells in the epithelium that process the protein and transport it from the intestinal lumen to the B and T lymphocytes in the mucosal Peyer's patches. Once stimulated, the lymphocytes migrate via the lymphatics into the systemic circulation and then return to the mucosal lamina propria, where they are primed for interaction with the sensitizing allergen. B lymphocytes in the intestinal mucosa secrete predominantly IgA, which acts to limit allergen absorption by the mucosa. Mucosal B cells also produce IgE against food antigens that penetrate the mucosal barrier. The IgE mediates the degranulation of mast cells in the gastrointestinal tract, causing an allergic reaction.[5]

A true food allergy, which involves an immune-mediated response to food, may be difficult to diagnose.[6] Valid diagnostic tests for food allergies include skin prick tests, radioallergosorbent tests (RASTs), and double-blind, placebo-controlled food challenges (DBPCFCs). Overall positive predictive accuracy of food skin prick tests is less than 50%, and therefore a positive result from a skin prick test for a specific food only suggests an allergy.[7] The RAST is an *in vitro* test for specific IgE antibodies in the individual's serum, which is a slightly less sensitive testing method than skin testing.[7] The DBPCFC is considered the "gold standard" test for the diagnosis of food allergies.[8] Foods to which the individual may be sensitive and placebos are given in lyophilized form in capsules or liquid, beginning with a low dose and doubling the dose every 15 to 60 minutes. False-negative results have been shown to occur in less than 5% of DBPCFCs and false-positive results in less than 1% of DBPCFCs.[7]

The number of atopic adults who believe themselves to have at least 1 food sensitivity has been found to be as high as 24%,[9] while as many as 28% of parents believe that their children have had an adverse reaction to a food.[10] However, the confirmed incidence of adverse reactions to food is probably less than 1% in adults, 1% to 2% in young children, and 4% to 6% in infants.[8] Infants have an increased incidence of true food allergies, which is believed to be the result of immaturity both of the gut, allowing the absorption of more antigen, and of the immune system, with less IgA to limit absorption.[11]

The role of food allergies in asthma is controversial. In a questionnaire study conducted by Adler et al,[12] 14.5% of parents of children with asthma stated that food provoked asthmatic symptoms in their children. Subsequently, Oehling et al[13] reviewed 25,000 clinical histories during a 5-year period and diagnosed 400 patients as having food allergy based on history, skin testing, and in vivo tests. Respiratory symptoms after food ingestion were reported by 18.5% and asthma was the main reaction in 15.5%. The foods that are most frequently implicated as causes of respiratory symptoms are eggs and milk. Other offenders include wheat, soy, peanuts, fish, and shellfish. In addition, although the majority of food additives have not been proven to cause respiratory symptoms, antioxidant sulfiting agents are known to exacerbate asthma in sensitive individuals.

Double-blind, placebo-controlled food challenges have been used to establish the true incidence of asthmatic symptoms caused by allergies to food. In general, studies have shown that although the overall effect of food allergies in asthma is minor, in a select group of patients food allergies can exacerbate asthma. For example, a 1986 study by Onorato et al[14] found food allergies in 25 of 300 asthmatic adults and children screened using a questionnaire, RASTs, and skin prick tests. During DBPCFCs, 6 (2%) of the screened patients experienced asthma, with 3 of these patients having asthma as their only reaction. Similarly, respiratory symptoms in response to DBPCFCs were demonstrated in 9.2% and asthma in 5.7% of children with asthma studied by Novembre et al.[15] Only 1 child in the study had asthma exclusively, with the remainder having associated cutaneous or gastrointestinal symptoms. The investigators in both studies concluded that IgE-mediated reactions to food are a minor cause of respiratory symptoms.

Bock[16] performed DBPCFs on 279 children with a history of induced asthma and 24% experienced wheezing; 5 children had wheezing as the only symptom. In addition, 10 (5%) of 188 children with a history of an adverse nonrespiratory reaction to food experienced wheezing during DBPCFCs. Similar results were obtained by James et al,[17] who studied children and adults with atopic dermatitis and found expiratory wheezing occurring in 17% of patients with positive

DBPCFC results. However, when one fourth of the patients were evaluated with spirometry during food challenges, only 7% experienced greater than a 20% decrease in forced expiratory volume in 1 second (FEV_1). Both of these studies demonstrate that food can cause wheezing, but it is uncommon even among children with histories of an adverse reaction to food. In addition, when respiratory symptoms do occur after food ingestion, significant objective changes in pulmonary function are not commonly seen.

In contrast to the aforementioned studies, Pelikan and Pelikan-Filipek[18] demonstrated a greater than 20% decrease in FEV_1 after open (unblinded) food challenges in 71% of adult patients with histories of food-induced asthma and in 56% of patients with asthma without such histories. The high rate of respiratory reactions to foods demonstrated in this study conflicts with the results of other similar studies. This may be because 80% of the food challenges were open and therefore not as well controlled as DBPCFCs.

The data presented herein suggest that in a small percentage of patients with asthma, food allergies may provoke respiratory symptoms. This effect may be particularly relevant in children. Large, well-controlled studies incorporating objective measures of pulmonary function are needed to identify other types of patients with asthma in whom this clinical effect is important.

Sodium Sensitivity

It has been hypothesized that diets high in salt may accentuate bronchial reactivity. Animal studies[19] have shown that passive *in vitro* sensitization of airway smooth muscle cells leads to increased sodium influx of the cells with the subsequent stimulation of Na^+, K^+-adenosinetriphosphatase, resulting in the sustained hyperpolarization of the airway smooth muscle cells. The contractile response of airway smooth muscle cells to specific antigen was demonstrated to be dependent on the level of hyperpolarization resulting from the sodium influx.

Several groups of researchers have investigated the relationship between sodium intake and asthma. The data have demonstrated a small adverse effect of increased sodium intake on bronchial reactivity, but no significant effect on clinical symptoms has been shown.

An epidemiological study by Burney[20] examined the relationship between asthma death rates and table salt purchases in regions of Britain. Using accumulated data from more than 37,000 households, Burney demonstrated that a significant proportion (64%) of the variance in asthma mortality among men was explained by table salt purchases. However, no such effect was seen for women. Although it raises some interesting issues, this research cannot prove cause and effect. In addition, the accuracy of using asthma death rates as a measure of asthma prevalence and table salt purchases as a measure of intake is questionable.

To investigate the effect of increasing salt intake on bronchial reactivity, Javaid et al[21] doubled baseline dietary salt intake in patients for 1 month and then performed histamine challenge tests. A significant increase in bronchial reactivity to histamine occurred in 9 of the 10 patients with asthma, but not in the 5 controls. This was a small, open, nonrandomized study in which an unspecified amount of salt was ingested. An observed difference in baseline sodium excretion between the 2 groups was not addressed and individual data were not shown.

Thirty-six adults with asthma were randomized by Burney et al[22] to receive either 80 mmol per day of sodium or a placebo for 2 weeks each in a crossover fashion. The bronchial response to histamine (measured as the dose causing a 10% decrease in FEV_1 [PD_{10}]) was found to be greater when the men were taking a sodium supplement than when they were taking the placebo. No such change was seen among the women. In addition, no significant change in FEV, was seen in either group during the study. While the investigators concluded that a high-sodium diet increases bronchial reactivity in men, in fact the statistically significant changes in PD_{10} are small and may lack clinical significance. Similarly, Medici et al[23] gave patients with asthma a low-salt diet plus an additional 6 g per day of sodium chloride or a placebo for 3 weeks each in a crossover protocol. Finally, all patients received sodium citrate supplementation (equivalent to 154 mmol of sodium) for 3 weeks. Forced expiratory volume in 1 second and peak expiratory flow rate (PEFR) significantly decreased with both sodium chloride and sodium citrate, but there was no effect on the dose causing a 20% decrease in FEV_1 (PD_{20}) as a sign of bronchial reactivity. Since the changes in pulmonary function test results were observed with both sodium chloride and sodium citrate, the effect appeared to be sodium mediated. This study used a low-salt diet that in fact contained 5 to 6 g per day of sodium chloride and demonstrated only small changes in FEV_1 and PEFR. In addition, only a limited number of patients were included and women were not analyzed separately.

Finally, an open trial was conducted by Lieberman and Heimer[24] with adults with asthma who received their normal diet for 2 weeks and were then randomly assigned to either a low- or high-salt diet for another 2 weeks each in a crossover protocol. Peak expiratory flow rates did not change during any of the 3 diet periods and no difference was demonstrated between men and women. From the data presented in this study, it is not known how much sodium the patients actually received. Since neither bronchial reactivity (PD_{20}) nor other pulmonary function tests such as FEV_1 were measured, the clinical relevance of these results is unclear.

It is not clear how much salt was actually ingested in all these studies and how this relates to the US average daily intake of 3 to 7 g. While the aforementioned studies lack concordance of results, they do suggest that increased sodium intake adversely affects the bronchopulmonary system. The pathogenesis of this effect is unknown and may or may not involve the airway smooth muscle cells as suggested by studies of animal tissues. Since the studies do not prove that there are clinical implications to these bronchopulmonary changes, there is currently little support for the adoption of low-salt diets by patients with asthma.

Magnesium

Magnesium plays a role in many enzymatic reactions, including those involved in the adenylate cyclase system, and acts with calcium to affect neuromuscular transmission and activity. The mechanism of magnesium's proposed effect on asthma is unknown, but may involve a direct action on bronchial smooth muscle, producing airway dilatation. Spivey *et al*[25] used an *in vitro* rabbit model to study this effect. In a series of experiments, they demonstrated that magnesium relaxes bronchial smooth muscle, not only when passively stretched, but also when contracted by different stimuli.

Clinical trials have been conducted to study the effect of magnesium infusion on asthma and have demonstrated a minor role for magnesium in the treatment of acute exacerbations of asthma. One such study by Skobeloff *et al*[26] involved patients who presented to the emergency department with an acute exacerbation of asthma and who did not respond to initial treatment. Patients were randomly assigned to receive either 1.2 g of magnesium sulfate or saline intravenously and were followed up for 45 minutes after the infusion. The group that received the magnesium infusion showed a significant increase in mean PEFR when compared with the saline group. In addition, only 7 of the 19 patients who received magnesium required admission to the hospital, while 15 of the 19 who received saline were admitted. Unfortunately, this study was short-term and the length of the beneficial effect attributed to magnesium was not reported.

The effect of intravenous magnesium in hospitalized patients with acute asthma was studied by Noppen *et al.*[27] On 2 consecutive days, 6 patients received infusions of 3 g of magnesium sulfate. In 10 of 12 trials, there was a significant improvement in FEV_1 immediately after the infusion with a decrease in FEV_1 toward baseline after 30 minutes. Inhalation of a ß$_2$-agonist after magnesium infusion resulted in an increase in FEV_1 in 11 of 12 trials, which was greater than the improvement seen after magnesium alone. Overall, the changes in FEV_1 after magnesium infusion were small and transient, especially when compared with the changes after ß$_2$-agonist inhalation.

Conflicting results were obtained by Tiffany *et al*[28] in a study of 48 patients who presented to the emergency department with asthma. Patients who did not improve after initial therapy were randomized to 1 of 3 treatment groups: an infusion group that received 2 g of intravenous magnesium sulfate followed by a continuous magnesium infusion of 2 g per hour over 4 hours; a bolus group that received 2 g of intravenous magnesium sulfate followed by a placebo infusion; and a placebo group that received a saline placebo both as bolus and infusion. Pulmonary function test results (PEFR and FEV_1) showed no difference between the 3 groups at any time during the 260-minute period following infusion.

In 1994, Britton *et al*[29] tested the hypothesis that magnesium is an independent determinant of lung function in the general population. The average daily intake of magnesium for 2644 subjects was estimated from semiquantitative food-frequency questionnaires. A 100-mg per day higher magnesium intake was found to be independently associated with a 27.7-mL higher FEV_1 and reduced airway reactivity to methacholine, even when adjusted for estimated daily intake of calcium or vitamin C, smoking, occupation, or social class. This study did not measure magnesium levels in serum or erythrocytes, and it did not analyze subjects with asthma separately. In addition, the increase in FEV_1 was small and may not have been clinically significant, making it difficult to draw any firm conclusions from this study.

Serum and erythrocyte magnesium levels have been measured in patients with asthma. Since magnesium is largely intracellular, it is thought that erythrocyte levels are a more accurate measure of magnesium status than serum levels. In 1992, Falkner *et al*[30] compared serum magnesium levels in patients during acute exacerbations of asthma with levels in nonasthmatic controls. Serum magnesium levels for both groups were within the normal range. Similary, magnesium levels in serum, erythrocytes, and mononuclear leukocytes were measured by de Valk *et al.*[31] There were no significant differences found in either extracellular or intracellular magnesium levels in asthmatic vs. normal patients.

Although magnesium infusion may cause an immediate improvement in pulmonary function in patients with acute asthma, it does not appear to be as effective as currently available standard therapy. Furthermore, its effectiveness over time, and therefore its clinical usefulness in managing chronic asthma, has not been proven. Finally, patients with asthma have not been shown to have even a marginal deficiency of magnesium. Therefore, all available evidence suggests that intravenous magnesium supplementation may have a minimal role in the treatment of acute asthma, but is of no value in the treatment of chronic asthma.

Vitamin C

Vitamin C acts as a reducing agent for hydroxylation reactions, such as those involved in collagen synthesis, and is important as an antioxidant. In asthma, vitamin C may act on airways by affecting arachidonic acid (AA) metabolites, particularly prostaglandins. The major prostaglandins (PGs) produced in the human lung are PGI_2, which causes pulmonary vasodilation; $PGF_2\alpha$ and PGD_2, which cause bronchoconstriction; and PGE_2, which causes bronchodilation. Work done by Puglisi *et al*[32] on guinea pig trachea showed an antagonistic effect of vitamin C on $PGF_2\alpha$-induced bronchoconstriction. Supporting these results, Ogilvy *et al*[33] demonstrated *in vivo* that ingestion of indomethacin, an inhibitor of PG synthesis, abolished the protective effect of vitamin C on methacholine-induced bronchoconstriction.

In search of a possible relationship between vitamin C and asthmatic symptoms, both vitamin C plasma levels and results of vitamin C supplementation have been studied. In these studies, supplemental vitamin C has been shown to cause an immediate decrease in airway responsiveness. One of the earlier studies by Olusi *et al*[34] found significantly higher concentrations of vitamin C in plasma and white blood cells in controls than in either treated or untreated patients with asthma. Similarly, in a study comparing plasma vitamin C levels in children with asthma with levels in healthy controls, Aderele *et al*[35] found significantly lower levels in children with asthma. However, no relationship was demonstrated between vitamin C levels and atopy or severity or duration of asthma. Unfortunately, this study did not quantify vitamin C intake in the diet or in supplements taken by approximately 50% of the children, making the results difficult to interpret.

In the first National Health and Nutrition Examination Survey, Schwartz and Weiss[36] assessed the relationship between dietary vitamin C intake and pulmonary function in 2526 randomly selected adults, of whom approximately 3% were asthmatic. Lower dietary vitamin C intakes were shown to be directly related to lower values of FEV_1. However, the difference in FEV_1 was only 40 mL between the highest and lowest tertiles of dietary vitamin C levels and occurred in patients with and without asthma, making the clinical relevance of these results suspect.

Ting et al[37] studied the effect of an intake of 2 g per day of vitamin C on the airways of adults with asthma. No change was demonstrated in any pulmonary function tests performed or in reported asthma symptoms after 4 days of supplementation. This was an unblinded short-term study with obvious limitations. A short-term study of adults with exercise-induced asthma was done by Schachter and Schlesinger.[38] After ingestion of 500 mg of vitamin C, the immediate postexercise PEFR in subjects was significantly improved, while 5 minutes after exercise only forced vital capacity showed significant improvement when compared with the placebo. The authors concluded that the results demonstrate partial protection by vitamin C against exercise-induced airway obstruction with a more prominent effect in the large airways. However, the lack of consistent changes in the pulmonary function test results and the very short follow-up make it difficult to draw any substantial conclusions.

A number of studies have been performed to assess the effect of vitamin C on bronchial challenge testing. Six ragweed-sensitive adults with asthma were studied by Kordansky et al[39] after a 1-week course of 500 mg per day of ingested vitamin C or a placebo. No protective effect of vitamin C against ragweed antigen-induced bronchospasm was demonstrated. In healthy adults studied by Ogilvy et al,[33] ingestion of 1 g of vitamin C caused a 25% reduction in the duration and intensity of methacholine-induced bronchoconstriction. However, responses to methacholine were similar to baseline after the ingestion of indomethacin, indicating that indomethacin abolished the protective effect of vitamin C. In a similar study, Mohsenin et al[40] found that vitamin C decreased airway responses to methacholine and indomethacin significantly reduced this effect in 11 of 14 adults with asthma. The effect of indomethacin in the latter 2 studies supports previous work that shows vitamin C enhancing the production of a bronchodilator PG.

Placebo-controlled studies involving histamine bronchial challenges have been performed with vitamin C. Zuskin et al[41] measured changes in airway response to histamine in healthy adults after ingestion of 500 mg of vitamin C or a placebo. Less histamine-induced reduction in flow rates occurred following the ingestion of vitamin C than after the placebo. Similar results were obtained by Bucca et al[42] using 2 g of vitamin C or a placebo. Vitamin C was shown in this study to acutely decrease airway responsiveness to inhaled histamine. In contrast, Malo et al[43] demonstrated that ingestion of 2 g per day of vitamin C for 4 days had no effect on histamine-induced bronchoconstriction in adults with asthma. In all 3 studies, observed changes in bronchial challenge test results secondary to vitamin C use were small. In none of them did vitamin C prevent histamine-induced bronchoconstriction.

Two long-term studies on the effects of vitamin C on pulmonary function test results and immunity have been done by Anderson et al.[44,45] During a 6-month period, Anderson et al[44] supplemented 10 children with asthma with histories of recurrent respiratory tract infections with 1 g per day of vitamin C and performed pulmonary function tests and immunologic studies. Six children demonstrated improved pulmonary function test results with return of peak flow and maximum midexpiratory flow to greater than 85% of normal; 9 children remained free of infection after 6 months. In addition, 2 patients with reduced neutrophil chemotaxis and 4 patients with decreased lymphocyte transformation had values increase to normal; 7 patients with increased antistreptolysin O levels had the levels decrease significantly. In 1983, Anderson et al[45] studied children with asthma, randomly assigning 7 patients to receive 1 g per day of vitamin C plus standard asthma therapy and 9 patients to receive standard asthma therapy alone for 6 months. Vitamin C supplementation was demonstrated to improve neutrophil motility and decrease antistreptolysin O levels. The acute effect of 1 g of intravenous vitamin C on exercise-induced bronchoconstriction was studied in the first 10 patients and no protective effect of vitamin C was seen. The clinical benefit of the demonstrated immunologic changes is not clear. In the first study by Anderson et al[44] the improvement in pulmonary function test results may have been related to the decreased rate of infections, rather than to a direct effect of vitamin C. In the second study by Anderson et al,[45] vitamin C had no effect on pulmonary function.

The majority of these studies suggest at least a short-term protective effect of vitamin C on airway responsiveness. It remains to be proven whether consistent use of vitamin C would have a positive effect on objective measures of pulmonary function. More long-term, controlled studies need to be done to clarify the possible role of vitamin C in the treatment of chronic asthma.

Selenium

Selenium acts as an antioxidant and thus interacts with other nutrients, such as vitamin E, that protect cells against oxidative stress. Selenium is an essential component of the enzyme glutathione peroxidase (GSH-Px), which reduces hydrogen peroxide and other organic peroxides to harmless substances. By detoxifying peroxides, GSH-Px prevents peroxidation and subsequent instability of cell membranes.

Inflammatory cells in asthmatic airways oxidize nicotinamideadenine dinucleotide phosphate, producing oxygen-derived free radicals and peroxides.[46] It has been proposed that selenium, as a component of GSH-Px, can protect membranes in asthmatic airways from damage caused by peroxides and can protect antiproteases in the lung from inactivation by toxic antioxidants.[47]

Studies performed to examine a possible relationship between low selenium levels and asthma have yielded inconsistent results. In New Zealand, Shaw et al[48] surveyed 708 children and found a prevalence of current wheezing of 21.3%. For 26 of the children with current wheezing and for 61 healthy control children, stored serum samples drawn 8 years prior were tested for IgE and selenium levels. It was found that current wheezing was more common in those with high levels of IgE or low levels of selenium. This type of study cannot assume cause and effect. It is possible that the high IgE level has more to do with current wheezing than the low selenium level, and it is unfortunate that current serum levels were not measured.

Selenium concentrations and GSH-Px activity were measured in both adults with asthma and healthy controls for a study by Stone et al.[49] Patients with asthma had lower concentrations of selenium in plasma and whole blood but not in platelets when compared with controls. There was no accompanying reduction in GSH-Px activity found in whole blood or platelets. The authors concluded that the reduced selenium status of the patients with asthma did not contribute to decreased antioxidant defenses. Somewhat different results were obtained by Flatt et al[50] who found that whole blood, but not plasma, selenium concentrations and GSH-Px activity were lower in adults with asthma than in controls. The authors conclude that whole blood levels reflect a longer term index of selenium status than plasma and that the study results are consistent with a role for lowered selenium concentrations in the pathogenesis of asthma. Similarly, reduced GSH-Px activity in whole blood was found by Powell et al[51] in 37 children with asthma when compared with controls. Although these studies showed some measurements of selenium levels to be lower in patients with asthma, the effect on GSH-Px activity was inconsistent. In addition, the mechanism for low selenium levels in the pathogenesis of asthma has not been shown.

Pearson *et al*[52] studied aspirin-sensitive patients with asthma who were thought to have an acetylsalicylic acid-induced release of oxygen radicals. They found aspirin-tolerant patients with asthma to have higher mean serum selenium concentrations than either aspirin-sensitive patients with asthma or normal patients. However, only aspirin-sensitive patients with asthma were found to have reduced platelet GSH-Px activity. The authors conclude that reduced GSH-Px activity in aspirin-sensitive patients with asthma must be dependent on another unknown factor in addition to lowered serum selenium levels. They could not explain, however, the higher selenium concentration seen in the aspirin-tolerant asthmatic population.

A therapeutic role for selenium in the management of asthma was suggested in a case report by Ahlrot-Westerlund and Norrby.[53] They treated a 35-year-old man with a posterior subcapsular cataract, keratoconus, atopic eczema, and asthma with daily supplements of selenium and vitamin E for 2 months. After treatment, the patient had no signs of atopic eczema or asthma. In 1993, Hasselmark *et al*[54] conducted a study of 24 adults with asthma in which half of the patients were randomized to receive 100 μg of selenium per day for 14 weeks, while the other half received a placebo. Six patients from the selenium-supplemented group and 1 from the placebo group noted significant subjective clinical improvement, although neither group showed improvement in pulmonary function test results or a histamine inhalation challenge. The authors are cautious in their interpretation of these inconsistent results.

There are no current data demonstrating a beneficial effect of selenium supplementation on objective tests of pulmonary function in patients with asthma. In addition, the data on whole blood selenium levels and GSH-Px activity are inconsistent. A possible correlation between low serum levels of selenium and wheezing is not sufficient to support the use of selenium supplements in the treatment of asthma.

Fish Oils

There are 2 classes of polyunsaturated fatty acids obtained from our diets: [omega]ω-6 fatty acids are represented by linoleic acid, which is metabolized in humans and animals to AA, and ω-3 fatty acids are represented by α-linolenic acid, which is metabolized in humans and animals to eicosapentaenoic acid (EPA) and docosahexaenoic acid (DHA). Arachidonic acid is obtained in our diet mainly from grain-fed animals, while EPA and DHA are obtained from fatty fish. Humans consume more α-6 fatty acids than α-3 fatty acids.

Arachidonic acid is incorporated into cell membranes from which it is released to act as the precursor for the 2 series of PGs and thromboxanes and the 4 series of leukotrienes (LTs). These metabolites promote such responses as smooth muscle contraction, bronchoconstriction, increased vascular permeability, and leukocyte chemotaxis. When humans ingest fish or fish oil, EPA and DHA replace AA in cell membranes. When EPA is released from cell membranes, it is the precursor for the 3 series of PGs and thromboxanes and the 5 series of LTs. Therefore, EPA leads to decreased production of the inflammatory metabolites of AA and replaces them with metabolites that have less inflammatory potential. It is this change in the pattern of metabolites and the potential effect on airway inflammation that have led to an interest in fish oil supplementation in the management of asthma. However, clinical studies have not shown the expected benefits on airway functioning.

Payan *et al*[55] and Kirsch *et al*[56] studied the effect of fish oil in adults with asthma who were randomized into 2 groups receiving either 0.1 g per day of EPA or 4 g per day of EPA for 8 weeks. Only the high-dose supplement decreased LTB_4 generation from AA by leukocytes and suppressed neutrophil but not mononuclear leukocyte chemotaxis to multiple stimuli. Neither dose led to any change in clinical status or pulmonary function test results in the 8-week testing period. In a study by Arm *et al*,[57] patients with asthma received either 3.2 g per day of EPA and 2.2 g per day of DHA or a placebo for a 10-week period. The neutrophils of the patients receiving EPA and DHA showed decreased LTB_4 generation and decreased chemotaxis in response to stimuli. There was, however, no change in reported symptoms, pulmonary function test results, or bronchial responsiveness to either histamine or exercise in either group. The authors suggest that since neutrophil function was suppressed without a concomitant change in severity of asthma, either neutrophils do not play a major role in the pathogenesis of asthma or the suppression of function was not adequate to see a clinical effect. Since neutrophils are believed to have a role in latephase reactions in asthma, the second explanation seems more likely than the first.

Twelve adults with asthma were randomized into 2 groups receiving either 1 g per day of EPA and DHA or a placebo for 1 year in a study by Dry and Vincent.[58] Pulmonary function test results showed an increased FEV_1 only at 9 months of supplementation. In this study, the baseline FEV, varied substantially between the 2 groups, making any claim of a significant effect of fish oil supplementation questionable. In another long-term study, Thien *et al*[59] supplemented adults with asthma with 3.2 g per day of EPA and 2.2 g per day of DHA or a placebo for 6 months and demonstrated no change in peak flow, bronchial responsiveness to histamine, symptom score, or medication use for either group.

The effect of fish oil supplementation on the early and late asthmatic responses to antigen has been studied by Arm *et al*.[60] Bronchial responses to allergen (measured as the dose causing a 35% decrease in FEV_1 [PD_{35}]) were measured in adults with asthma, 9 of whom received 3.2 g per day of EPA and 2.2 g per day of DHA and 8 of whom received a placebo for 10 weeks. In contrast to those receiving the placebo, the group taking the EPA and DHA demonstrated a smaller late asthmatic response to allergen when compared with baseline. They did not, however, show any change in clinical parameters, such as peak flows or symptom scores. In addition, the effect on the late-phase response of the EPA and DHA supplements could not be compared with that of the placebo since the baseline late-phase response was much greater in the EPA/DHA-supplemented group than in the placebo group.

It has been demonstrated by Picado *et al*[61] that fish oil supplementation might be detrimental to patients with asthma who are aspirin intolerant. Ten aspirin-intolerant adults with asthma received 6 weeks of a control diet containing placebo supplementation followed by 6 weeks of a diet enriched with 3 g per day of ω-3 fatty acids. While neither diet caused a change in symptom scores, peak expiratory flow values were significantly lower and bronchodilator use was greater during the last 2 weeks of the fish oil-supplemented diet.

These studies do not show clinical improvement in patients with asthma using fish oil supplementation, despite some changes seen in inflammatory cell functions. There is, at this time, no data to support the recommendation of using fish oil in the treatment of asthma.

Summary

It is clear from a review of the existing data that there is no proven role for nutritional therapy in the management of asthma. Food allergies may occasionally be involved in the exacerbation of asthma, particularly in children. Magnesium infusion may have a place in the acute treatment of asthma, but does not seem to have long-term benefits. The studies of sodium, selenium, and fish oils do not show convincing evidence of clinical benefits. Vitamin C, however, did demonstrate a possible effect on bronchial responsiveness and pulmonary function. Whether these changes have clinical importance can only be determined by further studies. Until more definitive studies are completed, the use of nutritional supplements for the treatment of asthma cannot be recommended.

References

1. Gergen PJ, Mullally DI, Evans R III. National survey of prevalence of asthma among children in the United States, 1976 to 1980. *Pediatrics*. 1988; 81:1-7.

2. McWhorter WP, Polis MA, Kaslow RA. Occurrence, predictors and consequences of adult asthma in NHANES 1 and follow-up survey. *Am Rev Respir Dis*. 1989;139:721-724.

3. Weiss ST, Sparrow D, O'Connor GT. The inter-relationship among allergy, airways responsiveness and asthma. *J Asthma*. 1993; 30:329-349.

4. Burrows B, Martinez FD, Halonen M, Barbee RA, Cline MG. Association of asthma with serum IgE levels and skin-test reactivity to allergens. *N Engl J Med*. 1989;320:271-277.

5. Murphy MS, Walker WA. Antigen absorption. In: Metcalfe DD, Sampson MA, Simon RA, eds. *Food Allergy: Adverse Reactions to Foods and Food Additives*. Cambridge, Mass: Blackwell Publishers; 1991:52-66.

6. Bjorksten B. *In vitro* diagnostic methods in the evaluation of food hypersensitivity. In: Metcalfe DD, Sampson MA, Simon RA, eds. *Food Allergy: Adverse Reactions to Foods and Food Additives*. Cambridge, Mass: Blackwell Publishers; 1991:67.

7. Sampson HA. Adverse reactions to foods. In: Middleton E Jr, Reed CE, Ellis EF, Adkinson NF Jr, Yunginger JW, Busse WW, eds. *Allergy Principles and Practice. 4th ed*. St Louis, Mo: Mosby-Year Book Inc; 1993:1676-1678.

8. Sampson HA. IgE-mediated food intolerance. *J Allergy Clin Immunol*. 1988;81:495-504.

9. Erickson NE. Food sensitivity reported by patients with asthma and hay fever. *Allergy*. 1978; 33:189-196.

10. Bock SA. Prospective appraisal of complaints of adverse reactions to foods in children during the first 3 years of life. *Pediatrics*. 1987;79:683-688.

11. Sampson HA, Metcalfe DD. Food allergies. *JAMA*. 1992;268:2840-2844.

12. Adler BR, Assadullahi T, Warner JA, Warner JO. Evaluation of a multiple food specific IgE antibody test compared to parental perception, allergy skin tests and RAST. *Clin Exp Allergy*. 1991; 21:683-688.

13. Oehling A, Garcia B, Santos F, *et al*. Food allergy as a cause of rhinitis and/or asthma. *J Investig Allergol Clin Immunol*. 1992;2:78-83.

14. Onorato J, Merland N, Terral C, Michel FB, Bousquet J. Placebo-controlled double-blind food challenge in asthma. *J Allergy Clin Immunol*.1986; 78:1139-1146.

15. Novembre E, de Martino M, Vierucci A. Foods and respiratory allergy. *J Allergy Clin Immunol*. 1988;81:1059-1065.

16. Bock SA. Respiratory reactions induced by food challenges in children with pulmonary disease. *Pediatr Allergy Immunol*. 1992;3:188-194.

17. James JM, Bernhisel-Broadbent J, Sampson HA. Respiratory reactions provoked by double-blind food challenges in children. *Am J Respir Crit Care Med*. 1994;149:59-64.

18. Pelikan Z, Pelikan-Filipek M. Bronchial response to the food ingestion challenge. *Ann Allergy*. 1987;58:164-172.

19. Souhrada M, Souhrada JF. Sensitization-induced sodium influx in airway smooth muscle cells. *Am Rev Respir Dis*. 1985;131:356. Abstract.

20. Burney P. A diet rich in sodium may potentiate asthma: epidemiologic evidence for a new hypothesis. *Chest* 1987;91:1435-1485.

21. Javaid A, Cushley MJ, Bone MF. Effect of dietary salt on bronchial reactivity to histamine in asthma. *BMJ*. 1988.297:454.

22. Burney PGJ, Neild JE, Twort CHC, et al. Effect of changing dietary sodium on the airway response to histamine, *Thorax*. 1989;44:36-41.

23. Medici TC, Zumster C, Zumstein-Schmid A, Hacki M, Vetter W. Are asthmatics salt sensitive? A premiliminary controlled study. *Chest*. 1993;104:1138-1143.

24. Lieberman D, Heimer D. Effect of dietary sodium on the severity of bronchial asthma. *Thorax*. 1992;47:360-362.

25. Spivey WH, Skobeloff EM, Levin RM. Effect of magnesium chloride on rabbit bronchial smooth muscle. *Ann Emerg Med*. 1990;19:1107-1112.

26. Skobeloff EM, Spivey WH, McNamara RM, Greenspon L. Intravenous magnesium sulfate for the treatment of acute asthma in the emergency department. *JAMA*. 1989;262:1210-1213.

27. Noppen M, Vanmaele L, Impens N, Schandevyl W. Bronchodilating effect of intravenous magnesium sulfate in acute severe bronchial asthma. *Chest* 1990;97:373-376.

28. Tiffany BR, Berk WA, Todd IK, White SR. Magnesium bolus or infusion fails to improve expiratory flow in acute asthma exacerbations. *Chest*. 1993;104:831-834.

29. Britton J, Pavord I, Richards K, *et al*. Dietary magnesium, lung function, wheezing and airway hyperreactivity in a random adult population sample. *Lancet*. 1994;344:357-362.

30. Falkner D, Glauser J, Allen M. Serum magnesium levels in asthmatic patients during acute exacerbations of asthma. *Am J Emerg Med*. 1992; 10:1-3.

31. de Valk HW, Kok PTM, Struyvenberg A, *et al*. Extracellular and intracellular magnesium concentrations in asthmatic patients. *Eur Respir J*. 1993;6:1122-1125.

32. Puglisi L, Berti F, Bosisio E, Longiave D, Nicosia S. Ascorbic acid and PGF_2-alpha antagonism on tracheal smooth muscle. In: Samuelsson B, Paoletti R, eds. *Advances in Prostaglandin and Thromboxane Research, Volume 1*. New York, NY: Raven Press; 1976:503-506.

33. Ogilvy CS, DuBois AB, Douglas JS. Effects of vitamin C and indomethacin on the airways of healthy male subjects with and without induced bronchoconstriction. *J Allergy Clin Immunot* 1981; 67:363-369.

34. Olusi SO, Ojutiku OO, Jessop WJE, Iboko MI. Plasma and white blood cell vitamin C concentrations in patients with bronchial asthma. *Clin Chim Acta*. 1979;92:161-166.

35. Aderele WI, Ette SI, Oduwole O, Ikpeme SJ. Plasma vitamin C (ascorbic acid) levels in asthmatic children. *Afr J Med Med Sci*. 1985;14: 115-120.

36. Schwartz J, Weiss ST. Relationship between dietary vitamin C intake and pulmonary function in the First National Health and Nutrition Examination Survey (NHANES 1). *Am J Clin Nutr*. 1994; 59:110-114.

37. Ting S, Mansfield LE, Yarbrough J. Effects of vitamin C on pulmonary functions in mild asthma. *J Asthma*. 1983;20:39-42.

38. Schachter EN, Schlesinger A. The attenuation of exercise: induced bronchospasm by vitamin C. *Ann Allergy*. 1982;49:146-151.

39. Kordansky DW, Rosenthal RR, Norman PS. The effect of vitamin C on antigen-induced bronchospasm. *J Allergy Clin Immunol* 1979; 63:61-64.

40. Mohsenin V, DuBois AB, Douglas JS. Effect of vitamin C on response to methacholine challenge in asthmatic subjects. *Am Rev Respir Dis*. 1983;127:143-147.

41. Zuskin E, Lewis AJ, Bouhuys A. Inhibition of histamine-induced airway constriction by vitamin C. *J Allergy Clin Immunol* 1973;51:218-226.

42. Bucca C, Rolla G, Oliva A, Farina JC. Effect of vitamin C on histamine bronchial responsiveness of patients with allergic rhinitis. *Ann Allergy*. 1990;65:311-314.

43. Malo JL, Cartier A, Pineau L, L'Archeveque J, Ghezzo H, Martin RR. Lack of acute effects of vitamin C on spirometry and airway responsiveness to histamine in subjects with asthma. *J Allergy Clin Immunol*. 1986;78:1153-1158.

44. Anderson R, Hay I, VanWyk H, Oosthuizen R, Theron A. The effect of ascorbate on cellular humoral immunity in asthmatic children. *S Afr Med J*. 1980;58:974-977.

45. Anderson R, Hay I, VanWyk HA, Theron A. Ascorbic acid in bronchial asthma. *S Afr Med J*. 1983;63:649-652.

46. Hogg JC. Pathology of asthma. *J Allergy Clin Immunol* 1993;92:1-5.

47. Beasley R, Thomson C, Pearce N. Selenium, glutathione peroxidase and asthma. *Clin Exp Allergy*. 1991;21:157-159.

48. Shaw R, Woodman K, Crane J, Moyes C, Kennedy J, Pearce N. Risk factors for asthma symptoms in Kawerau children. *N Z Med J*. 1994;107:387-391.

49. Stone J, Hinks LJ, Beasley R, Holgate ST, Clayton BA. Reduced selenium status of patients with asthma. *Clin Sci*. 1989;77:495-500.

50. Flatt A, Pearce N, Thomson CD, Sears MR, Robinson MF, Beasley R. Reduced selenium in asthmatic subjects in New Zealand. *Thorax*. 1990; 45:95-99.

51. Powell CVE, Nash AA, Powers HJ, Primhak RA. Antioxidant status in asthma. *Pediatr Pulmonol* 1994;18:34-38.

52. Pearson DJ, Suarez-Mendez VJ, Day JP, Miller PF. Selenium status in relation to reduced glutathione peroxidase activity in aspirin-sensitive asthma. *Clin Exp Allergy*. 1991;21:203-208.

53. Ahlrot-Westerlund B, Norrby A. Remarkable success of antioxidant treatment (selenomethionine and vitamin E) to a 35-year-old patient with posterior subcapsular cataract, keratoconus, severe atopic eczema, and asthma. *Acta Ophthalmol (Copenh)*. 1988;66:237-238.

54. Hasselmark L, Malmgren R, Zetterstrom O, Unge G. Selenium supplementation in intrinsic asthma. *Allergy*. 1993;48:3026.

55. Payan DG, Wong MYS, Chernov-Rogan T, *et al*. Alterations in human leukocyte function induced by ingestion of eicosapentaenoic acid. *J Clin Immunol* 1986;6:402-410.

56. Kirsch CM, Payan DG, Wong MYS, *et al*. Effect of eicosapentaenoic acid in asthma. *Clin Allergy*. 1988;18:177-187.

57. Arm JP, Horton CE, Mencia-huerta JM, *et al*. Effect of dietary supplementation with fish oil lipids on mild asthma. *Thorax*. 1988;43:84-92.

58. Dry J, Vincent D. Effect of a fish oil diet on asthma: results of a 1-year double blind study. *Int Arch Allergy Immunol*. 1991; 95:156-157.

59. Thien FCK, Mencia-Huerta JM, Lee TH. Dietary fish oil effects on seasonal hay fever and asthma in pollen-sensitive subjects. *Am Rev Respir Dis*. 1993;47:1138-1143.

60. Arm JP, Horton CE, Spur BW, Mencia-Huerta JM, Lee TH. The effects of dietary supplementation with fish oil lipids on

the airways response to inhaled allergen in bronchial asthma. *Am Rev Respir Dis.* 1989;139:1395-1400.

61. Picado C, Castillo JA, Schinca N, *et al.* Effects of a fish oil-enriched diet on aspirin-intolerant asthmatic patients: a pilot study. *Thorax.* 1988; 43:93-97.

— by Catherine A. Monteleone and Adria R. Sherman

From the Department of Medicine, University of Medicine and Dentistry of New Jersey, Robert Wood Johnson Medical School (Dr. Monteleone), and the Department of Nutritional Sciences, Cook College, Rutgers, The State University of New Jersey (Dr. Sherman), New Brunswick.

Chapter 55

Selenium and Cancer Prevention

A 10-year cancer prevention trial suggests that dietary supplements of the trace element selenium may significantly lower the incidence of prostate, colorectal, and lung cancers in people with a history of skin cancer. The supplements did not, however, affect the incidence of basal or squamous cell cancers of the skin, the original hypothesis of the study. The results are published in the December 25 [1996] issue of the *Journal of the American Medical Association*. The study is titled: "Effects of Selenium Supplementation for Cancer Prevention in Patients with Carcinoma of the Skin." The authors are Larry C. Clark, Gerald F. Combs Jr., Bruce W. Turnbull, Elizabeth H. Slate, Daniel K. Chalker, James Chow, Loretta S. Davis, Renee A. Glover, Gloria F. Graharn, Earl G. Gross, Arnon Krongrad, Jack Lesher, H. Kim Park, Beverly B. Sanders Jr., Cameron L. Smith, J. Richard Taylor.

The study began in 1983 and included a total of 1,312 skin cancer patients with a mean age of 63 seen at seven dermatology clinics in the eastern United States. At that time, the primary purpose of the study was to see if dietary supplements of selenium could lower the incidence of basal cell or squamous cell skin cancers. In 1990, secondary end points, including incidence of the most commonly occurring cancers, lung, prostate, and colorectal were added.

"The results of this study are exciting because they show the cancer prevention potential of a nutritional supplement to a normal diet,"

"Selenium Lowers Incidence of Lung. Colorectal, and Prostate Cancers," National Cancer Institute (NCI), Cancer Facts—Prevention, January 1997; available at http://cancernet.nci.nih.gov.

said Larry C. Clark, Ph.D., MPH, associate professor of epidemiology at the Arizona Cancer Center in Tucson, Ariz., and principal investigator of the study. "The study needs to be repeated in other populations before a public health recommendation can be made for selenium supplementation."

Patients in the double-blinded (neither patients nor doctors knew who was receiving the intervention), randomized study took a tablet containing 200 micrograms (μg) of selenium as brewer's yeast, or placebo, daily for 4.5 years and were followed for an additional 6.4 years. Three-quarters of the patients were men. The trial ended in January 1996, two years before the planned end of the trial.

American diets generally include enough grain, meat, and fish, the primary sources of selenium, to meet the recommended dietary allowance (RDA), 70 μg/day for men and 55 μg/day for women. (Although the EPA established a reference dose, 350 μg/day, as a measure of the maximum safe intake, the human toxicity levels for selenium have not been definitely established.)

The study population, however, was from a region of the eastern United States with relatively low selenium levels in soils and crops, and before treatment had a mean plasma selenium concentration in the lower range of the U.S. levels. The supplements increased the plasma concentration by 67 percent and the average daily intakes by 3-fold. The higher plasma concentrations were reached within six to nine months of supplementation and were maintained throughout the trial, although a small decline was seen over the course of the trial.

The results of the study showed that total cancer incidence was significantly lower in the selenium group than in the placebo group (77 cases versus 119), as was the incidence of some site-specific cancers: the selenium group had fewer prostate cancers (13 versus 35), fewer colorectal cancers (8 versus 19), and fewer lung cancers (17 versus 31). These differences were statistically significant. The number of cases at other sites were insufficient for a valid analysis.

The results also showed that over-all mortality was 17 percent less in the selenium versus the control group (108 versus 129) with this difference largely due to a 50 percent reduction in cancer deaths (29 versus 57). Lung cancer deaths were lower in the selenium-treatment group than in the placebo (12 versus 26). The number of deaths for other cancers were insufficient for meaningful statistical analysis. There was no significant difference between the two treatment groups for other causes of death.

Peter Greenwald, M.D., director of the National Cancer Institutes Division of Cancer Prevention and Control commented, "These results are interesting for several reasons. First, there was no detectable increase in adverse effects from the supplementation which is very important to know for future trials. Secondly, beneficial effects were seen for three major cancers."

"Having said all that," he added, "we need to be cautious." Greenwald noted that the study population was relatively small and consisted of people who live in low-selenium regions and are at high risk for non-melanoma skin cancer. The lower cancer rates were found for cancers that were secondary, not primary study endpoints. The work, he believes, needs to be confirmed in a larger population more representative of the U.S.

Selenium soil levels were first associated inversely with cancer mortality in the late 1960s. Similar results were found in prospective studies which measured selenium status by several methods; soil, blood, nails, hair. Some studies have also found inverse associations with the incidence of cancers of the lung, colon, bladder, rectum, breast, pancreas, and ovary. However, several studies have shown no association between selenium status and cancer and a few have shown a direct association—cancer risk increased with selenium status.

In animals, selenium administration has been shown to have antitumor activity, but at levels several times greater than the nutritional needs. Likewise, in tissue culture experiments, supplementation of cultured tumor cells with selenium at much higher doses than the cells normally require, has been shown to inhibit tumor growth and stimulate apoptosis, programmed cell death.

Three human intervention studies with selenium have had various outcomes. The low soil selenium content in Finland led the Finnish government to begin adding selenium to fertilizers in 1984 with an eye towards reducing cancer risk and cardiovascular disease. No significant effects on cancer incidence have been seen to date in the Finnish population of four million.

Two additional human intervention trials took place in Linxian, China from 1985-1991. In one trial, a daily supplement containing 50 μg selenium plus three other minerals and vitamins, had no effect on the high incidence of esophageal cancer or total cancer incidence or mortality. The second and largest trial showed a significant reduction in stomach cancer incidence (16 percent) and stomach cancer mortality (21 percent) using a daily mixture of antioxidants—one component of which was selenium.

The current study is the first double-blinded cancer prevention trial to test whether a nutritional supplement of selenium alone can reduce cancer risk. Participating dermatology clinics were located in

Augusta, Georgia; Macon, Georgia; Columbia, South Carolina; Miami, Florida; Wilson, North Carolina; Greenville, North Carolina; and Newington, Connecticut.

Greenwald commented on the possibility of future prevention trials. "This study highlights the value of clinical trials in cancer prevention. The interesting observation of a possible benefit of selenium needs to be assessed in a larger, more definitive trial."

Additional Resources

Telephone Service

Cancer Information Service (CIS)
Toll-free phone number: 1-800-4-CANCER (1-800-422-6237)
TTY: 1-800-332-8615.

The Cancer Information Service (CIS) is the National Cancer Institute's (NCI) national information and education network. The CIS is the source for the latest, most accurate cancer information for patients, the public, and health professionals. Specially trained staff provide scientific information in understandable language. CIS staff answer questions in English and Spanish and distribute NCI materials.

Electronic Services

National Cancer Institute (NCI)
Website: http://rex.nci.nih.gov

The NCI maintains a Web site that provides easy access to the most current information on cancer. Many of NCI's patient education resources are located on the Web site, including full-text publications and fact sheets for cancer patients and their families.

PDQ

The National Cancer Institute (NCI) has developed PDQ (Physician Data Query), a computerized database designed to give health professionals, patients, and the public quick and easy access to:

- the latest treatment, supportive care, screening, and prevention information for most types of cancer;

- descriptions of research studies (also known as clinical trials) that are open for enrollment including treatment, supportive care, screening, and prevention studies; and

- information on organizations and physicians who specialize in cancer care.

PDQ can be accessed through the National Library of Medicine, licensed vendors, the Information Associates Program (1-800-624-7890), or through a medical library with online searching capability. Staff at the Cancer Information Service (1-800-4-CANCER) can provide information from PDQ to callers. The PDQ Search Service also conducts PDQ searches for physicians and other health care professionals (1-800-345-3300).

CancerNet-R

You can use the Internet to acquire PDQ and other NCI information by computer. To access CancerNet through the Internet, use the World Wide Web at http://cancernet.nci.nih.gov/.

CancerMail

You can also use e-mail to acquire PDQ and other NCI information by computer. To obtain a CancerMail contents list, send e-mail to cancermail@icicc.nci.nih.gov with the word "help" in the body of the message.

CancerFax-R

For NCI information by fax, dial 301-402-5874 from the telephone on a fax machine and listen to recorded instructions.

Part Seven

Additional Help
and Information

Chapter 56

Dietary and Nutrition Terms

The words are listed in alphabetical order. Some words have many meanings; only those meanings that relate to diet, nutrition, and digestive diseases are included. The use of brand names is for identification purposes only; it does not constitute an endorsement.

A

absorption: The way nutrients from food move from the small intestine into the cells in the body.

acceptable daily intake (ADI)*: The amount of a chemical that, if ingested daily over a lifetime, appears to be without appreciable effect.

acesulfame K*: Acesulfame K, or acesulfame potassium, is a low-calorie sweetener approved for use in the United States in 1988. It is an organic salt consisting of carbon, nitrogen, oxygen, hydrogen, sulfur and potassium atoms. it is 200 times sweeter than sucrose, has a synergistic sweetening effect with other sweeteners, has a stable shelf-life

This chapter includes terms excerpted from the following publications: *The Digestive Diseases Dictionary*, National Institute of Diabetes and Digestive and Kidney Diseases (NIDDK), NIH Pub. No. 97-2750, March 1997; "Fat Words," *FDA Consumer*, 1995; *Managing Your Child's Eating Problems During Cancer Treatment*, National Cancer Institute (NCI), 1994; and *Glossary of Food-Related Terms* International Food Information Council, an undated document located at http://ificinfo.health.org, selected terms reprinted with permission; copyrighted definitions are marked with an asterisk (*).

and is heat stable. It is excreted through the human digestive system unchanged, and is therefore non-caloric.

additives (food additives)*: Any natural or synthetic material, other than the basic raw ingredients, used in the production of a food item to enhance the final product. Any substance that may affect the characteristics of any food, including those used in the production, processing, treatment, packaging, transportation or storage of food.

alactasia: An inherited condition causing the lack of the enzyme needed to digest milk sugar.

allergen (food allergen)*: A food allergen is the part of a food (a protein) that stimulates the immune system of food allergic individuals. A single food can contain multiple allergens. Carbohydrates or fats are not allergens.

allergy (food allergy)*: A food allergy is any adverse reaction to an otherwise harmless food or food component (a protein) that involves the body's immune system. To avoid confusion with other types of adverse reactions to foods, it is important to use the terms "food allergy" or "food hypersensitivity" only when the immune system is involved in causing the reaction.

amino acids: The basic building blocks of proteins. The body makes many amino acids. Others come from food and the body breaks them down for use by cells. (*See also* protein.)

anemia: Not enough red blood, red blood cells, or hemoglobin in the body. Hemoglobin is a protein in the blood that contains iron.

anorexia: Loss of appetite for food.

anorexia nervosa*: An eating disorder characterized by refusal to maintain a minimally normal weight for height and age. The condition includes weight loss leading to maintenance of body weight 15 percent below normal; an intense fear of weight gain or becoming fat, despite the individual's underweight status; a disturbance in the self-awareness of one's own body weight or shape; and in females, the absence of at least three consecutive menstrual cycles that would otherwise be expected to occur.

antacids: Medicines that balance acids and gas in the stomach. Examples are Maalox, Mylanta, and Di-Gel.

antidiarrheals: Medicines that help control diarrhea. An example is loperamide (Imodium).

antiemetics: Medicines that prevent and control nausea and vomiting. Examples are promethazine (Phenergan) and prochlorperazine (Compazine).

antioxidant*: Antioxidants protect key cell components by neutralizing the damaging effects of "free radicals," natural byproducts of cell metabolism. Free radicals form when oxygen is metabolized, or burned by the body. They travel through cells, disrupting the structure of other molecules, causing cellular damage. Such cell damage is believed to contribute to aging and various health problems.

aspartame*: Aspartame is a low-calorie sweetener used in a variety of foods and beverages and as a tabletop sweetener. It is about 200 times sweeter than sugar. Aspartame is made by joining two protein components, aspartic acid and phenylalanine.

atherosclerosis*: A condition that exists when too much cholesterol builds up in the blood and accumulates in the walls of the blood vessels.

B

biotechnology*: The simplest definition of biotechnology is "applied biology." The application of biological knowledge and techniques to develop products. It may be further defined as the use of living organisms to make a product or run a process. By this definition, the classic techniques used for plant and animal breeding, fermentation and enzyme purification would be considered biotechnology. Some people use the term only to refer to newer tools of genetic science. In this context, biotechnology may be defined as the use of biotechnical methods to modify the genetic materials of living cells so they will produce new substances or perform new functions. Examples include recombinant DNA technology, in which a copy of a piece of DNA containing one or a few genes is transferred between organisms or "recombined" within an organism.

bloating: Fullness or swelling in the abdomen that often occurs after meals.

bulking agents: Laxatives that make bowel movements soft and easy to pass.

bulimia nervosa*: An eating disorder characterized by rapid consumption of a large amount of food in a short period of time, with a sense of lack of control during the episode and self-evaluation unduly influenced by body weight and shape. There are two forms of the condition, purging and non-purging. The first type regularly engages in purging through self-induced vomiting or the excessive use of laxatives or diuretics. Alternatively, the non-purging type controls weight through strict dieting, fasting or excessive exercise.

C

calorie: Calories measure the energy your body gets from food. Your body needs calories as "fuel" to perform all of its functions such as breathing, circulating the blood, and physical activity.

caffeine*: Caffeine is a naturally-occurring substance found in the leaves, seeds, or fruits of over 63 plant species worldwide and is part of a group of compounds known as methylxanthines. The most commonly known sources of caffeine are coffee and cocoa beans, cola nuts and tea leaves. Caffeine is a pharmacologically active substance and, depending on the dose, can be a mild central nervous system stimulant. Caffeine does not accumulate in the body over the course of time and is normally excreted within several hours of consumption.

carbohydrates: One of the three main classes of food and a source of energy. Carbohydrates are the sugars and starches found in breads, cereals, fruits, and vegetables. During digestion, carbohydrates are changed into a simple sugar called glucose. Glucose is stored in the liver until cells need it for energy.

celiac disease: Inability to digest and absorb gliadin, the protein found in wheat. Undigested gliadin causes damage to the lining of the small intestine. This prevents absorption of nutrients from other foods. Celiac disease is also called celiac sprue, gluten intolerance, and nontropical sprue.

chloride: A mineral the body needs for fluid balance and other essential functions.

cholesterol: A fat-like substance in the body. The body makes and needs some cholesterol, which also comes from foods such as butter and egg yolks. Too much cholesterol may cause gallstones. It also may cause fat to build up in the arteries. This may cause a disease that slows or stops blood flow.

chronic: A term that refers to disorders that last a long time, often years.

colic: Attacks of abdominal pain, caused by muscle spasms in the intestines. Colic is common in infants.

colostomy: An operation that makes it possible for stool to leave the body after the rectum has been removed. The surgeon makes an opening in the abdomen and attaches the colon to it. A temporary colostomy may be done to let the rectum heal from injury or other surgery.

constipation: A condition in which the stool becomes hard and dry. A person who is constipated usually has fewer than three bowel movements in a week. Bowel movements may be painful.

continence: The ability to hold in a bowel movement or urine.

D

dehydration: When the body loses too much water; severe diarrhea or vomiting can cause dehydration.

diabetes*: Diabetes is the name for a group of medical disorders characterized by high blood sugar levels. Normally when people eat, food is digested and much of it is converted to glucose—a simple sugar— which the body uses for energy. The blood carries the glucose to cells where it is absorbed with the help of the hormone insulin. For those with diabetes, however, the body does not make enough insulin, or cannot properly use the insulin it does make. Without insulin, glucose accumulates in the blood rather than moving into the cells. High blood sugar levels result.

diet: The food you eat each day, including both liquids and solids.

dietary cholesterol: Cholesterol found in animal products that are part of the human diet. Egg yolks, liver, meat, some shellfish, and whole-milk dairy products are all sources of dietary cholesterol. (*See also* cholesterol.)

digestants: Medicines that aid or stimulate digestion. An example is a digestive enzyme such as Lactaid for people with lactase deficiency.

digestion: The process the body uses to break down food into simple substances for energy, growth, and cell repair.

digestive system: The organs in the body that break down and absorb food. Organs that make up the digestive system are the mouth, esophagus, stomach, small intestine, large intestine, rectum, and anus. Organs that help with digestion but are not part of the digestive tract are the tongue, glands in the mouth that make saliva, pancreas, liver, and gallbladder.

Digestive System

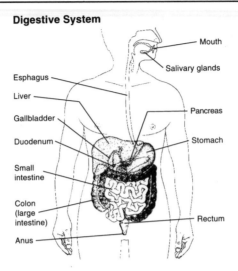

Mouth
Salivary glands
Esphagus
Liver
Gallbladder
Duodenum
Small intestine
Colon (large intestine)
Anus
Pancreas
Stomach
Rectum

Figure 56.1. Organs of the digestive system and organs that aid digestion.

diuretics: Medication that helps the body get rid of water and salt.

dyspepsia/indigestion: Upset stomach.

dysphagia: Difficulty in swallowing.

E

electrolytes: Chemicals such as salts and minerals needed for various functions in the body.

enteral nutrition: A way to provide food through a tube placed in the nose, the stomach, or the small intestine. A tube in the nose is called a nasogastric or nasoenteral tube. A tube that goes through the skin into the stomach is called a gastrostomy or percutaneous endoscopic gastrostomy (PEG). A tube into the small intestine is called a jejunostomy or percutaneous endoscopic jejunostomy (PEJ) tube. Also called tube feeding. (*See also* gastrostomy and jejunostomy.)

esophagus: The organ that connects the mouth to the stomach. Also called gullet.

F

failure to thrive: A condition that occurs when a baby does not grow normally.

fats: One of the three main classes of food and a source of energy in the body. Bile dissolves fats, and enzymes break them down. This process moves fats into cells.

fatty acid: A molecule composed mostly of carbon and hydrogen atoms. Fatty acids are the building blocks of fats.

fatty liver: The buildup of fat in liver cells. The most common cause is alcoholism. Other causes include obesity, diabetes, and pregnancy. Also called steatosis.

fecal fat test: A test to measure the body's ability to break down and absorb fat. The patient eats a fat-free diet for 2 to 3 days before the test and collects stool samples for examination.

fiber: A substance in foods that come from plants. Fiber helps with digestion by keeping stool soft so that it moves smoothly through the colon. Soluble fiber dissolves in water. Soluble fiber is found in beans, fruit, and oat products. Insoluble fiber does not dissolve in water. Insoluble fiber is found in whole-grain products and vegetables.

fortified: A food is fortified when extra nutrients are added.

flatulence: Excessive gas in the stomach or intestine. May cause bloating.

fluoride*: Fluoride is a natural component of minerals in rocks and soils. Widespread use of fluoride in water supplies and oral health products is credited with the dramatic decline in dental caries among children and adults alike. All water contains fluoride, but it is sometimes necessary to add it to some public supplies to attain the optimal amount for dental health. Fluoride makes tooth enamel stronger and more resistant to decay. It also prevents the growth of harmful bacteria and interferes with converting fermentable carbohydrates to acids in the mouth.

folic acid*: Folic acid, folate, folacin, all form a group of compounds functionally involved in amino acid metabolism and nucleic acid synthesis. Good dietary sources of folate include leafy, dark green vegetables, legumes, citrus fruits and juices, peanuts, whole grains and fortified breakfast cereals. Recent studies show, if all women of childbearing age consumed sufficient folic acid (either through diet or supplements), 50 to 70 percent of birth defects of the brain and spinal cord could be prevented, according to the U.S. Centers for Disease Control and Prevention (CDC.) Folic acid is critical from conception through the first four to six weeks of pregnancy when the neural tube is formed. This means adequate diet or supplement use should begin before pregnancy occurs. Recent research findings also show low blood folate levels can be associated with elevated plasma homocysteine and increased risk of coronary heart disease.

Food Guide Pyramid*: The Food Guide Pyramid is a graphic design used to communicate the recommended daily food choices contained in the Dietary Guidelines for Americans. The information provided was developed and promoted by the U.S. Department of Agriculture and the U.S. Department of Health and Human Services.

fructose*: Fructose is a monosaccharide found naturally in fruits, as an added sugar in a crystalline form and as a component of high-fructose corn syrup (HFCS).

fruit*: Fruit is the usually edible reproductive body of a seed plant, especially one having a sweet pulp associated with the seed.

functional disorders: Disorders such as irritable bowel syndrome. These conditions result from poor nerve and muscle function. Symptoms such as gas, pain, constipation, and diarrhea come back again and again, but there are no signs of disease or damage. Emotional stress can trigger symptoms. Also called motility disorders.

functional foods*: Foods that may provide health benefits beyond basic nutrition. Examples include tomatoes with lycopene, thought to help prevent the incidence of prostate and cervical cancers; fiber in wheat bran and sulfur compounds in garlic also believed to prevent cancer.

G

galactose: A type of sugar in milk products and sugar beets. The body also makes galactose.

gastrin: A hormone released after eating. Gastrin causes the stomach to produce more acid.

gastroesophageal reflux disease (GERD): Flow of the stomach's contents back up into the esophagus. Happens when the muscle between the esophagus and the stomach (the lower esophageal sphincter) is weak or relaxes when it shouldn't. May cause esophagitis. Also called esophageal reflux or reflux esophagitis.

gastrointestinal (GI) tract: The large, muscular tube that extends from the mouth to the anus, where the movement of muscles and release of hormones and enzymes digest food. Also called the alimentary canal or digestive tract.

gastronomy*: The study and appreciation of good food and good eating, and a culture's culinary customs, style and lore. Any interest or study of culinary pursuits as relates essentially to the kitchen and cookery, and to the higher levels of education, training and achievement of the chef apprentice or professional chef.

gastrostomy: An artificial opening from the stomach to a hole (stoma) in the abdomen where a feeding tube is inserted. (*See also* enteral nutrition.)

glucose: A simple sugar the body manufactures from carbohydrates in the diet. Glucose is the body's main source of energy. (*See also* carbohydrates.)

gluten: A protein found in wheat, rye, barley, and oats. In people who can't digest it, gluten damages the lining of the small intestine or causes sores on the skin.

glutamate*: Glutamate is an amino acid. It is necessary for metabolism and brain function, and is manufactured by the body. Glutamate is found in virtually every protein food we eat. In food, there is "bound" glutamate and "free" glutamate. Glutamate serves to enhance flavors in foods when it is in its free form and not bound to other amino acids in protein. Some foods have greater quantities of glutamate than others. Foods that are rich in glutamate include tomatoes, mushrooms, parmesan cheese, milk and mackerel.

gluten intolerance: *See* celiac disease.

gluten sensitive enteropathy: A general term that refers to celiac disease and dermatitis herpetiformis.

glycerol*: A colorless, odorless, syrupy liquid—chemically, an alcohol—that is obtained from fats and oils and used to retain moisture and add sweetness to foods.

glycogen: A sugar stored in the liver and muscles. It releases glucose into the blood when cells need it for energy. Glycogen is the chief source of stored fuel in the body.

grains*: Grains are the seeds or fruits of various food plants including cereal grasses. The examples of wheat, corn, oats, barley, rye, and rice provide a partial list. Grain foods include foods such as bread, cereals, rice and pasta.

GRAS (Generally Recognized as Safe)*: GRAS is the regulatory status of food ingredients not evaluated by the FDA prescribed testing procedure. It also includes common food ingredients that were already in use when the 1959 Food Additives Amendment to the Food, Drug and Cosmetic Act was enacted.

H

heartburn: A painful, burning feeling in the chest. Heartburn is caused by stomach acid flowing back into the esophagus. Changing the diet and other habits can help to prevent heartburn. Heartburn may be a symptom of GERD. See also Gastroesophageal Reflux Disease (GERD).

high-fructose corn syrup (HFCS)*: HFCS are formulations generally containing 42 percent, 55 percent, or 90 percent fructose (the remaining carbohydrate being primarily glucose) depending on the product application. HCFS are used in products such as soft drinks or cake mixes.

hormone: A substance in the body that regulates certain organs. Hormones such as gastrin help in breaking down food. Some hormones come from cells in the stomach and small intestine.

hydrochloric acid: An acid made in the stomach. Hydrochloric acid works with pepsin and other enzymes to break down proteins.

hydrogen breath test: A test for lactose intolerance. It measures breath samples for too much hydrogen. The body makes too much hydrogen when lactose is not broken down properly in the small intestine.

hydrogenation*: Hydrogenation is the process of adding hydrogen molecules directly to an unsaturated fatty acid from sources such as vegetable oils to convert it to a semi-solid form such as margarine or shortening. Hydrogenation contributes important textural properties to food. The degree of hydrogenation influences the firmness and spreadability of margarines, flakiness of pie crust and the creaminess of puddings. Hydrogenated oils are sometimes used in place of other fats with higher proportions of saturated fatty acids such as butter or lard.

hydrogenated fat: A fat that has been chemically altered by the addition of hydrogen atoms (*see* hydrogenation; trans fatty acid). Vegetable oil and margarine are hydrogenated fats.

I

ileostomy: An operation that makes it possible for stool to leave the body after the colon and rectum are removed. The surgeon makes an opening in the abdomen and attaches the bottom of the small intestine (ileum) to it.

indigestion: Poor digestion. Symptoms include heartburn, nausea, bloating, and gas. Also called dyspepsia.

J

jejunostomy: An operation to create an opening of the jejunum to a hole (stoma) in the abdomen. (*See also* enteral nutrition.)

L

lactase: An enzyme in the small intestine needed to digest milk sugar (lactose).

lactase deficiency: Lack of the lactase enzyme. Causes lactose intolerance.

lactose: The sugar found in milk. The body breaks lactose down into galactose and glucose.

lactose intolerance: Being unable to digest lactose, the sugar in milk. This condition occurs because the body does not produce the lactase enzyme.

lactose tolerance test: A test for lactase deficiency. The patient drinks a liquid that contains milk sugar. Then the patient's blood is tested; the test measures the amount of milk sugar in the blood.

large intestine: The part of the intestine that goes from the cecum to the rectum. The large intestine absorbs water from stool and changes it from a liquid to a solid form. The large intestine is 5 feet long and includes the appendix, cecum, colon, and rectum. Also called colon.

laxatives: Medicines to relieve long-term constipation. Used only if other methods fail. Also called cathartics.

lipid: A chemical compound characterized by the fact that it is insoluble in water. Both fat and cholesterol are members of the lipid family.

lipoprotein: A chemical compound made of fat and protein. Lipoproteins that have more fat than protein are called low-density lipoproteins

(LDLs). Lipoproteins that have more protein than fat are called high-density lipoproteins (HDLs). Lipoproteins are found in the blood, where their main function is to carry cholesterol.

low-calorie sweetener*: Low-calorie sweeteners are non-nutritive sweeteners, also referred to as intense sweeteners. Low-calorie sweeteners can replace nutritive sweeteners in most foods at a caloric savings of approximately 16 calories per teaspoon. Thus, caloric reduction may be achieved when low-calorie sweetened foods and beverages are substituted for their full-calorie counterparts. Examples of low-calorie sweeteners in use in the U.S. food supply are saccharin, aspartame, and acesulfame K.

lycopene*: Lycopene is a carotenoid related to the better known beta-carotene. Lycopene gives tomatoes and some other fruits and vegetables their distinctive red color. Nutritionally, it functions as an antioxidant. Research shows lycopene is best absorbed by the body when consumed as tomatoes that have been heat-processed using a small amount of oil. This includes products such as tomato sauce and tomato paste. (*See* also functional foods.)

M

malabsorption syndromes: Conditions that happen when the small intestine cannot absorb nutrients from foods.

malnutrition: A condition caused by not eating enough food or not eating a balanced diet.

metabolism: The way cells change food into energy after food is digested and absorbed into the blood.

minerals: Nutrients required by the body in small amounts such as iron, calcium, and potassium.

monosodium glutamate (MSG)*: MSG is the sodium salt of glutamic acid. Glutamic acid, or glutamate, is one of the most common amino acids found in nature. (*See also* glutamate.) In the early part of the century, MSG was extracted from seaweed and other plant sources. Today, MSG is produced in many countries around the world through a fermentation process of molasses from sugar cane or sugar beets, as well as starch and corn sugar.

monounsaturated fat: A fat made of monounsaturated fatty acids. Olive oil and canola oil are monounsaturated fats. Monounsaturated fats tend to lower levels of LDL-cholesterol in the blood.

monounsaturated fatty acid: A fatty acid that is missing one pair of hydrogen atoms in the middle of the molecule. The gap is called an "unsaturation." Monounsaturated fatty acids are found mostly in plant and sea foods.

morbid obesity*: This is a state of adiposity or overweight, in which body weight is 100 percent above the ideal and a body mass index of 45 or greater.

motility: The movement of food through the digestive tract.

mucosal lining: The lining of GI tract organs that makes mucus.

mucus: A clear liquid made by the intestines. Mucus coats and protects tissues in the GI tract.

N

Nationwide Food Consumption Survey (NFCS)*: A survey conducted by the USDA roughly every ten years that monitors the nutrient intake of a cross-section of the U.S. public.

National Health and Nutrition Examination Survey (NHANES)*: A series of surveys that include information from medical history, physical measurements, biochemical evaluation, physical examination and dietary intake of population groups within the United States. The NHANES is conducted by the U.S. Department of Health and Human Services approximately every five years.

nausea: The feeling of wanting to throw up (vomit).

neural tube defect*: In simple terms, a neural tube defect (NTD) is a malformation of the brain or spinal cord (neurological system) during embryonic development. Infants born with spina bifida, where the spinal cord is exposed, can grow to adulthood but usually suffer from paralysis or other disabilities. Babies born with anencephaly, where most or all of the brain is missing, usually die shortly after birth. These NTDs make up about 5 percent of all U.S. birth defects each year. According to the CDC, the use of sufficient folic acid is enough to eliminate the risk of NTDs. (*See also* folic acid)

nitrite*: Nitrite is a safe food additive that has been used for centuries to preserve meats, fish and poultry. It also contributes to the characteristic flavor, color and texture of processed meats such as hot dogs. Because nitrite safeguards cured meats against the most deadly foodborne bacterium of all, *Clostridium botulinum*, its use is supported by the public health community. The human body generates much greater nitrite levels than are added to food. Nitrates consumed in foods such as carrots and green vegetables are converted to nitrite during digestion. Nitrite in the body is instrumental in promoting blood clotting, healing wounds and burns, and boosting immune function to kill tumor cells.

nitrosamines*: Nitrosamines are a digestive reaction-product of nitrite, a food additive used to preserve meats, fish and poultry. (*See also* nitrite.)

nutraceuticals*: One term used to describe substances in or parts of a food that may be considered to provide medical or health benefits beyond basic nutrition, including disease prevention. Research indicates this term might not appeal to consumers. (*See also* functional foods.)

nutrient: The form food takes after being broken down during digestion. The major classes of nutrients that the body needs are proteins, minerals, fats, carbohydrates, and vitamins.

nutrition: A three-part process that gives the body the nutrients it needs. First, you eat or drink food. Second, the body breaks the food down into nutrients. Third, the nutrients travel through the bloodstream to different parts of the body where they are used as "fuel." To give your body proper nutrition, you have to eat or drink enough of the foods that contain key nutrients.

O

obesity, or overweight*: Although precise definitions vary among experts, overweight has been traditionally defined as 10 percent to 20 percent above an optimal weight for height derived from statistics. Obesity is defined as body weight being 20% above normal. Some scientists argue that the amount and distribution of an individual's body fat is a significant indicator of health risk and therefore should be considered in defining overweight. Abdominal fat has been linked to more adverse health consequences than fat in the hips or thighs. Thus, calculations of waist-to-hip ratio are preferred by some health experts to help determine if an individual is overweight.

obstruction: A blockage in the GI tract that prevents the flow of liquids or solids.

oral rehydration therapy: The use of specially formulated solutions to replace the water and other essential minerals lost as a results of severe diarrhea or vomiting.

organic*: Organic defines agricultural products that are grown using cultural, biological and mechanical methods prior to the use of synthetic, non-agricultural substances to control pests, improve soil quality an/or enhance processing. The USDA is currently addressing the issue of organic products, and aims to have official rules for what may be considered organic ready for the 1999 spring planting season. Currently organic defines an agricultural process in which farmers use techniques such as crop rotation, cultivation, mulching, soil enrichment and the "encouragement" of predators and microorganisms which naturally keep pests away. The now widely accepted definition allows farmers to use natural pesticides, but nothing synthetic.

ostomy: An operation that makes it possible for stool to leave the body through an opening made in the abdomen. An ostomy is necessary when part or all of the intestines are removed. Colostomy and ileostomy are types of ostomy.

P

pancreas: A gland that makes enzymes for digestion and the hormone insulin.

parenteral nutrition: A way to provide a liquid food mixture through a special tube in the chest. Also called hyperalimentation or total parenteral nutrition.

partial parenteral nutrition (PPN): When a person receives some of the nutrients he or she needs through a needle in his or her vein.

pepsin: An enzyme made in the stomach that breaks down proteins.

pernicious anemia: Anemia caused by a lack of vitamin B_{12}. The body needs B_{12} to make red blood cells.

pharynx: The space behind the mouth. Serves as a passage for food from the mouth to the esophagus and for air from the nose and mouth to the larynx.

phytochemical*: Phytochemicals are substances found in edible fruits and vegetables that may be ingested by humans daily in gram quantities and that exhibit a potential for modulating the human metabolism in a manner favorable for reducing risk of cancer. (*See* functional foods.)

polyunsaturated fat: A fat made of polyunsaturated fatty acids. Safflower oil and corn oil are polyunsaturated fats. Polyunsaturated fats tend to lower levels of both HDL-cholesterol and LDL-cholesterol in the blood.

polyunsaturated fatty acid: A fatty acid that is missing more than one pair of hydrogen atoms. Polyunsaturated fatty acids are mostly found in plant and sea foods.

potassium: A mineral the body needs for fluid balance and other essential functions.

protein: One of the three main classes of food. Protein is found in meat, eggs, and beans. The stomach and small intestine break down proteins into amino acids. The blood absorbs amino acids and uses them to build and mend cells. (*See also* amino acids.)

R

reflux: A condition that occurs when gastric juices or small amounts of food from the stomach flow back into the esophagus and mouth. Also called regurgitation.

S

saccharin*: Saccharin, the oldest of the non-nutritive sweeteners, is currently produced from purified, manufactured methyl anthranilate, a substance occurring naturally in grapes. It is 300 times sweeter than sucrose, heat stable and does not promote dental caries. Saccharin has a long shelf life, but a slightly bitter aftertaste. It is not metabolized in the human digestive system, is excreted rapidly in the urine and does not accumulate in body.

saliva: A mixture of water, protein, and salts that makes food easy to swallow and begins digestion.

saturated fat: A fat made of saturated fatty acids. Butter and lard are saturated fats. Saturated fats tend to raise levels of LDL-cholesterol ("bad" cholesterol) in the blood. Elevated levels of LDL-cholesterol are associated with heart disease.

saturated fatty acid: A fatty acid that has the maximum possible number of hydrogen atoms attached to every carbon atom. It is said to be "saturated" with hydrogen atoms. Saturated fatty acids are mostly found in animal products such as meat and whole milk.

secretin: A hormone made in the duodenum. Causes the stomach to make pepsin, the liver to make bile, and the pancreas to make a digestive juice.

short bowel syndrome: Problems related to absorbing nutrients after removal of part of the small intestine. Symptoms include diarrhea, weakness, and weight loss. Also called short gut syndrome.

sigmoid colon: The lower part of the colon that empties into the rectum.

small intestine: Organ where most digestion occurs. It measures about 20 feet and includes the duodenum, jejunum, and ileum.

sodium: A mineral required by the body to keep body fluids in balance; too much sodium can cause you to retain water.

somatostatin: A hormone in the pancreas. Somatostatin helps tell the body when to make the hormones insulin, glucagon, gastrin, secretin, and renin.

steatorrhea: A condition in which the body cannot absorb fat. Causes a buildup of fat in the stool and loose, greasy, and foul bowel movements.

stoma: An opening in the abdomen that is created by an operation (ostomy). Must be covered at all times by a bag that collects stool.

stomach: The organ between the esophagus and the small intestine. The stomach is where digestion of protein begins.

stool: The solid wastes that pass through the rectum as bowel movements. Stools are undigested foods, bacteria, mucus, and dead cells. Also called feces.

sucralose*: Sucralose is the only low-calorie sweetener that is made from sugar. It is approximately 600-times sweeter and does not contain calories. Sucralose is highly stable under a wide variety of processing conditions. Thus, it can be used virtually anywhere sugar can, including cooking and baking, without losing any of its sugar-like sweetness. Currently, sucralose is approved in over 25 countries around the world for use in food and beverages. In the US, the FDA has been petitioned to approve the use of sucralose in 15 different food and beverage categories.

sucrose*: Sucrose, a type of sugar, is a diglyceride composed of glucose and fructose. (*See also* carbohydrates.)

sugar*: Although the consumer is confronted by a wide variety of sugars—sucrose, raw sugar, turbinado sugar, brown sugar, honey, corn syrup—there is no significant difference in the nutritional content or energy each provides, and therefore no advantage of one nutritionally over another. There also is no evidence that the body can distinguish between naturally occurring or added sugars in food products.

T

total parenteral nutrition (TPN): When a person receives all the nutrients he or she needs through a needle in his or her vein. TPN may be used when the mouth, the stomach, or the bowel is sore from cancer treatment, or when a person is unable to eat solid foods, such as right after surgery.

trans fatty acid: A polyunsaturated fatty acid in which some of the missing hydrogen atoms have been put back in a chemical process called hydrogenation. Trans fatty acids are the building blocks of hydrogenated fats.

tropical sprue: A condition of unknown cause. Abnormalities in the lining of the small intestine prevent the body from absorbing food normally.

U

umami*: In addition to the four main taste components (sweet, sour, salty, and bitter), there is the additional taste characteristic called "umami" or savory. One of the food components responsible for the umami flavor in foods is glutamate, an amino acid. (See also glutamate; monosodium glutamate.)

V

villi: The tiny, fingerlike projections on the surface of the small intestine. Villi help absorb nutrients.

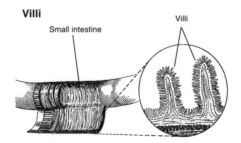

Figure 56.2. Villi help absorb nutrients in the small intestine.

vitamins*: Vitamins are organic compounds that are nutritionally essential in small amounts to control metabolic processes and cannot be synthesized by the body. Vitamins are usually classified by their solubility, which to some degree determines their stability; occurrence in foodstuffs; distribution in body fluids, and tissue storage capacity. Each of the fat-soluble vitamins A, D, E and K has a distinct and separate physiologic role. Several have antioxidant properties to depress the effects of metabolic byproducts called free radicals, which are thought to cause degenerative changes related to aging. Most of the water-soluble vitamins are components of essential enzyme systems. Many are involved in the reactions supporting energy metabolism. These vitamins are not normally stored in the body in appreciable amounts and are normally excreted in the urine. Thus, a daily supply is desirable to avoid depletion and interruption of normal physiologic functions.

vomiting: The release of stomach contents through the mouth.

W

water*: Although deficiencies of energy or nutrients can be sustained for months or even years, a person can survive only a few days without water. Experts rank water second only to oxygen as essential for life. In addition to offering true refreshment for the thirsty, water plays a vital role in all bodily processes. It supplies the medium in which various chemical changes of the body occur, aiding in digestion, absorption, circulation, and lubrication of body joints. For example, as a major component of blood, water helps deliver nutrients to body cells and removes waste to the kidneys for excretion.

Chapter 57

Federal Nutritional Support Programs

National School Lunch Program

What Is the National School Lunch Program?

The National School Lunch Program (NSLP) is a federally assisted meal program operating in nearly 94,000 public and nonprofit private schools and residential child care institutions. It provides nutritionally balanced, low-cost or free lunches to more than 26 million children each school day. Established under the National School Lunch Act, signed by President Harry Truman in 1946, the program celebrated its 50th anniversary in 1996.

The U.S. Department of Agriculture, through its Food and Nutrition Service (FNS—formerly the Food and Consumer Service), administers the program at the Federal level. At the State level, the NSLP is usually administered by State education agencies, which operate the program through agreements with local school districts. School districts and independent schools that choose to take part in the lunch program receive cash reimbursement and donated commodity assistance from USDA for each meal they serve. In return, they must serve

This chapter contains text from the U.S. Department of Agriculture's Food and Nutrition Service (FNS), Nutrition Program Facts: National School Lunch Program, December 1997; Special Milk Program, December 1997; The School Breakfast Program, February 1998; Summer Food Service Program, December 1997; Child and Adult Care Food Program, December 1997; WIC: The Special Supplemental Nutrition Program for Women, Infants, and Children, February 1998; Nutrition Program for the Elderly, December 1997.

lunches that meet Federal nutrition requirements, and they must offer free and reduced-price lunches to eligible children.

In 1994, FNS launched the School Meals Initiative for Healthy Children to teach children the importance of making healthy food choices, and to support school food service professionals in delivering healthy school meals. Supported by legislation passed in 1994 and 1996, the initiative updated nutrition standards so that all school meals meet the recommendations of the Dietary Guidelines for Americans. New regulations implementing the initiative became final in June, 1995, and took effect at the beginning of school year 1996-97.

How Does the National School Lunch Program Work?

Schools in the lunch program get cash subsidies and donated commodities from the U.S. Department of Agriculture for each meal they serve. In return, they must serve lunches that meet Federal requirements, and they must offer free or reduced-price lunches to eligible children.

How Do Children Qualify for Free and Reduced-Price Meals?

Any child at a participating school may purchase a meal through the National School Lunch Program. Children from families with incomes at or below 130 percent of the poverty level (currently $20,865 for a family of four) are eligible for free meals. Those between 130 percent and 185 percent of the poverty level (currently $29,693 for a family of four) are eligible for reduced-price meals, for which students can be charged no more than 40 cents.

Children from families with incomes over 185 percent of poverty pay a full price, though their meals are still subsidized to some extent. Local school food authorities set their own prices for full-price meals.

How Many Schools Take Part in the School Lunch Program?

Nearly 94,000 schools and residential child care institutions participate in the National School Lunch Program. Public schools or nonprofit private schools of high school grade or under, and residential child care institutions are eligible. The program is available in almost 99 percent of all public schools, and in many private schools as well. About 92 percent of all students nationwide have access to meals through the NSLP. On a typical day, about 58 percent of the school children to whom the lunch program is available participate.

How Much Reimbursement Do Schools Get?

Most of the support USDA provides to schools in the National School Lunch Program comes in the form of a cash reimbursement for each meal served. The current cash reimbursement rates are:

- Free meals: $1.89
- Reduced-price meals: $1.49
- Paid meals: 18 cents

Higher reimbursement rates are in effect for Alaska and Hawaii, and for some schools in special circumstances.

What Other Support Do Schools Get from USDA?

In addition to cash reimbursements, schools are entitled by law to receive commodity foods, called "entitlement" foods, at a value of 15 cents for each meal served. Schools can also get "bonus" commodities as they are available from surplus stocks. Under the School Meals Initiative, USDA also provides schools with technical training and assistance to help school food service staffs prepare healthy meals, and with nutrition education to help children understand the link between diet and health.

What Types of Foods Do Schools Get from USDA?

States select entitlement foods for their schools from a list of more than 60 different kinds of food purchased by USDA and offered through the school lunch program. The list includes fresh, canned, and frozen fruits and vegetables; meats; fruit juices; vegetable shortening; peanut products; vegetable oil; and flour and other grain products.

Bonus foods are offered only as they become available through agricultural surplus. The variety of both entitlement and bonus commodities schools can get from USDA depends on quantities available and market prices.

About 17 percent of the total dollar value of the food that goes on the table in school lunch programs is provided directly by USDA as commodities. Schools purchase the remaining 83 percent from their own vendors. As a part of its School Meals Initiative, USDA has placed special emphasis on improving the quality of commodities donated to the school lunch program, including a great increase in the amount and variety of fresh produce available to schools.

What Foods Are Schools Required to Serve in a School Lunch?

USDA does not require schools to serve—or not serve—any particular foods. School meals must meet Federal nutrition requirements, but decisions about what foods to serve and how they are prepared are made by local school food authorities.

Until the School Meals Initiative for Healthy Children, the Federal nutritional requirements for school meals had not changed significantly since the school lunch program began in 1946. As part of the initiative, USDA published regulations to help schools bring their meals up to date to meet the Dietary Guidelines for Americans. The Dietary Guidelines recommend that no more than 30 percent of an individual's calories come from fat, and no more than 10 percent from saturated fat.

The new regulations require schools to have met the Dietary Guidelines by school year 1996-1997, unless they received a waiver to allow an extension for up to two years. They also establish a standard for school meals to provide one-third of the Recommended Daily Allowances of protein, Vitamin A, Vitamin C, iron, calcium, and calories. Schools' compliance with both the Dietary Guidelines and the RDA's is measured over a week's menu cycle.

Schools have the option to choose one of five systems for their menu planning: NuMenus, Assisted NuMenus, traditional meal pattern, enhanced meal pattern, and other "reasonable approaches." Both the NuMenus and Assisted NuMenus systems base their planning on a computerized nutritional analysis of the week's menu. The traditional and enhanced meal pattern options base their menu planning on minimum component quantities of meat or meat alternate; vegetables and fruits; grains and breads; and milk. The fifth menu option allows schools to develop other "reasonable approaches" to meeting the Dietary Guidelines, using menu planning guidelines from USDA.

How Many Children Have Been Served Over the Years?

The National School Lunch Act in 1946 created the modern school lunch program, though USDA had provided funds and food to schools for many years prior to that. In signing the 1946 act, President Harry S Truman said, "Nothing is more important in our national life than the welfare of our children, and proper nourishment comes first in attaining this welfare."

About 7.1 million children were participating in the National School Lunch Program by the end of its first year, 1946-47. By 1970, 22 million children were participating, and by 1980 the figure was nearly 27 million. In 1990, an average of 24 million children ate school lunch every day. In Fiscal Year 1997, more than 26 million children each day got their lunch through the National School Lunch Program. Since the program began, more than 180 billion lunches have been served.

How Much Does the Program Cost?

The Fiscal Year 1998 appropriation for the National School Lunch Program is $4.2 billion. That figure is less than the $5.2 billion that was appropriated for 1997, but additional FY 98 funding will be available from carried-over 1997 money.

By comparison, the lunch program's total cost in 1947 was $70 million; in 1950, $119.7 million; 1960, $225.8 million; 1970, $565.5 million; 1975, $1.7 billion; 1980, $3.2 billion; 1985, $3.4 billion; and 1990, $3.8 billion.

Special Milk Program

What Is the Special Milk Program?

The Special Milk Program (SMP) provides milk to children in schools and child care institutions that do not participate in other Federal child nutrition meal service programs. The program reimburses schools for the milk they serve.

Schools in the National School Lunch or School Breakfast Programs may also participate in the SMP to provide milk to children in half-day pre-kindergarten and kindergarten programs where children do not have access to the school meal programs.

Begun in 1955, the Special Milk Program is administered at the Federal level by the U.S. Department of Agriculture through its Food and Nutrition Service (FNS), formerly the Food and Consumer Service.

Who May Participate?

Any child at a participating school or kindergarten program can get milk through the SMP. Children may buy milk or receive it free, depending on the school's choice of program options.

Who Is Eligible for Free Milk?

When local school officials offer free milk under the program, any child from a family that meets income guidelines for free meals and milk is eligible. Each child's family must apply annually for free milk eligibility.

How Does the SMP Operate?

Participating schools and institutions receive reimbursement from USDA for each half-pint of milk served. They must operate their milk programs on a non-profit basis. They agree to use the Federal reimbursement to reduce the selling price of milk to all children.

What Is the Federal Reimbursement?

The Federal reimbursement for each half-pint of milk sold to children in school year 1997-98 is 12.5 cents. For children who receive their milk free, the USDA reimburses schools the net purchase price of the milk.

What Types of Milk Can Be Offered?

Schools or institutions may choose unflavored or flavored whole milk, low-fat milk, skim milk, and cultured buttermilk that meet State and local standards. All milk should contain vitamins A and D at levels specified by the Food and Drug Administration.

How Much Milk Is Served Annually in the Special Milk Program?

In 1997, more than 140 million half-pints of milk were served through the Special Milk Program. Expansion of the National School Lunch and School Breakfast Programs, which include milk, has led to a substantial reduction in the SMP since its peak in the late 1960s. The program served nearly 3 billion pints of milk in 1969; 1.8 billion in 1980; and 181 million in 1990.

How Many Institutions Participate in the Special Milk Program?

In 1997, almost 8,000 schools and residential child care institutions participated, along with 1,400 summer camps and 500 non-residential child care institutions.

How Much Does the Program Cost?

Congress appropriated $18.2 million for the Special Milk Program in Fiscal Year 1998, down from $19.2 million for the program in FY 1997. By comparison, the program cost $101.2 million in 1970; $145.2 million in 1980; and $19.2 million in 1990.

The School Breakfast Program

What Is the School Breakfast Program?

Some 6.9 million children in more than 68,000 schools start their day with the School Breakfast Program, a Federal program that provides States with cash assistance for non-profit breakfast programs in schools and residential child care institutions.

Teachers have reported that their students are more alert and perform better in class if they eat breakfast. Studies support that notion. Most recently, a 1998 Tufts University statement on the link between nutrition and cognitive development in children cited new findings: "Children who participated in the School Breakfast Program were shown to have significantly higher standardized achievement test scores than eligible non-participants. Children getting school breakfast also had significantly reduced absence and tardiness rates."

Two other recent studies, by the State of Minnesota and by Harvard Medical/Massachusetts General Hospital, found that students who ate school breakfast had improved math grades, reduced hyperactivity, decreased absences and tardiness rates, and improved psycho-social behaviors. A 1989 study published in the *American Journal of Diseases of Children* found that "participation in the School Breakfast Program is associated with significant improvements in academic functioning among low-income elementary school children."

The School Breakfast Program began as a pilot project in 1966, and was made permanent in 1975. The program is administered at the Federal level by the U.S. Department of Agriculture through its Food and Nutrition Service (FNS), formerly the Food and Consumer Service (FCS). State education agencies and local school food authorities administer the program at the local level.

Recognizing the importance of a nutritious breakfast, USDA has actively promoted the School Breakfast Program, and at the same time has made a commitment to improve the nutritional quality of all school meals.

In 1994, in an effort to improve the nutritional quality of school meals, USDA launched the School Meals Initiative for Healthy Children.

The centerpiece of the initiative was new regulations to update nutrition standards so that all school meals will meet the recommendations of the Dietary Guidelines for Americans. Other elements of the initiative will teach and motivate children to make healthy food choices, cut administrative red tape, and continue to improve the quality of the commodities USDA provides to schools. The new regulations became final in June, 1995, and took effect at the beginning of school year 1996-97.

What Schools and Institutions Can Participate?

Public schools or non-profit private schools of high school grade or under, and residential child care institutions are eligible to participate in the School Breakfast Program.

Participating schools and institutions must serve breakfasts that meet Federal nutrition standards, and must provide free and reduced-price breakfasts to eligible children.

Who May Buy a Meal? Who Gets Free or Reduced-Price Breakfasts?

Any child at a participating school may purchase a meal through the School Breakfast Program. A child whose family meets income criteria may receive a free or reduced-price breakfast. The Federal government then reimburses the schools for each meal served that meets program nutritional requirements.

Children from families with incomes at or below 130 percent of the poverty level (currently $20,865 for a family of four) are eligible for free meals. Those between 130 percent and 185 percent of the poverty level (currently $29,693 for a family of four) are eligible for reduced-price meals. Children from families over 185 percent of poverty pay a full price, though their meals are still subsidized to some extent.

How Do Schools Get Reimbursed for Meals?

Schools submit a claim to their State agency for meals served. USDA reimburses the State, which in turn reimburses the local school food authority. For school year 1997-1998, the Federal government reimburses schools at the following rates:

- $1.045 per meal for free breakfasts.
- 74.5 cents for reduced-price breakfasts.
- 20 cents for paid breakfasts.

Schools may qualify for higher "severe-need" reimbursements if a specified percentage of their meals are served free or at a reduced price. Severe-need payments are 20 cents higher than the normal reimbursements for free and reduced-price breakfasts. More than 70 percent of the breakfasts served in the School Breakfast Program receive the severe-need subsidy. Reimbursement payments for all meals are higher in Alaska and Hawaii.

Schools may charge no more than 30 cents for a reduced-price breakfast. Schools set their own prices for breakfasts served to students who pay the full meal price.

How Many Children Participate? At What Cost?

For Fiscal Year 1998, Congress appropriated $1.3 billion for the School Breakfast Program, up from $1.2 billion in FY 1997.

In FY 1997, an average of 6.9 million children participated every day. Of those, 5.5 million received their meals free or at a reduced price.

By comparison, participation and cost in previous years:

- 1995: 6.3 million children at a cost of $1.05 billion
- 1990: 4.1 million children at a cost of $596.2 million
- 1985: 3.4 million children at a cost of $379.3 million
- 1980: 3.6 million children at a cost of $287.8 million
- 1975: 1.8 million children at a cost of $86.1 million
- 1970: 500,000 children at a cost of $10.8 million

Summer Food Service Program

What Is the Summer Food Service Program?

The Summer Food Service Program provides free, nutritious meals to low-income children during school vacations. The SFSP served 2.3 million children a day at more than 28,000 sites across the country during the summer of 1997.

How Does the Program Operate?

The program is administered at the Federal level by the Food and Nutrition Service (formerly the Food and Consumer Service), an agency of the U.S. Department of Agriculture. State education agencies administer most programs at the State level, but other State agencies may also be designated. Food and Nutrition Service regional offices administer a few state programs. Locally, it is operated by approved sponsors, which receive reimbursement from USDA through their State agencies for the meals they serve and for their documented operating costs. Sponsors can include units of local government, camps, nonprofit private organizations, and schools.

Sponsors provide meals at a central site, such as a school or community center. All meals are served free to eligible participants.

Where Does the Program Operate?

States designate SFSP feeding sites as either "open" or "enrolled" sites. Open sites operate in low-income areas where half or more of the children are from households with income at or below 185 percent of the Federal poverty guideline (currently $29,693 a year for a family of four). Meals are provided free to any child at the open site. Enrolled sites provide meals only to children who are enrolled in an activity program, such as a day camp, at the site. In order for the enrolled site to participate in the SFSP, at least half of the children enrolled must be from households with incomes at or below 185 percent of the poverty level.

Homeless feeding sites that primarily serve homeless children may participate regardless of location. Residential camps also may get reimbursement for eligible children through the SFSP.

Who Is Eligible to Get Meals?

Children 18 and under, and people over 18 who are determined by a State educational agency to be mentally or physically handicapped, and who participate in a school program for the mentally or physically handicapped, may receive meals through the Summer Food Service Program.

How Many Meals do Participants Receive Each Day?

At most sites, participants receive either one or two meals a day. Residential camps and sites that primarily serve children from migrant households may be approved to serve up to three meals per day.

How Much Reimbursement Does the Government Provide?

For summer 1998, the maximum reimbursement rate per meal will be:

- Breakfast $1.16
- Lunch/supper $2.0825

- Snack/supplement 54.3 cents

Sponsors also receive Federal funds for administrative costs. Depending on the type of site, sponsors can receive up to 10.75 cents for each breakfast, 19.75 cents for each lunch or supper, and 5.25 cents for each snack.

How Long Has the SFSP Been in Existence?

SFSP was first created as part of a larger pilot program in 1968, and became a separate program in 1975. By 1980, 1.9 million children were participating. Participation dropped to 1.5 million in 1985, and grew to 1.7 million again by 1990. More than 2.3 million children participated at more than 28,000 sites in the summer of 1997.

How Much Does the Program Cost?

Congress appropriated $272.3 million for SFSP in Fiscal year 1998, up from $250 million for the program in FY 1997.

By comparison, the program cost $110.1 million in 1980; $111.5 million in 1985; and $164.5 million in 1990.

Child and Adult Care Food Program

What Is the Child and Adult Care Food Program?

The Child and Adult Care Food Program (CACFP) is a Federal program that provides healthy meals and snacks in child and adult day care facilities.

CACFP reimburses participating day care operators for their meal costs and provides them with USDA commodity food. The program generally operates in child care centers, outside-school-hours care centers, family and group day care homes, and some adult day care centers. Day care providers in the CACFP must serve meals that meet federal guidelines, and must offer free or reduced-price meals to eligible people.

First authorized as a pilot project in 1975, the program was formerly known as the Child Care Food Program. It was made a permanent program in 1978, and the name was changed in 1989 to reflect the addition of an adult component. CACFP is administered at the Federal level by the Food and Nutrition Service (FNS), an agency of the U.S. Department of Agriculture. State agencies or FNS regional offices oversee the program at the local level.

What Types of Institutions Provide Benefits?

Child Care Centers. Includes licensed or approved non-residential, public or private non-profit child care centers; and Head Start centers, settlement houses, and neighborhood centers. For-profit child care centers may also participate if they meet certain criteria for serving low-income children.

Family Day Care Homes. Generally, family day care homes provide care in a licensed or approved private home for a small group of children. Family or group day care homes must be administered by a sponsoring organization that maintains Federal and State regulations, and prepares a monthly food reimbursement claim. The sponsor also receives Federal reimbursement for administrative expenses, based on the number of homes it sponsors.

Adult Day Care Centers. Licensed day care centers that are operated by public agencies for functionally impaired adults may receive cash reimbursements and commodity foods under the adult component of the CACFP. Private organizations, both non-profit and for-profit, are also eligible if they meet certain criteria for serving low-income people.

Who Gets Free or Reduced-Price Meals?

At child and adult day care centers, participants may pay full price for their meals, or they may qualify for free or reduced-price meals. Those from families with income at or below 130 percent of the poverty level may qualify for free meals; those from families with income between 130 percent and 185 percent of the poverty level may qualify for reduced-price meals; and those from families with income above 185 percent of the poverty level pay full price. Currently, for a family of four, 130 percent of the poverty level is $20,865 a year; 185 percent is $29,693 a year.

For family day care homes, Congress instituted a two-tier system of reimbursements under the welfare reform act of 1996. Under the new system, which went into effect July 1, 1997, day care providers located in low-income areas, or whose own households are low income, are reimbursed at a single rate (tier 1 reimbursement). Other providers will be reimbursed at a lower rate (tier 2 reimbursement) unless they choose to have their sponsoring organizations identify income-eligible children through use of income applications similar to those used in day care centers. Meals served to such income-eligible children will be reimbursed at the higher tier 1 level.

How Much Reimbursement Does the Federal Government Provide?

The Tables 57.1 shows how much reimbursement the Federal government provides to child and adult day care centers and family day care homes for breakfasts, lunches, suppers, and supplements (snacks).

Table 57.1. Federal Government Reimbursement for meals provided under the Child and Adult Care Food Program

Child and adult day care centers:

	Free	Reduced price	Paid
Breakfast	$1.045	74.5 cents	20 cents
Lunch/Supper	$1.89	$1.49	18 cents
Supplement (snack)	51.75 cents	26 cents	4 cents

Family day care homes:

	Tier 2 rate	Tier 1 rate
Breakfast	33 cents	88 cents
Lunch/Supper	98 cents	$1.62
Supplement (snack)	13 cents	48 cents

Higher rates apply in Alaska and Hawaii. These rates do not include the average 14 cents value of commodities (or cash in lieu of commodities) that institutions receive as additional assistance for each lunch or supper served to program participants.

Family day care home sponsors also receive reimbursement for their administrative costs. The current administrative rates per home per month are:

- 1–50 homes: $75
- 51–200 homes: $57
- 201–1,000 homes: $45
- Each home over 1,000: $39

How Much Does the Child and Adult Care Food Program Cost, and How Many People Does It Serve?

Congress appropriated $1.6 billion for the CACFP in both Fiscal Year 1997 and FY 1996. In June 1997, CACFP provided meals to nearly 2.3 million children and more than 58,000 adults.

By comparison, participation and costs from earlier years:

- 1995: 2.3 million children and 44,000 adults participated at a cost of $1.5 billion.

- 1990: 1.5 million children and 18,000 adults participated at a cost of $812.9 million

- 1985: 1 million children participated at a cost of $452.1 million.

- 1980: 663,000 children participated at a cost of $236.4 million.

- 1975: 375,000 children participated at a cost of $51 million.

What Is the Homeless Children Nutrition Program?

The Homeless Children Nutrition Program is designed to provide free food service throughout the year to homeless children under the age of 6 in emergency shelters. Sponsoring organizations are reimbursed for the meals that they serve. First established as a demonstration project by the Child Nutrition and WIC Reauthorization Act of 1989, the Homeless Children Nutrition Program was made permanent by the Healthy Meals for Healthy Americans Act of 1994. A total of 86 sponsoring organizations operate the program in 117 shelters, providing meals to more than 2,500 preschool-age children every month.

Public and private nonprofit organizations that operate emergency shelters may participate in the Homeless Children Nutrition Program, but they may operate no more than five food service sites and may feed no more than 300 children per day at each site. Sponsors are reimbursed at a rate of $1.8375 for each lunch or supper served; $1.0175 for each breakfast served; and 50.5 cents for each supplement (snack).

For FY 1997, Congress appropriated $3.1 million for the Homeless Children Nutrition Program. For 1996, the appropriation was $2.6 million.

WIC: The Special Supplemental Nutrition Program for Women, Infants, and Children

What Is WIC?

Food, nutrition counseling, and access to health services are provided to low-income women, infants, and children under the Special Supplemental Nutrition Program for Women, Infants, and Children, popularly known as WIC.

WIC provides Federal grants to States for supplemental foods, health care referrals, and nutrition education for low-income pregnant, breastfeeding, and non-breastfeeding postpartum women, and to infants and children who are found to be at nutritional risk.

Established as a pilot program in 1972 and made permanent in 1974, WIC is administered at the Federal level by the Food and Nutrition Service of the U.S. Department of Agriculture. Formerly known as the Special Supplemental Food Program for Women, Infants, and Children, WIC's name was changed under the Healthy Meals for Healthy Americans Act of 1994, in order to emphasize its role as a nutrition program.

Most State WIC programs provide vouchers that participants use at authorized food stores. A wide variety of State and local organizations cooperate in providing the food and health care benefits, and 46,000 merchants nationwide accept WIC vouchers.

WIC is effective in improving the health of pregnant women, new mothers, and their infants. A 1990 study showed that women who participated in the program during their pregnancies had lower Medicaid costs for themselves and their babies than did women who did not participate. WIC participation was also linked with longer gestation periods, higher birth weights and lower infant mortality.

Who Is Eligible?

Pregnant or postpartum women, infants, and children up to age 5 are eligible. They must meet income guidelines, a State residency requirement, and be individually determined to be at "nutritional risk" by a health professional.

To be eligible on the basis of income, applicants' income must fall below 185 percent of the U.S. Poverty Income Guidelines (currently $29,693 for a family of four). While most States use the maximum guidelines, States may set lower income limit standards. A person who participates in certain other benefits programs such as the Food Stamp Program or Medicaid automatically meets the income eligibility requirement.

What Is "Nutritional Risk"?

Two major types of nutritional risk are recognized for WIC eligibility:

- Medically-based risks (designated as "high priority") such as anemia, underweight, maternal age, history of pregnancy complications, or poor pregnancy outcomes.
- Diet-based risks such as inadequate dietary pattern.

Nutritional risk is determined by a health professional such as a physician, nutritionist, or nurse, and is based on Federal guidelines. This health screening is free to program applicants.

How Many People Does WIC Serve?

More than 7 million people get WIC benefits each month. Participation has risen steadily since the program began. In 1974, the first year WIC was permanently authorized, 88,000 people participated. By 1980, participation was at 1.9 million; by 1985 it was 3.1 million; and by 1990 it was 4.5 million. Average monthly participation for Fiscal Year 1997 was 7.4 million.

Children have always been the largest category of WIC participants. Of the average 7.4 million people who received WIC benefits each month in FY 1997, 3.8 million were children, 1.9 million were infants, and 1.7 million were women.

What Percent of Eligible People Does WIC Reach?

About 45 percent of all babies born in the United States, and 98 percent of eligible infants, are estimated to be served by WIC. Of all eligible women, infants, and children, the program is estimated to serve about 60 percent.

Where Is WIC Available?

The WIC program is available in each State, the District of Columbia, 32 Indian Tribal Organizations, Puerto Rico, the Virgin Islands, American Samoa, and Guam.

What Food Benefits Do WIC Participants Receive?

WIC participants receive vouchers that allow them to purchase a monthly food package designed to supplement their diets. The foods provided are high in protein, calcium, iron, and vitamins A and C. These are the nutrients frequently lacking in the diets of the program's target population. Different food packages are provided for different categories of participants.

WIC foods include iron-fortified infant formula and infant cereal, iron-fortified adult cereal, vitamin C-rich fruit or vegetable juice, eggs, milk, cheese, and peanut butter or dried beans or peas. Special therapeutic infant formulas are provided when prescribed by a physician for a specified medical condition.

Who Gets First Priority for Participation?

WIC cannot serve all eligible people, so a system of priorities has been established for filling program openings. Once a local WIC agency has reached its maximum caseload, vacancies are filled in the order of the following priority levels:

Pregnant women, breastfeeding women, and infants determined to be at nutritional risk because of a nutrition-related medical condition. Infants up to 6 months of age whose mothers were at nutritional risk during pregnancy. Children at nutritional risk because of a nutrition-related medical condition. Pregnant or breastfeeding women and infants at nutritional risk because of an inadequate dietary pattern. Children at nutritional risk because of an inadequate dietary pattern. Non-breastfeeding, postpartum women at nutritional risk.

What Is the WIC Infant Formula Rebate System?

Mothers participating in WIC are encouraged to breastfeed their infants if possible, but State WIC agencies still provide formula for mothers who choose to use it. By negotiating rebates with formula manufacturers, States greatly increase the amount of formula they can provide, and help WIC funds go further to serve more people. States take bids or negotiate with manufacturers for the highest rebate for each can of formula purchased. For FY 1996, WIC state agencies spent $620 million on infant formula, after rebate savings totaling $1.18 billion.

What Is the WIC Farmers Market Nutrition Program?

The WIC Farmers' Market Nutrition Program (FMNP), established in 1992, provides additional coupons to WIC participants that they can use to purchase fresh fruits and vegetables at participating farmers' markets. FMNP is funded through a Congressionally mandated set-aside in the WIC appropriation. The program has two goals: To provide fresh, nutritious, unprepared food, such as fruits and vegetables, from farmers' markets to WIC participants who are at nutritional risk; and to expand consumers' awareness and use of farmers' markets.

This program, operated in conjunction with the regular WIC Program, is offered in 32 States, the District of Columbia, and two Indian tribal organizations. State agencies may limit FMNP sales to specific foods that are locally grown to encourage participants to support the farmers in their own State. The amount set aside in the WIC appropriation for FMNP for Fiscal Year 1998 is $12 million, up from $6.75 million in FY 1997.

How Much Does WIC Cost?

Congress appropriated $3.9 billion for WIC in FY 1998, up from $3.7 billion in 1997. The appropriation includes $12 million for the WIC Farmers' Market Nutrition Program.

By comparison, the WIC program cost $10.4 million in 1974; $727.7 million in 1980; $1.5 billion in 1985; and $2.1 billion in 1990.

Nutrition Program for the Elderly

What Is the Nutrition Program for the Elderly?

The Nutrition Program for the Elderly helps provide elderly persons with nutritionally sound meals through meals-on-wheels programs or in senior citizen centers and similar settings.

The NPE is administered by the U.S. Department of Health and Human Services, but receives commodity foods and financial support from the U.S. Department of Agriculture's Food and Nutrition Service under provisions of the Older Americans Act of 1965.

Who Is Eligible?

Age is the only factor used in determining eligibility. People age 60 or over and their spouses, regardless of age, are eligible for NPE benefits. Indian tribal organizations may select an age below 60 for defining an "older" person for their tribes.

There is no income requirement to receive meals under NPE. Each recipient can contribute as much as he or she wishes toward the cost of the meal, but meals are free to those who cannot make any contribution.

What Does the Program Provide?

Under NPE, the Department of Agriculture provides cash reimbursements and/or commodity foods to state agencies, which pass them on to agencies or organizations that serve meals through Department of Health and Human Services programs. In order to qualify for cash or commodity assistance, meals served must meet a specified percentage of the nutrients prescribed by the Recommended Dietary Allowances.

Is NPE a Commodity or Cash Subsidy Program?

States can take all or part of their subsidies in cash, rather than commodity foods. Although it was originally established as a program to distribute USDA commodities to senior citizen meal sites, the NPE has evolved primarily into a cash subsidy program. Approximately 94 percent of program resources are distributed to meal providers in cash.

How Much Reimbursement Do the States Get?

When Congress provides sufficient funds, states are reimbursed at whichever is greater: a flat rate, which is adjusted annually; or the current appropriation divided by the number of meals served in the preceding year. However, actual reimbursement for meals may be limited by the appropriation level set by Congress.

How Many Meals Are Served and At What Cost?

Congress appropriated $140 million for NPE for FY 1998, the same as for FY 1997. USDA provided reimbursement for an average of more than 20 million meals a month in FY 1997.

Nutrition Education and Training (NET) Program

What Is the NET program?

FNS operates the Nutrition Education and Training (NET) Program to support nutrition education in the food assistance programs for children: the National School Lunch Program, School Breakfast, Summer Food Service, and Child and Adult Care Food Programs. The Secretary of Agriculture allocates NET funds to States each year in the form of grants. Congress appropriated $3.75 million for NET in FY 1998.

For More Information

For more information, contact the USDA Food and Nutrition Service Public Information Staff at 703-305-2286, or by mail at 3101 Park Center Drive, Room 819, Alexandria, Virginia 22302.

The Food and Nutrition Service was formerly known as the Food and Consumer Service. Information on FNS programs is available on the World Wide Web at www.usda.gov/fcs, and will be available soon on a new web site: www.usda.gov/fns.

Chapter 58

Health and Nutrition Information On-Line

Cautions about Health Information On-Line

Consumers are using the Internet to get information about health. How reliable is this information? That's not an easy question to answer.

A survey by CDB Research & Consulting indicates that consumers are showing a growing interest in obtaining information about health and beauty aids on-line as a means of supplementing traditional medical counsel.

However, easy access to virtually limitless health and medical information has pitfalls, experts caution. "My advice to consumers about information on the Internet is the same as it is for other media: You can't believe everything you see, whether it's in a newspaper, on TV, or on a computer screen," says Bill Rados, director of FDA's Communications Staff. Since anyone—reputable scientist or quack—who has a computer, a modem (the device that permits a computer to dial and connect to the Internet or an on-line service), and the necessary software can publish a Web page, post information to a newsgroup, or proffer advice in an on-line chat room, "you must protect yourself by carefully checking out the source of any information you obtain."

This chapter contains excerpts from "Health Information On-Line," FDA Publication No. (FDA) 98-1253, updated January 1998 and excerpts from "Sensible Nutrition Resource List for Consumers," U.S. Department of Agriculture (USDA), August 1998.

World Wide Web

By far, the most consumer-friendly part of the Internet is the World Wide Web. While the rest of the Internet displays text only, the Web, as it has come to be called, has the ability to display colorful graphics and multimedia (sounds, video, virtual reality).

Many legitimate providers of reliable health and medical information, including FDA and other government agencies, are taking advantage of the Web's popularity by offering brochures and in-depth information on specific topics on their websites. Material may be geared to consumers as well as industry and medical professionals.

But con artists have also infiltrated the Web. "A physician was browsing the Web when he came across a site that contained a fraudulent drug offering. He called us to report it," says Roma Jeanne Egli, a compliance officer in FDA's division of labeling and nonprescription drug compliance. "The person who maintains the site claimed he had a cure for a very serious disease, and advised those with the disease to stop taking their prescription medication. Instead, they were told to buy the product he was selling, at a cost of several hundred dollars."

Egli advises consumers to be skeptical when someone advocates a purported "cure" to be purchased and taken in lieu of prescribed medicine.

Although the Internet can be a reliable source of information, it is important to be aware that what is found there is only as good as the quality and integrity of the original information. What you find cannot be taken as gospel. It should be checked out and supported by other sources. (See "Is This Site Reliable?")

If you come across a suspected fraudulent nonprescription drug on the Internet, alert FDA by E-mail: otcfraud@cder.fda.gov.

FDA On-Line

The FDA home page provides an excellent jumping off point for those who want to learn more about the agency and the drugs, food supplements, and medical devices it regulates. It includes a detailed index and special menus for such groups as consumers, health professionals, and industry representatives.

Warning letters from FDA to regulated companies, inspection manuals, monthly import detention lists, medical device problem reports, and other often-requested materials are available without having to go through the time and paperwork of filing a traditional Freedom of Information request. Users can reach the Electronic FOI

Reading Room directly from the FDA home page. Because it is expensive to print and mail materials, FDA offers many of its publications on the Internet. "Our goal is to have virtually all consumer education material available on the Internet," says Rados. "We now have more than a hundred different publications to choose from."

In addition to providing consumer education materials, the FDA site also offers technical information to help industry professionals file regulatory materials. Material can be downloaded to a computer and then printed out. Those who don't have a personal computer can try accessing the Internet from their local library or from a community organization.

FDA also has a "comments" button on many of its Web pages so that visitors can offer suggestions and feedback. However, questions about specific drugs, devices, or food supplements should be addressed to the agency in writing at "FDA" (HFE-88), Rockville, MD 20857, or by calling your local public affairs specialist. A list of FDA Public Affairs Specialists is available on the FDA website (at http://www.fda.gov/ora/fed_state/dfsr_activities/dfsr_pas.html). Before beginning any particular therapy, however, consult with your doctor or pharmacist.

Exchanging Information

In Internet "newsgroups," such as Usenet groups, people post questions and read messages much as they would on regular bulletin boards. Through "mailing lists," messages are exchanged by E-mail, and all messages are sent to all group subscribers. In "chat" areas on some services and on the Internet's IRC (Internet Relay Chat) users can communicate with each other live.

Assessing the value and validity of health and medical information in news and chat groups demands at least the same—and maybe more—discrimination as for websites, because the information is more ephemeral and you often can't identify the source. Although these groups can provide reliable information about specific diseases and disorders, they can also perpetuate misinformation.

Other information services are commercial on-line services, fee-charging companies that provide vast amounts of proprietary information. They often include health and medical databases, electronic versions of popular newspapers and magazines, and their own chats and newsgroups, as well as Internet access.

The fact that information may be screened by a commercial service does not necessarily make it more reliable than other sources.

And most services do not verify what is posted in their newsgroups, nor control what is "said" in chat rooms. Health and medical material obtained through services also should be corroborated by your physician or other medical sources.

Regulatory Concerns

The fact that it is easy to publish health and medical information and reach vast audiences without having the information verified by other sources presents potential issues for FDA and other government agencies. Product information on the Internet is unlike traditional forms of advertising and labeling. Current regulations on prescription drug advertising differ between print and broadcast media. The Internet presents additional challenges.

While regulatory agencies try to devise ways of ensuring that accurate and well-balanced health and medical information is presented on the Internet, consumers will have to use a lot more discretion in evaluating what they see. A Web page can be changed very quickly. It is easy to put up, and easy to take down. There is no guarantee that what you see one day will be there the next." So on the Internet, as elsewhere, "*caveat emptor*"—let the buyer beware—are watchwords for the foreseeable future.

Is This Site Reliable?

FDA staff and others familiar with Internet medical offerings suggest asking the following questions to help determine the reliability of a Website:

Who maintains the site? Government or university-run sites are among the best sources for scientifically sound health and medical information. Private practitioners or lay organizations may have marketing, social or political agendas that can influence the type of material they offer on-site and which sites they link to.

Is there an editorial board or another listing of the names and credentials of those responsible for preparing and reviewing the site's contents? Can these people be contacted if visitors to the site have questions or want additional information?

Does the site link to other sources of medical information? A reputable organization will not position itself as the sole source of information on a particular health topic. On the other hand, links alone are not a guarantee of reliability. Since anyone with a Web page can create links to any other site on the Internet—and the owner of the site that is "linked to" has no say over who links to it—then a person offering suspect medical advice could conceivably try to make his or her advice appear legitimate by, say, creating a link to FDA's website. What's more, health information produced by FDA or other government agencies is not copyrighted; therefore, someone can quote FDA information at a site and be perfectly within his or her rights. By citing a source such as FDA, experienced marketers using careful wording can make it appear as though FDA endorses their products.

When was the site last updated? Generally, the more current the site, the more likely it is to provide timely material. Ideally, health and medical sites should be updated weekly or monthly.

Are informative graphics and multimedia files such as video or audio clips available? Such features can assist in clarifying medical conditions and procedures. Bear in mind, however, that multimedia should be used to help explain medical information, not substitute for it. Some sites provide dazzling "bells and whistles" but little scientifically sound information.

Does the site charge an access fee? Many reputable sites with health and medical information, including FDA and other government sites, offer access and materials for free. If a site does charge a fee, be sure that it offers value for the money. Use a searcher to see whether you can get the same information without paying additional fees.

If you find something of interest at a site—say, a new drug touted to relieve disease symptoms with fewer side effects—write down the name and address of the site, print out the information, and bring it to your doctor. Your doctor can help determine whether the information is supported by legitimate research sources, such as journal articles or proceedings from a scientific meeting.

In addition, your doctor can determine if the drug is appropriate for your situation. Even if the information comes from a source that is reputed to be reliable, you should check with your doctor to make sure that it is wise for you to begin a certain treatment. Specific situations (such as taking other drugs) may make the therapy an inadvisable choice. Your doctor can decide whether the drug is suitable for you and may be able to offer more appropriate alternatives.

Search Programs

Because the Internet contains no central indexing system, getting the information you want quickly can be a major challenge. That's where search engines come in. These powerful tools can help narrow the field if you have a specific topic to pursue, or the name of a specific organization but no address for its site. Input a few words that describe what you're looking for, and the searcher returns a list of sites related to your query.

Be aware, however, that although a searcher can point the way, it does not evaluate the information it points to. For example, a search on the words "breast cancer" is just as likely to point to a page advertising a reconstructive surgeon or a health food store's article on the purported benefits of phytochemicals as it is to the National Cancer Institute. It is up to the visitor to evaluate the information the site contains. Here are a few of the many search engines:

- Alta Vista: http://www.altavista.digital.com/
- Excite: http://www.excite.com/
- Lycos: http://www.lycos.com/
- Webcrawler: http://www.webcrawler.com/
- Yahoo: http://www.yahoo.com/Health/Medicine/

Selected Nutrition Resources Available on the World Wide Web

The American Dietetic Association (ADA)
National Center for Nutrition and Dietetics
216 West Jackson Blvd.
Chicago, IL 60606-6995
(312) 899-0040 x4750
Fax: (312) 889-4739
Consumer Nutrition Hotline (800) 877-1600 x4821
Website: http://www.eatright.org/ncnd.html
Contents: Provides information about the variety of nutrition resources and programs that the NCND offers.

American Institute for Cancer Research (AICR)
1759 R Street, NW
Washington, DC 20009
(800) 843-8114

(202) 328-7744 (in the Washington, DC Metropolitan area)
Fax: (202) 328-7226
E-mail: aicrweb@aicr.org
Website: http://www.aicr.org/
Contents: Provides a variety of nutrition information, particularly those topics relating to cancer.

The Blonz Guide to Nutrition
E-mail: ed@blonz.com
Website: www.wenet.net/blonz/
Contents: Information on news in the fields of nutrition, food science, foods, fitness, and health. Also includes a selection of search engines and other important links.

Center for Science in the Public Interest (CSPI)
1875 Connecticut Ave., NW, Suite 300
Washington, DC 20009-5728.
(202) 332-9110
Fax: (202) 265-4954
E-mail: cspi@cspinet.org
Website: http://www.cspinet.org/
Contents: Provides a variety of nutrition information including the Nutrition Action Healthletter, nutrition quizzes, and a section for kids.

Children's Nutrition Research Center
Baylor College of Medicine, Public Affairs Office
Children's Nutrition Research Center
1100 Bates St., Houston, TX 77030
E-mail: cnrc@bcm.tmc.edu
Website: http://www.bcm.tmc.edu/cnrc/newsletter/
Contents: Provides newsletters for parents on child nutrition topics in an easy to read format.

Food & Drug Administration
Center for Food Safety & Applied Nutrition
200 C Street SW
Washington, DC 20204
(800) 332-4010 (Food Information & Seafood Hotline)
Website: http://www.fda.gov/
Contents: Provides information on dietary supplements, food additives, foodborne illness, food labeling and nutrition, and seafood.

Food Marketing Institute
800 Connecticut Ave., NW
Washington, DC 20006-2701
(202) 452-8444
Fax: (202) 429-4519
E-mail: fmi@fmi.org
Website: http://www.fmi.org/
Contents: Provides information on FMI publications, industry resources, consumer information, and FMI events.

Food and Nutrition Information Center
National Agricultural Library
Agricultural Research Service, USDA
10301 Baltimore Ave., Room 304
Beltsville, MD 20705-2351
(301) 504-5755
E-mail: arsweb@nal.usda.gov
Website: http://www.nal.usda.gov/fnic
Contents: Contains a variety of nutrition information, including an index that connects to the other addresses on this list. Also has a search mechanism to search the FNIC website.

Food Safety and Inspection Service
FSIS Food Safety Education and Communications Staff
Room 1175-South Bldg.
1400 Independence Ave. SW
Washington DC 20250
(202) 720-7943
Fax: (202) 720-1843
E-mail: fsis.webmaster@usda.gov
Website: http://www.fsis.usda.gov
Contents: Food safety information.

International Food Information Council
Publications Department (IFIC/www) IFIC Foundation
1100 Connecticut Ave., NW, Suite 430
Washington, DC 20036
E-mail: foodinfo@ific.health.org
Website: http://www.ificinfo.health.org/
Contents: Provides food safety and nutrition information and pamphlets on a variety of nutrition topics.

Iowa State University, University Extension
Food Science and Human Nutrition Extension
1127 Human Nutritional Sciences Bldg.
Iowa State University
Ames, IA 50011-1120
E-mail: xlschafe@exnet.iastate.edu
Website: http://www.exnet.iastate.edu/Pages/families/fshn/
Contents: Provides a variety of topics related to nutrition and your health. Need Adobe Acrobat reader to view most of the publications.

The Kellogg's Nutrition University
P.O. Box CAMB
Battle Creek, MI 49016-1986
(800) 962-1413
Website: http://www.kelloggsnu.com/
Contents: Provides up-to-date information about healthy eating, including nutrition courses, a risk assessment quiz, product information, and corporate news.

National Council Against Health Fraud, Inc.
P.O. Box 1276
Loma Linda, CA 92354
(909) 824-4690
Fax: (909) 824-4838
Website: http://www.ncahf.org/whatis.html
Contents: Provides information about suspected health frauds and other resources for pursuing health frauds.

National Heart, Lung, and Blood Institute (NHLBI) Information Center
PO Box 30105
Bethesda, MD 20814
Fax: (301) 251-1223
E-mail: NHLBIIC@dgsys.com
Website: http://www.nhlbi.nih.gov/nhlbi/nhlbi.htm
Contents: Contains information about NHLBI's research and educational activities.

NIDDK Weight Control Information Network
1 WIN Way
Bethesda, MD 20892-3665

(301) 984-7378
(800) WIN-8098
Fax: (301) 984-7196
E-mail: win@info.niddk.nih.gov
Website: http://www.niddk.nih.gov/health/nutrit/win.htm
Contents: Provides patient information documents on nutrition and obesity such as: choosing a safe and successful weight-loss program, nutrition and your health, physical activity and weight control, understanding adult obesity, weight cycling, etc.

Nutrient Data Laboratory
USDA Agricultural Research Service
Beltsville Human Nutrition Research Center
4700 River Rd., Unit 89
Riverdale, MD 20737
(301) 734-8491
Fax: (301) 734-5643
E-mail: ndlinfo@rbhnrc.usda.gov
Website: http://www.nal.usda.gov/fnic/foodcomp/
Contents: Provides information about the USDA Nutrient Database. Includes answers to frequently asked questions, a glossary of terms, facts about food composition, and useful links.

Tufts University Health and Nutrition Letter
6 Beacon St., Suite 1110
Boston, MA 02108
(800) 274-7581
E-mail: healthletter@tufts.edu
Website: http://www.healthletter.tufts.edu/
Contents: Contains a summary of articles from the most recent newsletter.

U.S. Department of Health and Human Services
Consumer Information Center
Department WWW
P.O. Box 100
Pueblo, CO 81009
(719) 948-9724
(888) 878-3256
Fax: (719) 948-9724
Website: http://www.pueblo.gsa.gov/food.htm

Contents: Provides a list of food and nutrition publications that can be ordered form DHHS and directions for ordering.

U.S. Food and Drug Administration
Center for Food Safety and Applied Nutrition Food Labeling
5600 Fishers Ln. (HFE-88), Room 1685
Rockville, MD 20847
(301) 443-9767
Website: http://www.fda.gov/
Contents: Contains information on food labeling, nutrition, and dietary supplements.

USDA Food and Nutrition Service
3101 Park Center Dr., Room 819
Alexandria, VA 22302
(703) 305-2286
Fax: (703) 305-2230
Website: http://www.usda.gov/fcs/fcs.htm
Contents: Provides information about the nutrition assistance programs offered by the USDA.

USDA Food Safety and Inspection Service (FSIS)
FSIS Food Safety Education and Communications Staff
Room 1175-South Bldg.
1400 Independence Ave. SW
Washington, DC 20250
(202) 720-7943
Fax: (202) 720-1843
E-mail: fsis.webmaster@usda.gov
Website: http://www.fsis.usda.gov/
Contents: Explains the mission and activities of FSIS, and provides news and information, publications, and consumer education and information.

University of California at Berkeley Wellness Letter
Ask the Experts
48 Shattuck Square, Suite 43
Berkeley, CA 94704-1140
Website: http://www.dc.enews.com/magazines/ucbwl/
Contents: Features the latest news from the world of preventive medicine and practical advice on all aspects of healthy living.

University of Minnesota

Department of Food Science and Nutrition
Nutritionist's Tool Box
1334 Eckles Ave.
Saint Paul, MN 55108
(612) 624-1290
Website: http://www.fsci.umn.edu/
Contents: Contains a calorie calculator for determining your energy needs, and a Nutrition Analysis Tool to analyze the foods you eat for a variety of nutrients.

Chapter 59

Nutrition Resource List

Opinions expressed in the publications listed in this chapter do not necessarily reflect the views of the U.S. Department of Agriculture, the Weight-Control Information Network (WIN), or Omnigraphics. Your local library or bookstore can help you locate these books and journals. Other items can be obtained from the source listed.

General Nutrition Books (in alphabetical order by title)

The American Dietetic Association's Complete Food & Nutrition Guide
Roberta Larson Duyff
The American Dietetic Association, 216 W. Jackson Blvd., Suite 800, Chicago, IL 60606-6995, (312) 899-0040; (312) 899-1979 fax

The American Heart Association Diet: An Eating Plan for Healthy Americans. Revised edition
Dallas, TX: American Heart Association, 1991, 18 p.
Local Affiliates; American Heart Association National Center, 7272 Greenville Ave., Dallas, TX 75231-4596; (214) 373-6300

Beyond Food Labels: Eating Healthy with the % Daily Values
Roberta Schwartz Wennik
New York: Berkley Pub. Group, 1996, 398 p.
Berkley Pub. Group, 200 Madison Ave., New York, NY 10016; (212) 951-8800; (212) 545-8917 fax

Information in this chapter was compiled from *Diet and Nutrition Materials for Consumers*, Weight-Control Information Network (WIN), August 1997; and *Sensible Nutrition Resource List for Consumers*, U.S. Department of Agriculture, August 1998.

The Buddy Diet
H. A. Tedder and M. Johnson
New York, NY: Warner Books, 1992, 194 p.
Warner Books, 1271 Avenue of the Americas, New York, NY 10020;
(212) 522-7200; (212) 522-7991 fax

Complete Book of Vitamins & Minerals
Editors of Consumer Guide; contributing writers: Arline McDonald,
Annette Natow, Jo-Ann Heslin, and Susan Male Smith
Lincolnwood, IL: Publications International, 1996, 560 p.
Publications International, 7373 N. Cicero Ave., Lincolnwood, IL
60646; (800) 745-9299

Computerized Health Diet (computer program)
R. A. Morreale
Overland Park, KS: INPS 1992
INPS, P.O. Box 7847, Overland Park, KS 66207-0847; (800) 798-6419

*Cut the Fat!: More than 500 Easy and Enjoyable Ways to Reduce the
Fat from Every Meal*
New York: HarperPerennial, 1996, 211 p.
The American Dietetic Association, 216 W. Jackson Blvd., Suite 800,
Chicago, IL 60606-6995; (312) 899-0040, (312) 899-1979 fax

DietAid (computer program)
Shannon Software
Falls Church, VA: Shannon Software, Ltd., 1991
Shannon Software, Ltd., P.O. Box 6126, Falls Church, VA 22040; (703)
573-9274

Diet Balancer (computer program)
R. J. Antonellis and B. Langston
Wappingers Falls, NY: Nutridata Software Corporation, 1992
Nutridata Software Corporation, 1211 Rt 9, Suite C, Wappingers
Falls, NY 12590; (914) 298-1308 or (800) 922-2988

Eat for the Health of It
Martha A. Erickson
Lancaster, PA: Starburst Publishers, 1997, 317 p.
Starburst Publishers, P.O. Box 4123, Lancaster, PA 17604; (800) 441-
1456; (717) 203-1945 fax

Eating Healthy (Videotape series)
C. O'Neil
Atlanta, GA: Turner Multimedia, 1990

CNN Library Tapes Sales, P.O. Box 105366, Atlanta, GA 30348; (800) 344-6219; (404) 827-3954 fax

Encyclopedia of Vitamins, Minerals and Supplements
Tova Navarra and Myron A. Lipkowitz
New York: Facts on File, 1996, 281 p.
Facts on File, 11 Penn Plaza, 15th Floor, New York, NY 10001; (212) 967-8800; (202) 322-8755 fax

Everywoman's Guide to Nutrition
J. E. Brown
Minneapolis, MN: University of Minnesota Press, 1991, 364 p.
University of Minnesota Press, 111 3rd Ave., Suite 290, Minneapolis, MN 55404; (612) 627-1970

The Fast Food Diet
M. Donkersloot
New York, NY: Simon and Schuster, 1991, 269 p.
Simon and Shuster, 1230 Avenue of the Americas, New York, NY 10020; (212) 698-7000

G-Index Diet: Missing Link That Makes Permanent Weight Loss Possible
R. N. Podell, W. Proctor, and J. Burani
New York, NY: Warner Books, Inc., 1993, 292 p.
Warner Books, 1271 Avenue of the Americas, New York, NY 10020; (212) 522-7200

Nutrition for Dummies
Carol Ann Rinzler
Chicago, IL: IDG Books Worldwide, 1997, 410 p.
IDG Books Worldwide, 919 E. Hillsddale Blvd., Suite 400, Foster City CA 94404-2112; (800) 434-3422

Nutrition in Women's Health
Debra A. Krummel and Penny M. Kris-Etherton (editors)
Gaithersburg, MD: Aspen Publisher's, 1996, 582 p.
Aspen Publisher's, 200 Orchard Ridge Dr., Suite 200, Gaithersburg, MD 20878; (301) 417-7500

Power of Your Plate: A Plan for Better Living
N. D. Barnard
Summertown, TN: Book Publishing Company, 1995, 255 p.
Book Publishing Company, Mail Order Catalog, P.O. Box 180, Summertown, TN 38483; (800) 695-2241

Personal Nutrition
Marie A. Boyle and Gail Zyla
Minneapolis: West Pub. Co., 1996, 1 volume
West Group, 610 Opperman Dr., Eagan, MN 55123; (612) 687-7000

Restaurant Companion: A Guide to Healthier Eating Out. 2nd edition
H. S. Warshaw
Chicago, IL: Surrey Books, 1995, 360 p.
Surrey Books, 230 East Ohio Street, Suite 120, Chicago, IL 60611;
(312) 751-7330 or (800) 326-4430

Safe Food for You and Your Family
Mildred M. Cody
The American Dietetic Association, 216 W. Jackson Blvd., Suite 800,
Chicago, IL 60606; (312) 899-0040, (312) 899-1979 fax

The Stanford Life Plan for a Healthy Heart
Helen Cassidy Page, John Speer Schroeder, and Tara C. Dickson
San Francisco, CA: Chronicle Books, 1996, 595 p.
Chronicle Books, 901 Mission St., San Francisco, CA 94103; (415) 777-1111

Cookbooks (in alphabetical order by title)

American Heart Association Cookbook, 5th edition
M. Winston
New York, NY: Random House, 1991, 643 p.
Random House, 1540 Broadway, New York, NY 10036; (212) 782-9000;
(212) 302-7985 fax

American Medical Association Family Health Cookbook
Melanie Barnard and Brooke Dojny
New York, NY: Pocket Books, 1997, 513 p.
Pocket Books, 1230 Avenue of the Americas, New York, NY 10020;
(212) 698-7000

Cooking for Few: A Guide to Easy Cooking for One or Two
Australia: National Heart Foundation of Australia, 1991, 116 p.
National Heart Foundation of Australia, Cnr. Dennison St. & Geils
Court, Deakin, A.C.T. 2606

Free and Equal Dessert Cookbook
C. Kruppa
Chicago, IL: Surrey Books, 1992, 167 p.
Surrey Books, 230 East Ohio Street, Suite 120, Chicago, IL 60611;
(800) 326-4430 or (312) 751-7330

Fun with Fruits and Vegetables: Kids Cookbook
Dole Food Company
Thousand Oaks, CA: Dole Food Company, 1994, 44 p.
Dole Consumer Center, P.O. Box 5700, Thousands Oaks, CA 91359; (800) 232-8888

The Guilt-Free Comfort Food Cookbook
Georgia Kostas with Robert A. Barnett
Nashville: T. Nelson Publishers, 1996, 301 p.
T. Nelson Publishers, 501 Nelson Pl., Nashville, TN 37214; (615) 889-9000

Healthy Weeknight Meals in Minutes
David Joachim (editor)
Emmaus, PA: Rodale Press, Inc., 1997, 312 p.
Rodale Press, Inc., 33 E. Minor St., Emmaus, PA 18098; (610) 967-8154

Kitchen Fun for Kids: Healthy Recipes and Nutrition Facts for 7 to 12 Year Old Cooks
M. Jacobson and L. Hill
New York, NY: Henry Holt and Company, 1991, 136 p.
Henry Holt and Company, 115 W 18th St., New York, NY 10011; (212) 886-9200

Lowfat Cooking for Dummies
Lynn Fischer
Foster City, CA: IDG Books Worldwide, Inc., 1997, 408 p.
IDG Books Worldwide, Inc., 919 E. Hillsdale Blvd., Suite 400, Foster City, CA 94404; (650) 655-3000

Low-fat & Luscious: Breakfasts, Snacks, Main Dishes, Side Dishes, Desserts
Kristi Fuller (editor)
Des Moines, IA: Meredith Corp., 1996, 160 p.
Meredith Corp., 1716 Locust St., Des Moines, IA 50309; (515) 284-3000

Meals Without Squeals: Child Care Feeding Guide and Cookbook
C. Berman and J. Fromer
Palo Alto, CA: Bull Publishing Company, 1991, 240 p.
Bull Publishing Company, P.O. Box 208, Palo Alto, CA 94302-0208, (650) 322-2855

New Low-fat Favorites
Ruth Spear
New York, NY: Little, Brown and Company, 1998, 306 p.
Little, Brown and Company, 3 Center Plaza, Boston, MA 02108; (617) 277-0730

Secrets of Fat-free Italian Cooking
Sandra Woodruff, R.D.
Garden City Park, NY: Avery Publishing Group, 1996, 230 p.
Avery Publishing Group, 120 Old Broadway, Garden City Park, NY 11040; (516) 741-2155

Simple Vegetarian Pleasures
Jeanne Lemlin
New York, NY: HarperCollins Publishers, 1998, 319 p.
HarperCollins Publishers, 10 E. 53rd St., New York, NY 10022; (212) 207-7000

Skinny Mexican Cooking
Sue Spitler
Chicago, IL: Surrey Books, 1996, 147 p.
Surrey Books, 230 East Ohio Street, Suite 120, Chicago, IL 60611; (800) 326-4430

Skinny Pizzas: Over 100 Low-fat, Easy-to-Make, Delicious Recipes for America's Favorite Fun Food—From an Original Roman Pizza to Trendy California-style Dishes
Barbara Grunes
Chicago, IL: Surrey Books, 1996, 174 p.
Surrey Books, 230 East Ohio Street, Suite 120, Chicago, IL 60611; (800) 326-4430

Skinny Spices: 50 Nifty Homemade Spice Blends That Can Make Any Diet Delicious
E. L. Klein
Chicago, IL: Surrey Books, 1990, 204 p.
Surrey Books, 230 East Ohio Street, Suite 120, Chicago, IL 60611; (800) 326-4430

Food Composition Books (in alphabetical order by title)

Bowes & Church's Food Values of Portions Commonly Used, 17th edition, revised
Jean A. T. Pennington
Philadelphia, PA: J.B. Lippincott, 1998, 481 p.
J.B. Lippincott, 227 E. Washington Sq., Philadelphia, PA 19106; (215) 238-4200

The Complete Book of Food Counts
Corinne T. Netzer

New York, NY: Dell Publishing, 1997, 770 p.
Dell Publishing, 1270 6th Ave., New York, NY 10020; (212) 698-1313

The Complete Food Count Guide
Editors of Consumer Guide, with the Nutrient Analysis Center, Chicago Center for Clinical Research
Lincolnwood, IL: Publications, Ltd., 1996, 704 p.
Publications, Ltd., 7373 N. Cicero Ave., Lincolnwood, IL 60646; (847) 676-3470

The Complete and Up-To-Date Fat Book. A Guide to the Fat Calories, and Fat Percentages in Your Food
Karen J. Bellerson
New York, NY: Avery Publishing Group, 1997, 870 p.
Avery Publishing Group, 120 Old Broadway, Garden City Park, NY 11040; (516) 741-2155

Fast Food Facts. The Original Guide for Fitting Fast Food into a Healthy Lifestyle
Marion J. Franz, MS, RD, LD, CDE
Minneapolis, MN: IDC Publishing, 1998, 243 p.
IDC Publishing, 3800 Park Nicollet Blvd., Minneapolis, MN 55416; (612) 993-3874

The Fat Counter. The Revised and Updated 4th edition
Annette B. Natow and Jo-Ann Heslin
New York, NY: Pocket Books, 1998, 661 p.
Pocket Books, 1230 Avenue of the Americas, New York, NY 10020; (212) 698-7000

Magazines/Newsletters (in alphabetical order by title)

Cooking Light. Southern Living, Inc., PO Box 80119, Birmingham, AL 35282-9562; (800) 336-0125

Environmental Nutrition. P.O. Box 420235, Palm Coast, FL 32142-0235; (800) 829-5384

Health Magazine. P.O. Box 56863, Boulder, CO 80322-6863

Healthy Weight Journal. Healthy Living Institute, 402 S. 14th St., Hettinger, ND 58639; (800) 663-0023

Mayo Clinic Health Letter. Subscription Services, P.O. Box 53889, Boulder, CO 80322-3889; (800) 333-9037

Nutrition Action Health Letter. Center for Science in the Public Interest (CSPI), 1875 Connecticut Ave., NW, Suite 300, Washington, DC 20009-5728; (202) 332-9110

Tufts University Health & Nutrition Letter. P.O. Box 57843, Boulder CO 80321; (800) 274-7581

University of California, Berkeley Wellness Letter. Health Letter Associates, P.O. Box 420-235, Palm Coast, FL 32142-0235; (800) 829-9080

Booklets/Pamphlets (in alphabetical order by producer)

American Dietetic Association
216 West Jackson Blvd., Suite 800
Chicago, IL 60606-6995
(800) 366-1655
Website: http://www.eatright.org

- Food Strategies for Men (1997)
- Good Nutrition Reading List (1996)
- The New Cholesterol Countdown (1997)
- Staying Healthy—A Guide for Elder Americans (1997)

American Heart Association
National Center
7272 Greenville Ave.
Dallas, TX 75231-4596
(214) 373-6300
Website: http://www.amhrt.org

- Easy Food Tips for Heart Healthy Eating (1996)
- AHA Diet, An Eating Plan for Healthy Americans (1996)
- Nutritious Nibbles: A Guide to Healthy Snacking (1996)

American Institute for Cancer Research
Attn: Publications Department
1759 R Street, NW
Washington, DC 20069-2012
Designate Agency #0808
(202) 328-7744
E-mail: aicrweb@capcon.net
Website: http://www.aicr.org

- AICR Diet and Health Guidelines for Cancer Prevention (1998)

- Cooking Solo (1996)
- Healthy Flavors of the World: India (1997)
- Healthy Flavors of the World: Mediterranean (1997)
- No Time to Cook (1998)

American Institute of Nutrition

American Society for Clinical Nutrition, Inc.
9650 Rockville Pike
Bethesda, MD 20814-3998
(301) 530-7050
E-mail: meyersp@ain.faseb.org
Website: http://www.faseb.org/ain/

- Guide to Experts With Specialized Knowledge in Nutrition and Clinical Nutrition (1991)

Iowa State University, Cooperative Extension Services

Publication Distribution
1119 Printing & Pub. Bldg.
Iowa State University
Ames, IA 50011-3171
(515) 294-5247
E-mail: pubdist@exnet.iastate.edu
Website: http://www.exnet.iastate.edu

- Cancer and Your Diet: Quiz (1996)
- Cholesterol in Your Body (1996)
- Family Nutrition Guide (1997)
- How to Eat without Raising Your Cholesterol (1996)
- Vegetarian Diets (1996)

Consumer Information Center

Pueblo, CO 81009
(719) 948-3334
Website: http://www.pueblo.gsa.gov

- Critical Steps Towards Safer Seafood (1997)
- Fight BAC! Four Simple Steps to Food Safety (1998)
- Fruits & Vegetables: Eating Your Way to 5 a Day (1997)
- Growing Older, Eating Better (1997)
- How to Help Avoid Foodborne Illness in the Home (1997)
- A Pinch of Controversy Shakes Up Dietary Salt (1997)

Egg Nutrition Center
1819 H Street, NW, Suite 520
Washington, DC 20006
(202) 833-8850

- Healthy Habits for the Best of Your Life! (nd)

Food Marketing Institute
800 Conneticut Ave., NW, Suite 400
Washington, DC 20006-2394
(202) 452-8444
E-mail: fmi@fmi.org
Website: http://www.fmi.org

- Eating Right With the Dietary Guidelines (1991)

National Cancer Institute
9000 Rockville Pike, Bldg. 31
Bethesda, MD 20892
(800) 4-CANCER
Website: www.nci.nih.gov

- Action Guide for Healthy Eating (1997)
- Eat 5 Fruits and Vegetables Every Day (1997)
- Tips on How to Eat Less Fat (1997)
- Time to Take Five: Eat 5 Fruits and Vegetables a Day (1997)

National Institute on Aging
NIA Information Center
P.O. Box 8057
Gaithersburg, MD 20898-8057
(800) 222-2225
Website: adobe.nia.nih.gov

- Hints for Shopping, Cooking, and Enjoying Meals (1991)
- Nutrition: A Lifelong Concern (1991)

Sugar Association, Inc.,
1101 Fifteenth Street, NW, Suite 600
Washington, DC 20005
(202) 785-1122

- Questions Most Frequently Asked About Nutrition and Aging

United States Department of Agriculture (USDA)
14th St. and Independance Ave., SW
Washington, DC 20250
(202) 720-2791
Website: http://www.usda.gov

- Eating Right The Dietary Guidelines Way (1990)
- Food Facts for Older Adults: Information on How to Use the Dietary Guidelines (1993)
- Team Nutrition's Food, Family and Fun: A Seasonal Guide to Healthy Eating: Commemorating 50 Years of School Lunch (1996)

University of Illinois, Cooperative Extension Services
Ag. Publication Office
1917 S Wright St
University of Illinois
Champaign, IL 61820
(217) 333-2007
E-mail: acespubs@uiuc.edu
Website: http://www.ag.uiuc.edu/~vista/catalog/catintro.html

- Food & Water: Partners for Survival (1996)
- Keeping Energy Levels Up (1996)
- Keeping Fluid Levels Up (1997)
- The Winning Connection: Sports & Nutrition (1997)

University of Minnesota, Educational Development System
Minnesota Extension Service
University of Minnesota
167 FSCN Building
1334 Eckles Avenue
St. Paul, MN 55108
(612) 624-7479
(612) 625-5272 fax

- Choosing Good Foods for Good Health (1992)

Weight-Control Information Network
1 WIN Way
Bethesda, MD 20892-3665
(301) 984-7378

E-mail: win@matthewsgroup.com
Website: http://www.niddk.nih.gov/health/nutrit/win.htm

• Dietary Guidelines for Americans, Fifth Edition (1995)

Chapter 60

Sources of Nutrition Materials

This text includes a list of organizations that provide free or low-cost food and nutrition materials for consumers. The Food and Nutrition Information Center (FNIC) receives many requests for materials to distribute at health fairs, classes, physicians' offices, wellness programs, and other locations. Since FNIC is not a clearinghouse and has a limited number of publications to distribute in bulk, the Center has developed this publication to help others locate free and low-cost food and nutrition materials.

FNIC recommends that you call or write the organization(s) for a publication list or order form. FNIC also suggests that you make your request(s) for materials as far in advance as possible to allow for processing and mailing time. Some organizations may take up to eight weeks to fill your request. There are fees for some of the materials distributed by these organizations.

Inclusion of an organization on this list does not indicate endorsement by the U.S. Department of Agriculture (USDA), nor does the USDA ensure the accuracy of all information provided by these organizations.

Excerpted from *Sources of Free or Low-Cost Food and Nutrition Materials*, Food and Nutrition Information Center, Agricultural Research Service, USDA, May 1998. To obtain the complete report, please write to the address given at the end of this chapter or visit the Food and Nutrition Information Center's website at: http://www.nal.usda.gov/fnic/.

National Nutrition, Medical, and Health Organizations

Aging

American Association of Retired Persons
601 E. Street, NW
Washington, DC 20049
(202) 434-2277
(800) 424-3410
(202) 434-2277 TTY
(202) 434-6466 Fax
E-mail: member@aarp.org
Website: http://www.aarp.org/

National Institute on Aging
Information Office
P.O. Box 8057
Gaithersburg, MD 20898-8057
(800) 222-2225
(800) 222-4225 TTY
(301) 589-3014 fax
E-mail: nianfo@access.digex.com
Website: http://www.nih.gov/nia

Alcohol and Drugs

National Clearinghouse for Alcohol and Drug Information
Information Specialist
P.O. Box 2345
Rockville, MD 20847-2345
(301) 468-2600
(800) 487-4889 TTY
(301) 468-6433 Fax
Website: http://www.health.org

Allergies

American Academy of Allergies—Asthma and Immunology
611 E. Wells Street
Milwaukee, WI 53202
(414) 272-6071
(800) 822-2762
Website: http://www.aaaai.org

The Food Allergy Network
10400 Eaton Place, Suite 107
Fairfax, VA 22030-2208
(703) 691-3179
(800) 929-4040
Fax: (703) 691-2713
Website: http://www.foodallergy.org

Arthritis

Arthritis Foundation Information Line
1330 West Peachtree Street
Atlanta, GA 30309
(404) 872-7100
(800) 283-7800
(404) 872-0457 Fax
Website: http://www.arthritis.org

Cancer

American Cancer Society
1599 Clifton Road, NE
Atlanta, GA 30329
(404) 320-3333
(800) 227-2345
TTY: (804) 527-3661 TTY
(404) 225-2217 Fax
Website: http://www.cancer.org

American Institute for Cancer Research
1759 R Street, NW
Washington, DC 20009
(202) 328-7744
(800) 843-8114
(202) 328-7226 Fax
E-mail: aicrweb@aicr.org
Website: http://www.aicr.org/

National Cancer Institute
Office of Cancer Communications
31 Center Dr., MSC 2580
Building 31, Room 10A-29
Bethesda, MD 20892-2580

(800) 4-CANCER
(800) 638-6070 in Alaska
(800) 524-1234 in Hawaii
(301) 402-5874 Fax
E-mail: cancermail@icicc.nci.nih.gov
Website: http://cancernet.nci.nih.gov

Dental Health

National Institute of Dental Research
Public Information and Reports Section
Building 31, Room 5-B49
31 Center Dr. MSC 2190
Bethesda, MD 20892-2190
(301) 496-4261
(301) 496-9988 Fax
E-mail: nidrinfo@od31.nidr.nih.gov
Website: http://www.nidr.nih.gov/

Diabetes

American Diabetes Association
National Service Center
1660 Duke Street
Alexandria, VA 22314
(703) 549-1500
(800) 232-3472
(703) 549-6995 Fax
Website: http://www.diabetes.org/

National Diabetes Information Clearinghouse
Box NDIC
1 Information Way
Bethesda, MD 20892-3560
(301) 654-3327
(301) 907-8906 Fax
Website: http://www.niddk.nih.gov

Dietary Supplements

American Botanical Council
P.O. Box 144345
Austin, Texas 78714-4345

(512) 926-4900
(512) 926-2345 Fax
E-mail: abc@herbalgram.org
Website: http://www.herbalgram.org

Functional Foods for Health
Program Department of Food Science and Human Nutrition
University of Illinois at Urbana-Champaign
103 Agricultural Bioprocessing Lab
1302 W. Pennsylvania Avenue
Urbana, IL 61801
(217) 333-6364
(217) 333-7386 Fax
Website: http://www.ag.uiuc.edu

Herb Research Foundation
1007 Pearl Street, Suite 200
Boulder, CO 80302
(303) 449-2265
Fax: (303) 449-7849
E-mail: info@herbs.org
Website: http://www.herbs.org

Digestive Diseases

National Digestive Diseases Information Clearinghouse
2 Information Way
Bethesda, MD 20892-3570
(301) 654-3810
(301) 907-8906 Fax
E-mail: nddic@aerie.com
Website: http://www.niddk.nih.gov

Celiac Disease Foundation
13251 Ventura Blvd., Suite 1
Studio City, CA 91604-1838
(818) 990-2354
(818) 990-2379 Fax
E-mail: cdf@celiac.org
Website: http://www.celiac.org/cdf

Celiac Sprue Association/United States of America, Inc. (CSA/USA)
P.O. Box 31700

Omaha, NE 68131-0700
(402) 558-0600
(402) 558-1347 Fax
E-mail: celiacs@csaceliacs.org
Website: http://csaceliacs.org/

Crohn's and Colitis Foundation of America, Inc.
386 Park Avenue, South, 17th Floor
New York, NY 10016-8804
(212) 685-3440
(800) 932-2423
(212) 779-4098 Fax
E-mail: info@ccfa.org
Website: http://www.ccfa.org

The Gluten Intolerance Group of North America
P.O. Box 23053
Seattle, WA 98102-0353
(206) 325-6980
(206) 850-2394 Fax

Eating Disorders (Disordered Eating)

American Anorexia/Bulimia Association
165 W. 65th Street, Suite 1108
New York, NY 10036
(212) 575-6200
(212) 501-0342 Fax
E-mail: amanbu@aol.com
Website: http://members.aol.com/AmAnBu/index.html

Anorexia Nervosa and Related Eating Disorders, Inc.
P.O. Box 5102
Eugene, OR 97405
(541) 344-1144
E-mail: jarinor@rio.com
Website: http://www.anred.com/

National Association of Anorexia Nervosa and Associated Disorders
Box 7
Highland Park, IL 60035
(847) 831-3438

(847) 433-4632 Fax
E-mail: anad20@aol.com

National Eating Disorders Organization
6655 South Yale
Tulsa, OK 74136
(918) 481-4044
Fax: (918) 481-4076

Fitness and Sports

Aerobics and Fitness Foundation
15250 Ventura Blvd., Suite 200
Sherman Oaks, CA 91403
(818) 905-0040
(800) 445-5950 ext. 628
(818) 990-5468 Fax
E-mail: /@aimnet.com
Website: http://www.afa.com

International Center for Sports Nutrition
502 South 44th Street, Suite 3012
Omaha, NE 68105
(402) 559-5505
(402) 559-7302 Fax

The President's Council on Physical Fitness and Sports
HHH Building, Room 738 H
200 Independence Avenue, SW
Washington, DC 20201
(202) 690-9000
(202) 690-5211 Fax

Women's Sports Foundation
Eisenhower Park
East Meadow, NY 11554
(516) 542-4700
(800) 227-3988
(516) 542-4716 Fax
E-mail: wosport@aol.com
Website:http://lifetimetv.com/WoSport/stage/INTERACT/index.
html

Food and Nutrition

Center for Nutrition Policy and Promotion
1120 20th Street, NW
Suite 200, North Lobby
Washington, DC 20036
(202) 418-2312
(202) 208-2321 Fax
E-mail: john.webster@usda.gov
Website: http://www.usda.gov/cnpp/

Food and Drug Administration
Office of Consumer Affairs
Department of Health and Human Services
5600 Fishers Lane (HFE-88), Room 16-85
Rockville, MD 20857
(800) 532-4440
(301) 443-9767 Fax
Website: http://www.fda.gov/

Food and Nutrition Information Center
National Agricultural Library/ARS/USDA
10301 Baltimore Avenue, Room 304
Beltsville, MD 20705-2351
(301) 504-5755
Website: http://www.nal.usda.gov/

National Center for Nutrition and Dietetics
The American Dietetic Association
216 W. Jackson Blvd., Suite 800
Chicago, IL 60606-6995
(312) 899-0040
(800) 366-1655
(312) 899-4817 Fax
E-mail: hotline@eatright.org
Website: http://www.eatright.org/ncnd

Penn State Nutrition Center
The Pennsylvania State University
Ruth Building
5 Henderson Bldg.
University Park, PA 16802-5663

(814) 865-6323
(814) 865-5870 Fax

Nutrition Information Center
NY Hospital-Cornell Medical Center
Memorial Sloan-Kettering Cancer Center
515 East 71st Street
New York, NY 10021
(212) 746-1617
(212) 746-8310 fax
E-mail: pssenat@mail.med.cornell.edu
Website: http://www.mskcc.org/
Garlic Information: (800) 330-5922
Calcium Information: (800) 321-2681
Olive Oil Information: (800) 232-6548

Food Safety

Food and Drug Administration
Consumer Food Information Hotline
(202) 205-2314
(800) FDA-4010 (M-F 12PM-4PM EST)
(202) 401-3532 Fax
Website: http://vm.cfsan.fda.gov/~lrd/advice.html

Food Safety and Inspection Service
Meat and Poultry Hotline/USDA
1400 Independence Avenue, SW Rm. 1175-S
Washington, DC 20250
(202) 720-7943
(800) 535-4555
(202) 720-1843 Fax
Website: http://www.usda.gov/fsis

Partnership for Food Safety Education
Fight Bac! Campaign
Website: http://www.fightbac.org

General Health

American Medical Association
515 N. State Street

Chicago, IL 60610
(312) 464-5000
(800) 621-8335
(312) 464-5600 Fax
Website: http://www.ama-assn.org/

Bureau of Refugee Services
Iowa Department of Human Services
1200 University, Suite D
Des Moines, IA 50314
(515) 283-7999
(515) 283-9160 Fax
(800) 362-2780 (in IA)
E-mail: djones4@dhs.state.ia.us
(publishes bibliography of sources of non-English language health resources)

Center for Science in the Public Interest
1875 Connecticut Avenue, NW, Suite 300
Washington, DC 20009-5728
(202) 332-9110
(202) 265-4954 Fax
E-mail: cspi@cspinet.org
Website: http://www.cspinet.org

Consumer Information Center
Dept. WWWW
Pueblo, CO 81009
(719) 948-3334
(888) 8-PUEBLO
(719) 948-9724 (credit card orders)
Website: http://www.pueblo.gsa.gov/

National Council Against Health Fraud, Inc.
P.O. Box 1276
Loma Linda, CA 92354
(909) 824-4690
(909) 824-4838 Fax
Website: http://www.ncahf.org/

New Mexico Department of Health
Health Promotion Bureau

P.O. Box 26110
Santa Fe, NM 87502-6610
(505) 827-0240

ODPHP National Health Information Center
(Office of Disease Prevention and Health Promotion)
P.O. Box 1133
Washington, DC 20013-1133
(301) 565-4167
(800) 336-4797
(301) 984-4256 Fax
E-mail: nhicinfo@health.org
Website: http://www.nhic-nt.health.org

Office of Alternative Medicine Clearinghouse
PO Box 8218
Silver Spring, MD 20907
(888) 644-6226
(301) 495-4957 Fax
Website: http://altmed.od.nih.gov/oam/clearinghouse/

Public Voice For Food and Health Policy
36 Western Avenue
Burlington, Vermont 05401
E-mail: info@publicvoice.org
Website: http://www.publicvoice.org/pvoice.html

Heart Disease

American Heart Association National Center
7272 Greenville Avenue
Dallas, TX 75231
(214) 373-6300
(800) AHA-USA-1
(800) 242-8721
(410) 685-5761 Fax
Website: http://www.amhrt.org

American Heart Association
Florida Affiliate, Inc.
600 Brickell Avenue
Miami, FL 33131

(305) 373-5119
Website: http://www.amhrt.org/affili/FL/index_fl.htm

NHLBI Information Center
(National Heart, Lung, and Blood Institute)
P.O. Box 30105
Bethesda, MD 20824-0105
(301) 251-1222
(800) 575-WELL
(301) 251-1223 Fax
Website: http://www.nhlbi.nih.gov/nhlbi/con-ed/ches_ce.thm

Maternal and Child Health

Allegheny County Health Department
Nutrition Service WIC Program
Investment Building
239 4th Avenue, 21st Floor
Pittsburgh, PA 15222
(412) 350-4000
Fax: (412) 350-4424

American College of Obstetricians and Gynecologists
Office of Public Information
409 12th Street, SW
P.O. Box 96920
Washington, DC 20090-6920
(202) 638-5577
(202) 484-1595 Fax
Website: http://www.acog.org

La Leche League International
1400 N. Meacham Road
P.O. Box 4079
Schaumburg, IL 60168-4079
(847) 519-7730
(800) LALECHE
(847) 519-0035 Fax
Website: http://www.lalecheleague.org/

March of Dimes Birth Defects Foundation
1275 Mamaroneck Avenue

White Plains, NY 10605
(914) 428-7100
(914) 997-4720
(800) 367-6630 (multiple copies)
Website: http://www.modimes.org

National Center for Education in Maternal and Child Health Clearinghouse
2000 15th Street, North, Suite 701
Arlington, VA 22201
(703) 524-7802
(703) 524-9335 Fax

National Maternal and Child Health Clearinghouse
2070 Chain Bridge Road, Suite 450
Vienna, VA 22182
(703) 821-8955
Fax: (703) 821-2098
E-mail: info@ncemch.org

Oncology

Oncology Nutrition Dietetics Practice Group of ADA
216 W. Jackson Blvd., Suite 800
Chicago, IL 60606
(312) 899-0040
Website: http://www.eatright.org/dpg20.html

Other Organizations of Interest

North American Menopause Society
University Hospitals
Department of OB/GYN
PO Box 94527
Cleveland, OH 44101
(216) 844-8748
(216) 844-8708 Fax
E-mail: info@menopause.org
Website: http://www.menopause.org/

Osteoporosis & Related Bone Disease
National Resource Center

1150 17th Street, NW, Suite 500
Washington, DC 20036-4603
(202) 223-0344
(800) 624-BONE
(202) 466-4315 TTY
E-mail: orbdnrc@nof.org
Website: http://www.osteo.org/

Weight Control Information Network
1 WIN Way
Bethesda, MD 20892-3665
(301) 984-7378
(800) 946-8098
(301) 984-7196 Fax
E-mail: win@info.niddk.nih.gov
Website: http://www.niddk.nih.gov/health/nutrit/win.htm

Other Food Related Organizations

Calorie Control Council
5775 Peachtree-Dunwoody Road
Suite 500-G
Atlanta, GA 30342
(404) 252-3663
(404) 252-0774 Fax
Website: http://www.caloriecontrol.org

Food Marketing Institute
800 Connecticut Avenue, NW, Suite 400
Washington, DC 20006
(202) 452-8444
(202) 429-4519 Fax
E-mail: fmi@fmi.org
Website: http://www.fmi.org/

The Glutamate Association
555 13th Street, NW
Washington, DC 20004-1109
(202) 738-6135
(202) 637-5910 Fax
Website: http://www.msgfacts.com

Infant Formula Council
5775 Peachtree-Dunwoody Road
Suite 500-G
Atlanta, GA 30342
(404) 252-3663
(404) 252-0774 Fax

International Food Additives Council
5775 Peachtree-Dunwoody Road
Suite 500-G
Atlanta, GA 30342
(404) 252-3663
(404) 252-0774 Fax

International Food Information Council
1100 Connecticut Avenue, NW, Suite 430
Washington, DC 20036
(202) 296-6540
(202) 296-6547 Fax
E-mail: foodinfo@ific.health.org
Website: http://www.ificinfo.health.org

The Sugar Association, Inc.
1101 15th Street, NW, Suite 600
Washington, DC 20005
(202) 785-1122
(202) 785-5019
E-mail: sugar@sugar.org
Website: http://www.sugar.org

Information about the Food and Nutrition Information Center

Food and Nutrition Information Center
Agricultural Research Service, USDA
National Agricultural Library
10301 Baltimore Avenue, Room 304
Beltsville, MD 20705-2351
Phone: 301-504-5719
(301) 504-6409 Fax
(301) 504-6856 TTY

E-mail: fnic@nal.usda.gov
Website: http://www.nal.usda.gov/fnic/

The United States Department of Agriculture (USDA) prohibits discrimination in all its programs and activities on the basis of race, color, national origin, gender, religion, age, disability, political beliefs, and marital or familial status. (Not all prohibited bases apply to all programs). Persons with disabilities who require alternative means for communication of program information (braille, large print, audiotape, etc.) should contact the USDA's TARGET Center at (202) 720-2600 (voice and TDD).

Index

Index

597

604

Contagious & Non-Contagious Infectious Diseases Sourcebook

Basic Information about Contagious Diseases like Measles, Polio, Hepatitis B, and Infectious Mononucleosis, and Non-Contagious Infectious Diseases like Tetanus and Toxic Shock Syndrome, and Diseases Occurring as Secondary Infections Such as Shingles and Reye Syndrome, Along with Vaccination, Prevention, and Treatment Information, and a Section Describing Emerging Infectious Disease Threats

Edited by Karen Bellenir and Peter D. Dresser. 566 pages. 1996. 0-7808-0075-3. $78.

Death & Dying Sourcebook

Basic Information for the Layperson about End-of-Life Care and Related Ethical and Legal Issues, Including Chief Causes of Death, Autopsies, Pain Management for the Terminally Ill, Life Support Systems, Coma, Euthanasia, Assisted Suicide, Hospice Programs, Living Wills, Near-Death Experiences, Counseling, Mourning, Organ Donation, Cryogenics and Physician Training and Liability, Along with Statistical Data, a Glossary, and Listings of Sources for Additional Help and Information

Edited by Annemarie Muth. 600 pages. 1999. 0-7808-0230-6. $78.

Diabetes Sourcebook, 1st Edition

Basic Information about Insulin-Dependent and Noninsulin-Dependent Diabetes Mellitus, Gestational Diabetes, and Diabetic Complications, Symptoms, Treatment, and Research Results, Including Statistics on Prevalence, Morbidity, and Mortality, Along with Source Listings for Further Help and Information

Edited by Karen Bellenir and Peter D. Dresser. 827 pages. 1994. 1-55888-751-2. $78.

"...very informative and understandable for the layperson without being simplistic. It provides a comprehensive overview for laypersons who want a general understanding of the disease or who want to focus on various aspects of the disease." — *Bulletin of the MLA, Jan '96*

Diabetes Sourcebook, 2nd Edition

Basic Consumer Health Information about Type 1 Diabetes (Insulin-Dependent or Juvenile-Onset Diabetes), Type 2 (Noninsulin-Dependent or Adult-Onset Diabetes), Gestational Diabetes, and Related Disorders, Including Diabetes Prevalence Data, Management Issues, the Role of Diet and Exercise in Controlling Diabetes, Insulin and Other Diabetes Medicines, and Complications of Diabetes Such as Eye Diseases, Periodontal Disease, Amputation, and End-Stage Renal Disease; Along with Reports on Current Research Initiatives, a Glossary, and Resource Listings for Further Help and Information

Edited by Karen Bellenir. 725 pages. 1998. 0-7808-0224-1. $78.

Diet & Nutrition Sourcebook, 1st Edition

Basic Information about Nutrition, Including the Dietary Guidelines for Americans, the Food Guide Pyramid, and Their Applications in Daily Diet, Nutritional Advice for Specific Age Groups, Current Nutritional Issues and Controversies, the New Food Label and How to Use It to Promote Healthy Eating, and Recent Developments in Nutritional Research

Edited by Dan R. Harris. 662 pages. 1996. 0-7808-0084-2. $78.

"Useful reference as a food and nutrition sourcebook for the general consumer."
— *Booklist Health Sciences Supplement, Oct '97*

"Recommended for public libraries and medical libraries that receive general information requests on nutrition. It is readable and will appeal to those interested in learning more about healthy dietary practices."
— *Medical Reference Services Quarterly, Fall '97*

"With dozens of questionable diet books on the market, it is so refreshing to find a reliable and factual reference book. Recommended to aspiring professionals, librarians, and others seeking and giving reliable dietary advice. An excellent compilation." — *Choice, Feb '97*

Diet & Nutrition Sourcebook, 2nd Edition

Basic Consumer Health Information about Dietary Guidelines, Recommended Daily Intake Values, Vitamins, Minerals, Fiber, Fat, Weight Control, Dietary Supplements, and Food Additives; Along with Special Sections on Nutrition Needs throughout Life and Nutrition for People with Such Specific Medical Concerns as Allergies, High Blood Cholesterol, Hypertension, Diabetes, Celiac Disease, Seizure Disorders, Phenylketonuria (PKU), Cancer, and Eating Disorders, and Including Reports on Current Nutrition Research and Source Listings for Additional Help and Information

Edited by Karen Bellenir. 600 pages. 1999. 0-7808-0228-4. $78.

Domestic Violence Sourcebook

Basic Information about the Physical, Emotional and Sexual Abuse of Partners, Children, and Elders, Including Information about Hotlines, Safe Houses, Safety Plans, Resources for Support and Assistance, Community Initiatives, and Reports on Current Directions in Research and Treatment; Along with a Glossary, Sources for Further Reading, and Listings of Governmental and Non-Governmental Organizations

Edited by Helene Henderson. 600 pages. 1999. 0-7808-0235-7. $78.

Ear, Nose & Throat Disorders Sourcebook

Basic Information about Disorders of the Ears, Nose, Sinus Cavities, Pharynx, and Larynx, Including Ear Infections, Tinnitus, Vestibular Disorders, Allergic and Non-Allergic Rhinitis, Sore Throats, Tonsillitis, and Cancers That Affect the Ears, Nose, Sinuses, and Throat, Along with Reports on Current Research Initiatives, a Glossary of Related Medical Terms, and a Directory of Sources for Further Help and Information

Edited by Karen Bellenir and Linda M. Shin. 592 pages. 1998. 0-7808-0206-3. $78.

Endocrine & Metabolic Disorders Sourcebook

Basic Information for the Layperson about Pancreatic and Insulin-Related Disorders Such as Pancreatitis, Diabetes, and Hypoglycemia; Adrenal Gland Disorders Such as Cushing's Syndrome, Addison's Disease, and Congenital Adrenal Hyperplasia; Pituitary Gland Disorders Such as Growth Hormone Deficiency, Acromegaly, and Pituitary Tumors; Thyroid Disorders Such as Hypothyroidism, Graves' Disease, Hashimoto's Disease, and Goiter; Hyperparathyroidism; and Other Diseases and Syndromes of Hormone Imbalance or Metabolic Dysfunction, Along with Reports on Current Research Initiatives

Edited by Linda M. Shin. 632 pages. 1998. 0-7808-0207-1. $78.

Environmentally Induced Disorders Sourcebook

Basic Information about Diseases and Syndromes Linked to Exposure to Pollutants and Other Substances in Outdoor and Indoor Environments Such as Lead, Asbestos, Formaldehyde, Mercury, Emissions, Noise, and More

Edited by Allan R. Cook. 620 pages. 1997. 0-7808-0083-4. $78.

". . . a good survey of numerous environmentally induced physical disorders . . . a useful addition to anyone's library."
— *Doody's Health Science Book Reviews, Jan '98*

". . . provide[s] introductory information from the best authorities around. Since this volume covers topics that potentially affect everyone, it will surely be one of the most frequently consulted volumes in the *Health Reference Series*." — *Rettig on Reference, Nov '97*

"Recommended reference source."
— *Booklist, Oct '97*

Ethical Issues in Medicine Sourcebook

Basic Information about Controversial Treatment Issues, Genetic Research, Reproductive Technologies, and End-of-Life Decisions, Including Topics Such as Cloning, Abortion, Fertility Management, Organ Transplantation, Health Care Rationing, Advance Directives, Living Wills, Physician-Assisted Suicide, Euthanasia, and More; Along with a Glossary and Resources for Additional Information

Edited by Helene Henderson. 600 pages. 1999. 0-7808-0237-3. $78.

Fitness & Exercise Sourcebook

Basic Information on Fitness and Exercise, Including Fitness Activities for Specific Age Groups, Exercise for People with Specific Medical Conditions, How to Begin a Fitness Program in Running, Walking, Swimming, Cycling, and Other Athletic Activities, and Recent Research in Fitness and Exercise

Edited by Dan R. Harris. 663 pages. 1996. 0-7808-0186-5. $78.

"A good resource for general readers."
— *Choice, Nov '97*

"The perennial popularity of the topic . . . make this an appealing selection for public libraries."
— *Rettig on Reference, Jun/Jul '97*

Food & Animal Borne Diseases Sourcebook

Basic Information about Diseases That Can Be Spread to Humans through the Ingestion of Contaminated Food or Water or by Contact with Infected Animals and Insects, Such as Botulism, E. Coli, Hepatitis A, Trichinosis, Lyme Disease, and Rabies, Along with Information Regarding Prevention and Treatment Methods, and a Special Section for International Travelers Describing Diseases Such as Cholera, Malaria, Travelers' Diarrhea, and Yellow Fever, and Offering Recommendations for Avoiding Illness

Edited by Karen Bellenir and Peter D. Dresser. 535 pages. 1995. 0-7808-0033-8. $78.

"Targeting general readers and providing them with a single, comprehensive source of information on selected topics, this book continues, with the excellent caliber of its predecessors, to catalog topical information on health matters of general interest. Readable and thorough, this valuable resource is highly recommended for all libraries."
— *Academic Library Book Review, Summer '96*

"A comprehensive collection of authoritative information." — *Emergency Medical Services, Oct '95*

Continues next page

Gastrointestinal Diseases & Disorders Sourcebook

Basic Information about Gastroesophageal Reflux Disease (Heartburn), Ulcers, Diverticulosis, Irritable Bowel Syndrome, Crohn's Disease, Ulcerative Colitis, Diarrhea, Constipation, Lactose Intolerance, Hemorrhoids, Hepatitis, Cirrhosis, and Other Digestive Problems, Featuring Statistics, Descriptions of Symptoms, and Current Treatment Methods of Interest for Persons Living with Upper and Lower Gastrointestinal Maladies

Edited by Linda M. Ross. 413 pages. 1996. 0-7808-0078-8. $78.

". . . very readable form. The successful editorial work that brought this material together into a useful and understandable reference makes accessible to all readers information that can help them more effectively understand and obtain help for digestive tract problems." — *Choice, Feb '97*

Genetic Disorders Sourcebook

Basic Information about Heritable Diseases and Disorders Such as Down Syndrome, PKU, Hemophilia, Von Willebrand Disease, Gaucher Disease, Tay-Sachs Disease, and Sickle-Cell Disease, Along with Information about Genetic Screening, Gene Therapy, Home Care, and Including Source Listings for Further Help and Information on More Than 300 Disorders

Edited by Karen Bellenir. 642 pages. 1996. 0-7808-0034-6. $78.

"Provides essential medical information to both the general public and those diagnosed with a serious or fatal genetic disease or disorder." — *Choice, Jan '97*

"Geared toward the lay public. It would be well placed in all public libraries and in those hospital and medical libraries in which access to genetic references is limited." — *Doody's Health Sciences Book Review, Oct '96*

Head Trauma Sourcebook

Basic Information for the Layperson about Open-Head and Closed-Head Injuries, Treatment Advances, Recovery, and Rehabilitation, Along with Reports on Current Research Initiatives

Edited by Karen Bellenir. 414 pages. 1997. 0-7808-0208-X. $78.

Health Insurance Sourcebook

Basic Information about Managed Care Organizations, Traditional Fee-for-Service Insurance, Insurance Portability and Pre-Existing Conditions Clauses, Medicare, Medicaid, Social Security, and Military Health Care, Along with Information about Insurance Fraud

Edited by Wendy Wilcox. 530 pages. 1997. 0-7808-0222-5. $78.

"The layout of the book is particularly helpful as it provides easy access to reference material. A most useful addition to the vast amount of information about health insurance. The use of data from U.S. government agencies is most commendable. Useful in a library or learning center for healthcare professional students." — *Doody's Health Sciences Book Reviews, Nov '97*

Healthy Aging Sourcebook

Basic Consumer Health Information about Maintaining Health through the Aging Process, Including Advice on Nutrition, Exercise, and Sleep, Along with Help in Making Decisions about Midlife Issues and Retirement, Practical and Informed Choices in Health Consumerism, and Data Concerning the Theories of Aging, Aging Now, and Aging in the Future, Including a Glossary and Practical Resource Directory

Edited by Jenifer Swanson. 500 pages. 1999. 0-7808-0390-6. $78.

Immune System Disorders Sourcebook

Basic Information about Lupus, Multiple Sclerosis, Guillain-Barré Syndrome, Chronic Granulomatous Disease, and More, Along with Statistical and Demographic Data and Reports on Current Research Initiatives

Edited by Allan R. Cook. 608 pages. 1997. 0-7808-0209-8. $78.

Kidney & Urinary Tract Diseases & Disorders Sourcebook

Basic Information about Kidney Stones, Urinary Incontinence, Bladder Disease, End Stage Renal Disease, Dialysis, and More, Along with Statistical and Demographic Data and Reports on Current Research Initiatives

Edited by Linda M. Ross. 602 pages. 1997. 0-7808-0079-6. $78.

Learning Disabilities Sourcebook

Basic Information about Disorders Such as Dyslexia, Visual and Auditory Processing Deficits, Attention Deficit/Hyperactivity Disorder, and Autism, Along with Statistical and Demographic Data, Reports on Current Research Initiatives, an Explanation of the Assessment Process, and a Special Section for Adults with Learning Disabilities

Edited by Linda M. Shin. 579 pages. 1998. 0-7808-0210-1. $78.

Medical Tests Sourcebook

Basic Consumer Health Information about Medical Tests, Including Periodic Health Exams, General Screening Tests, X-ray and Radiology Tests, Electrical Tests, Tests of Body Fluids and Tissues, Scope Tests, Lung Tests, Gene Tests, Pregnancy Tests, Newborn Screening Tests, Sexually Transmitted Disease Tests, and Computer Aided Diagnoses; Along with a Section on Paying for Medical Tests, a Glossary, and Resource Listings

Edited by Joyce B. Shannon. 600 pages. 1999. 0-7808-0243-8. $78.

Men's Health Concerns Sourcebook

Basic Information about Health Issues That Affect Men, Featuring Facts about the Top Causes of Death in Men, Including Heart Disease, Stroke, Cancers, Prostate Disorders, Chronic Obstructive Pulmonary Disease, Pneumonia and Influenza, Human Immunodeficiency Virus and Acquired Immune Deficiency Syndrome, Diabetes Mellitus, Stress, Suicide, Accidents and Homicides; and Facts about Common Concerns for Men, Including Impotence, Contraception, Circumcision, Sleep Disorders, Snoring, Hair Loss, Diet, Nutrition, Exercise, Kidney and Urological Disorders, and Backaches

Edited by Allan R. Cook. 760 pages. 1998. 0-7808-0212-8. $78.

Mental Health Disorders Sourcebook

Basic Information about Schizophrenia, Depression, Bipolar Disorder, Panic Disorder, Obsessive-Compulsive Disorder, Phobias and Other Anxiety Disorders, Paranoia and Other Personality Disorders, Eating Disorders, and Sleep Disorders, Along with Information about Treatment and Therapies

Edited by Karen Bellenir. 548 pages. 1995. 0-7808-0040-0. $78.

"This is an excellent new book . . . written in easy-to-understand language."
— *Booklist Health Science Supplement, Oct '97*

". . . useful for public and academic libraries and consumer health collections."
— *Medical Reference Services Quarterly, Spring '97*

"The great strengths of the book are its readability and its inclusion of places to find more information. Especially recommended." — *RQ, Winter '96*

". . . a good resource for a consumer health library."
— *Bulletin of the MLA, Oct '96*

"The information is data-based and couched in brief, concise language that avoids jargon. . . . a useful reference source." — *Readings, Sept '96*

"The text is well organized and adequately written for its target audience." — *Choice, Jun '96*

". . . provides information on a wide range of mental disorders, presented in nontechnical language."
— *Exceptional Child Education Resources, Spring '96*

"Recommended for public and academic libraries."
— *Reference Book Review, '96*

Ophthalmic Disorders Sourcebook

Basic Information about Glaucoma, Cataracts, Macular Degeneration, Strabismus, Refractive Disorders, and More, Along with Statistical and Demographic Data and Reports on Current Research Initiatives

Edited by Linda M. Ross. 631 pages. 1996. 0-7808-0081-8. $78.

Oral Health Sourcebook

Basic Information about Diseases and Conditions Affecting Oral Health, Including Cavities, Gum Disease, Dry Mouth, Oral Cancers, Fever Blisters, Canker Sores, Oral Thrush, Bad Breath, Temporomandibular Disorders, and other Craniofacial Syndromes, Along with Statistical Data on the Oral Health of Americans, Oral Hygiene, Emergency First Aid, Information on Treatment Procedures and Methods of Replacing Lost Teeth

Edited by Allan R. Cook. 558 pages. 1997. 0-7808-0082-6. $78.

"Recommended reference source." — *Booklist, Dec '97*

Pain Sourcebook

Basic Information about Specific Forms of Acute and Chronic Pain, Including Headaches, Back Pain, Muscular Pain, Neuralgia, Surgical Pain, and Cancer Pain, Along with Pain Relief Options Such as Analgesics, Narcotics, Nerve Blocks, Transcutaneous Nerve Stimulation, and Alternative Forms of Pain Control, Including Biofeedback, Imaging, Behavior Modification, and Relaxation Techniques

Edited by Allan R. Cook. 667 pages. 1997. 0-7808-0213-6. $78.

"The information is basic in terms of scholarship and is appropriate for general readers. Written in journalistic style . . . intended for non-professionals. Quite thorough in its coverage of different pain conditions and summarizes the latest clinical information regarding pain treatment." — *Choice, Jun '98*

"Recommended reference source."
— *Booklist, Mar '98*

Continues next page

Physical & Mental Issues in Aging Sourcebook

Basic Consumer Health Information on Physical and Mental Disorders Associated with the Aging Process, Including Concerns about Cardiovascular Disease, Pulmonary Disease, Oral Health, Digestive Disorders, Musculoskeletal and Skin Disorders, Metabolic Changes, Sexual and Reproductive Issues, and Changes in Vision, Hearing, and Other Senses; Along with Data about Longevity and Causes of Death, Information on Acute and Chronic Pain, Descriptions of Mental Concerns, a Glossary of Terms, and Resource Listings for Additional Help

Edited by Heather E. Aldred. 625 pages. 1999. 0-7808-0233-0. $78.

Pregnancy & Birth Sourcebook

Basic Information about Planning for Pregnancy, Maternal Health, Fetal Growth and Development, Labor and Delivery, Postpartum and Perinatal Care, Pregnancy in Mothers with Special Concerns, and Disorders of Pregnancy, Including Genetic Counseling, Nutrition and Exercise, Obstetrical Tests, Pregnancy Discomfort, Multiple Births, Cesarean Sections, Medical Testing of Newborns, Breastfeeding, Gestational Diabetes, and Ectopic Pregnancy

Edited by Heather E. Aldred. 737 pages. 1997. 0-7808-0216-0. $78.

". . . for the layperson. A well-organized handbook. Recommended for college libraries . . . general readers."
— *Choice, Apr '98*

"Recommended reference source."
— *Booklist, Mar '98*

"This resource is recommended for public libraries to have on hand."
— *American Reference Books Annual, '98*

Public Health Sourcebook

Basic Information about Government Health Agencies, Including National Health Statistics and Trends, Healthy People 2000 Program Goals and Objectives, the Centers for Disease Control and Prevention, the Food and Drug Administration, and the National Institutes of Health, Along with Full Contact Information for Each Agency

Edited by Wendy Wilcox. 698 pages. 1998. 0-7808-0220-9. $78.

Rehabilitation Sourcebook

Basic Information for the Layperson about Physical Medicine (Physiatry) and Rehabilitative Therapies, Including Physical, Occupational, Recreational, Speech, and Vocational Therapy; Along with Descriptions of Devices and Equipment Such as Orthotics, Gait Aids, Prostheses, and Adaptive Systems Used during Rehabilitation and for Activities of Daily Living, and Featuring a Glossary and Source Listings for Further Help and Information

Edited by Theresa K. Murray. 600 pages. 1999. 0-7808-0236-5. $78.

Respiratory Diseases & Disorders Sourcebook

Basic Information about Respiratory Diseases and Disorders, Including Asthma, Cystic Fibrosis, Pneumonia, the Common Cold, Influenza, and Others, Featuring Facts about the Respiratory System, Statistical and Demographic Data, Treatments, Self-Help Management Suggestions, and Current Research Initiatives

Edited by Allan R. Cook and Peter D. Dresser. 771 pages. 1995. 0-7808-0037-0. $78.

"Designed for the layperson and for patients and their families coping with respiratory illness. . . . an extensive array of information on diagnosis, treatment, management, and prevention of respiratory illnesses for the general reader."
— *Choice, Jun '96*

"A highly recommended text for all collections. It is a comforting reminder of the power of knowledge that good books carry between their covers."
— *Academic Library Book Review, Spring '96*

"This sourcebook offers a comprehensive collection of authoritative information presented in a nontechnical, humanitarian style for patients, families, and caregivers."
— *Association of Operating Room Nurses, Sept/Oct '95*

Sexually Transmitted Diseases Sourcebook

Basic Information about Herpes, Chlamydia, Gonorrhea, Hepatitis, Nongonoccocal Urethritis, Pelvic Inflammatory Disease, Syphilis, AIDS, and More, Along with Current Data on Treatments and Preventions

Edited by Linda M. Ross. 550 pages. 1997. 0-7808-0217-9. $78.